HOW
WE
DID IT

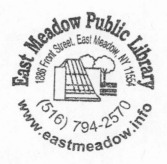

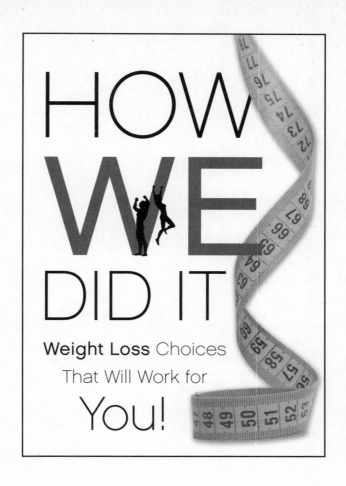

HOW WE DID IT

DID IT

Weight Loss Choices

That Will Work for

You!

NANCY B. KENNEDY

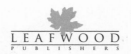

LEAFWOOD
PUBLISHERS

HOW WE DID IT

Weight Loss Choices That Will Work for You

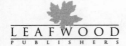

Copyright 2012 by Nancy B. Kennedy

ISBN 978-0-89112-293-7

Printed in the United States of America

Cover design by Marc Whitaker
Interior text design by Sandy Armstrong

Published in association with William K. Jensen Literary Agency. 119 Bampton Court, Eugene, Oregon 97404

Leafwood Publishers is an imprint of
Abilene Christian University Press
1626 Campus Court
Abilene, Texas 79601
1-877-816-4455
www.leafwoodpublishers.com

12 13 14 15 16 17 / 7 6 5 4 3 2 1

For everyone who has a goal—it is within reach!

Table of Contents

Chapter One

No Sweat

Weight Loss Your Own Way

"Mmm . . . mmm . . . mmm . . .," I stammered on the phone to the Lands' End lady.

I couldn't say it. *Mmm-edium.* Mee-dee-um. The concept was familiar to me, but I had little personal experience of it.

For close to twenty years, I'd been ordering clothes in that ugly next size up. Large. Grande. Even 1X at times. I once bought a pair of pants with the brand name of "Capacity." You can bet I cut *that* label out. But I still had to wear the pants.

The Lands' End lady waited patiently.

"It's just that I've recently lost weight, I've been swimming laps, and I'm not sure what size I am, maybe a 12, at least on top, and I'm worried that if I order the turtleneck in medium, it won't fit around my hips, which might be a 14, sadly, it's just the way all the women in my family are, unfortunately," I explained meekly, in a rush of words.

"If you'd like, I'll check the sweep of the garment for you," the Lands' End lady offered.

The *sweep*. What a lovely word. I didn't know it existed. The sweep of the garment. She checked the sweep. By her calculation, the shirt would fit with an inch to spare. Feeling positively giddy, I ordered the medium. And, incredibly, it *did* fit.

Today, I still wear my black, medium, Lands' End cotton turtleneck. And I relive this astounding moment every time I slip it on. An ordinary moment of catalog shopping turned extraordinary.

But soon, perhaps this season even, I'll need to call the Lands' End lady again. And this time, I might need to order a ssm. . . . I'm thinking about ordering a ssm. . . . Well, you know what I mean.

Sweet moments like that one don't come along very often when you wrestle with your weight, as I do. I'm sure you don't need me to point that out, if it's your struggle, too.

Far more often, the indelible moments of our lives are deeply painful. The moment we turn sideways so the camera catches us at a better angle. The moment we sink heavily into the couch, having overeaten once again. The moment we lean against the radiator on back-to-school night because we can't squeeze into a grade-school chair. The moment we buy the elastic-waist pants instead of the fitted jeans.

These moments make us miserable. They cause us to hate ourselves. They leave us feeling hopeless. And, although we know it isn't true, we begin to feel like we're the only one on the planet who can't control herself when it comes to food. I know that's how I have felt.

Where I live in central New Jersey, health and fitness are obsessive hobbies, much as mutual funds and day trading were hot pursuits here in the 1990s. Glam moms in exercise attire drop their kids at school and zip over to the gym for Zumba classes. Dads coach Babe Ruth baseball and enter 500-mile charity bike races. Organic farms and health food stores almost outnumber grocery stores. Rowing teams from Princeton University dot Lake Carnegie, and everywhere joggers pretty much own the roads. We exude robust health here.

That being the case, when I heard the statistic that two-thirds of Americans today are overweight, I just couldn't believe it. That's more than six out of ten people. I just don't see it here where I live. I wondered whether it was some sort of urban myth.

Like a good reporter, I decided to look into it. And sure enough, the statistic checks out. The Centers for Disease Control and Prevention (CDC) found in a 2010 survey that 68 percent of Americans are either overweight or obese. Of that number, the CDC reported that 34 percent are considered obese, a term that means they carry 20 percent or more of excess pounds over their ideal body weight.[1]

When I go on vacation, I can see the truth of these statistics. Perhaps it's because I have the leisure to take in my surroundings, or maybe I tend to see a broader cross section of the population in my travels, but that's when I notice how heavy we have become.

Sadly, vacations were also when I began to notice how heavy I had become. One year, my husband, John, and I rented an old stone cottage in Scotland on the brink of the North Sea. Behind the cottage, a steep, impossibly green hill rose up, beckoning us to take in the stunning countryside from the top of the cliff. At the time, I was newly pregnant and at my heaviest weight—about 170 pounds—and I'm only 5-foot-2. But when it comes to the British Isles, I am motivated! We started up.

I got about ten steps up the hill before I had to turn around and head back inside, huffing and panting, for a comforting cup of Yorkshire tea in front of our coal fire. As nice as that sounds, I was miserable. My mind was roiling in regret for the unseen view. I think of it even today.

Dr. C. Everett Koop, the U.S. Surgeon General during Ronald Reagan's presidency, has a unique perspective on this national epidemic. His tenure coincided with the burgeoning AIDS crisis, yet he was equally concerned about other looming threats to our national health. Among other measures, he forced the tobacco industry to include warning labels on its deadly products. Today, he sees a corollary.

"Obesity was not as urgent a problem as AIDS was at the time," Dr. Koop said in an email. "But in the future it will rank as a public health problem along with smoking."

Perhaps it's just the zeal of the newly converted, but I wish everyone could see the spare tires we carry around as the warning labels they are. Beyond the cosmetic argument for weight loss, the specters of heart disease, cancer, diabetes, sleep apnea, stroke, high blood pressure, gall-bladder disease, and osteoarthritis are all compelling reasons to keep the excess in check.

I wish, for myself, that I had decided sooner to do something about my excess.

I am not a serial dieter. I haven't spent my entire life chasing the elusive magic formula for weight loss, as I know many people have. I'd say I've given it a try maybe three or four times total. But I seem to have made a public spectacle of every halfhearted attempt.

In my junior year of college, my entire dorm went on a diet. I wrote an op-ed piece about it for Penn State's student paper, *The Daily Collegian*. Something about roaming dorm mates wielding menacing carrot sticks. I won't embarrass myself by going there! It went out on the Associated Press wire, and from there, a columnist from my hometown newspaper, the Rochester (NY) *Democrat and Chronicle*, picked up on the story and wrote a piece about the local Dieter-in-Chief.

Despite the fame and glory, I lived my life of quiet aspiration, always vaguely wanting to lose those 15 or 20 extra pounds but not really realizing that I needed to. It seems to me today that anyone under thirty is beautiful, and that's probably what I thought then. Or at least what I tried to convince myself.

During those years, my work as a journalist was so satisfying I didn't feel the need to deal with messy personal issues. It's ironic that even though my livelihood depended on ferreting out facts, I was willing to ignore the truth about my own problem.

It wasn't until I married and started lumbering through my thirties that I came back for more scrutiny.

My husband-to-be and I were separated during our engagement, he in London attending language school and me back in the States. When I visited John in April, we took the Tube to Bond Street to shop for a wedding dress. I know, I know. It's bad luck for the husband to see the dress before the big day. Maybe that explains why later we stumbled back out onto the street, all blue jeans and "gosh 'n golly!" into the middle of a nasty anti-American protest rally. But that's another story.

I ordered a dress in the size I thought corresponded to the correct American size, which would have been a size 12. It arrived by post about a month before the big day—one size too small. There was no time to exchange. FedEx wasn't even a speck on the horizon then.

At the time, I worked in a newsroom for Dow Jones, publisher of the *Wall Street Journal,* where daily donut and cheesesteak consumption was a point of pride. I began toting Tupperware containers of salad greens and diced watermelon. By combining the loss of about eight pounds with the skill of a dressmaker who found extra room in the seams, I was able to walk down the aisle tall—though a little breathless.

Like many newlywed couples, we packed on the pounds during those first few years. We were fond of dinner salads topped with blue cheese dressing and bacon. Burritos smothered in gooey cheese sauce. Cheeseburgers and fries. Onion rings. Chicken Kiev oozing butter and garlic. (OK, that last obsession was a little odd, but it reminded us of British pub food.)

Four years into our marriage, we decided to give Slim-Fast a try. The diet sounded right to us, slugging down chalky shakes during the day and settling down to what the program considered a "sensible dinner" in the evening. A dieter's take on the biblical interplay of suffering and reward.

And here, once again, I wasn't going to go quiet into that lousy diet. I wrote a piece about our odyssey for *U.S. 1,* a local newspaper, complete with a photo of me perched atop our open refrigerator, John leaning on the door. If I was going to lose 15 pounds, and lose them hard, you *bet* someone was going to hear about it.

Fast-forward many years. I'm in my forties. I have a young child and a closet full of size 16 clothes. Although I don't have a scale, I suspect I'm about 160 pounds. I catch sight of myself in a photo taken at a college reunion. I'm in a regrettable teal T-shirt that bunches around my middle before stretching over my ample hips, which are encased in a pair of "fat" pants. (No visuals needed for those pants. Sadly, we all know what they are.)

In fact, I suspect that, secretly, family photographers work for the diet industry.

My husband took a photo of our son Evan and me the day he entered kindergarten. That morning, we walked hand in hand down the sidewalk to the school, the crisp September sunlight virtually igniting Evan's blond head as he shouldered his Thomas the Tank Engine backpack. Needless to say, it was I and not Evan who wept like a baby when he pushed his way into the swarm of milling children on the playground without so much as a wave or a backward glance.

When we got our photos back, I impatiently tore open the pack, eager to relive that poignant mother-and-son moment on the sidewalk.

But when I got to the photo, I felt sick. What I saw had nothing to do with maternal bonds and everything to do with my backside. It blotted out everything in the photo, almost literally it seemed to me. *How can that possibly be me?* I thought in disbelief.

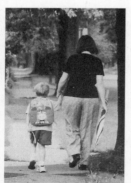

The shock was so great, I didn't even see my beautiful son in the photo. I could no longer remember my thoughts on that walk. Did we say anything to each other? Was he afraid? I don't know. Those sweet moments are forever lost to me.

I tore up the photo, as if it were that easy to destroy a memory.

Even with this heartache, I let another year go by. But with the coming of first grade—full days of school!—a friend offered me a one-week pass to her gym. Instinctively, I begged off. I was sure that I wouldn't be able to maintain a long-term interest in any fitness enterprise. I was eager just to get back to work; it had been five long years with Elmo and Little Critter.

But my friend persisted. And, miraculously, a niggling idea wormed its way to the fore. I thought: *What if I just go?* Just go, with no expectations. Ignore the scale. Nix the daily progress check. Just go. See what happens. Commit myself to the ragged, uneven—but possibly upward—path. *Could it all add up?* I wondered.

Besides, and it's not exaggerating to say this, I sensed God nudging me. Not in any mystical way, but in the practical, just-the-facts-ma'am way that I tend to experience things. The facts: I'm in my forties and overweight, and I haven't yet started vigorously walking my way to weight loss success. More facts: I have the time, a gym within reach, enough income for a membership, and an inkling of how I might be able to exercise without sweating. I hate sweating.

So I signed on and began swimming laps three times a week. At first the going was slow. I dragged myself to the gym. Once there, I swam in fits and starts, bored, easily tired, and in a constant argument with myself: *Can I stop now? It's been five minutes. It's been ten minutes. Can I stop NOW?* Seniors in surrounding lanes lapped me easily. Lifeguards made for the nearest chair, equipment at the ready. Once, a friend knifing through the water in full Speedo regalia shouted over, "Don't give up!" just when I thought I was doing pretty good.

And yet, three years went by, and it did add up. At 130 pounds, I'm 30 pounds lighter now. It doesn't sound like all that much, but at the grocery store recently, I picked up three ten-pound bags of flour and marveled at how heavy they were. I've dropped three dress sizes, and I'm even somewhat muscular. Buying my latest swimsuit, I felt almost dizzy taking size 10s into the dressing room.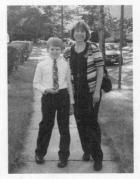

The lightness extends to my mood, too. I have a new relationship with food. It's not the enemy anymore. *I'm* not the enemy.

Not only that, but my enmity with my own body is over, too. My debilitating back troubles are gone. Even though all of Creation groans,

I don't anymore. And my stubbornly high blood pressure has dropped back to normal. When I read in the Psalms that I am "fearfully and wonderfully made," I have an easier time believing it.

Weight loss statistics are disheartening. I'm sure you've heard this one: 95 percent of people who lose weight eventually gain all of it back and more. Numbers, as I've learned from my work as a financial writer, can lie. So I thought I'd better check this one out, too.

Surprisingly, that depressing figure comes from a clinical study of just one hundred people treated for obesity at New York Hospital in 1959, more than fifty years ago. And you could almost have guaranteed the failure rate—the patients were simply given a written diet and sent home.[2]

Yet, newer studies don't show much progress. One study from 2007 suggests that within the first six months of a diet, people lose from five to 10 percent of their body weight, but that within four or five years, one- to two-thirds of dieters gain back even more weight than they lost.[3]

But again, how reliable are those figures? People who are tracked in obesity studies may have more intractable problems with weight than the average person. And, if a study relies on self-reporting, as many do, people who respond faithfully may not be representative of the entire group. Who's to say what the real numbers are?

What's clear is that anyone who makes a determined effort to drop the pounds—and keep them off—is in for a struggle. And yet, still we try. I believe our doggedness has something to do with the disharmony of the internal and the external. We see ourselves as one person, yet we must present an entirely different image to others. When the clash between the two identities becomes too painful for us, we are moved to action.

While interviewing dozens of people for this book, I discovered that my moment of truth—that photo from the sidewalk—is so common an epiphany that it has a name. It's called a *triggering event*. Something sets off an alarm. It can be a health scare, a cutting remark, an unflattering photo, a glance in a shop window. You have an almost instantaneous reaction of horror. And then a second, unbidden thought hits: *I can't live like this anymore.*

Without the internal motivation that flows from that moment, you're almost guaranteed to fail. But even with it, you're not guaranteed to succeed. You may be successful for the short term, but not over time. Onto the first blush of motivation you need to slap a healthy dose of reality. As I now know, you're embarking on a lifelong commitment, not a two-week fling.

It sounds grim, I know. As I thought about the magnitude of the struggle, that well-known quote from the writer G. K. Chesterton popped into my mind: "The Christian ideal has not been tried and found wanting. It has been found difficult; and left untried."[4] We in the weight loss wars haven't left our physical ideal untried—most of us have tried repeatedly—but we certainly have found it difficult to attain. When we feel we have tried and failed at everything, what happens to our souls?

The problem is not only that we battle daily with food but that our hunger bores much deeper. Our eating habits have to do not only with physical hunger but with kinds of hunger we may not even be aware of. Mind hunger, heart hunger, mouth hunger, God hunger, love hunger— the weight loss industry calls it by many names. What it boils down to is that we are complex creatures whose souls are needy and cry out for love, acceptance, harmony, and peace. We may eat to assuage a pain that has nothing to do with our growling stomachs.

Now, I may be coming late to the party, but here are some of the weight loss "secrets" I'm encountering on my journey. Weight loss emerges from a life change, not a short-term diet. Reaching for something that's good for you, and not something that's just plain good, is a learned response. It takes practice. It's all about good choices and portion control. Eat when you're hungry; stop before you're full. Go easy on the carbs, fats, and sweets. Calories count. Exercise counts. Muscle burns fat.

It sounds so simple, so universal that I'm surprised it's not an amendment to the Constitution. And yet, it's not simple at all. These may very well be irrefutable truths, yet each of us has to figure out how to make them work for us. I'm still trying to work this all out for myself.

On a deeper level, I'm learning how to find my comfort elsewhere, not in food. Starting to celebrate victories without the prize of food. Discovering that I must have strategies because my willpower will fail. I have been empowered by the realization that accomplishing the weight loss itself means more to me than the actual number of pounds lost or the amount of oversized clothes discarded.

Obviously, other people have learned these lessons long before I have—and perhaps more readily. I have always been riveted by magazine articles that chronicle the successes people have had with weight loss. Those before-and-after pictures? I can't take my eyes off them.

That's the reason I felt compelled to celebrate the victories with this book—because some doggedly determined people have triumphed against incredible odds.

For this book, I talked with people who have lost the weight and believe they've lost it for good. They triumphed on South Beach Diet, Body-*for*-LIFE, Weight Watchers, Thin Within, and Curves circuits. They've hired personal trainers, gone to gyms, and gotten out their running shoes. After years and years of trying, they finally found something that worked for them.

And do you know what? Something *can* work for you. In 2004, a group of researchers placed 160 people on four different weight loss plans—the Zone Diet, the Ornish Program, Atkins, and Weight Watchers—and asked them to stay on it for a year. Everyone who completed the study lost weight, regardless of which plan they followed! At the one-year mark, 25 percent of participants who stuck to their plan lost more than 5 percent of their body weight; 10 percent lost more than 10 percent. Researchers concluded that it was not the diet itself but *sticking with the diet* that worked—and they suggested that choosing a plan that matches a person's food preferences, lifestyle, and medical requirements may dramatically increase the likelihood of success.[5]

In this book, you'll hear from people who all had similar goals—to lose weight, get fit, stave off disease, or remain healthy—but who came to the task from many different places in life. Some had 20 pounds to lose, while some had 220. Some are teens, while others are in their six-ties. Some were motivated by personal reasons, and some professional reasons. But they all have one thing in common—they all succeeded.

For this book, I particularly sought out people whose weight loss stories weren't brand new. Weight loss is one thing; weight maintenance is another. I've read too many books whose authors trumpeted their suc-cess, only to see recent photos revealing that they have, sadly, regained their losses and then some. I'm only too aware that this can happen; there are no guarantees for any of us.

I also talked with a few people who are still on their quest for a healthy weight. When you've got a long road ahead, maybe 100 or more pounds to lose, you can become paralyzed by the seeming impossibility of the task. Yet people do succeed—they just start chipping away at the numbers, one day at a time, one pound at a time. To us, they may seem superhuman, more virtuous or more determined than we are. But they aren't any different than you or me. They just decide to start.

To help myself—and you—I asked each person not only to tell his or her story, but also to identify the people, books, and thoughts that influenced the transformation. They were pleased to have a way to pub-licly thank those who had supported them on their journeys. In addi-tion, I asked people to list their top tips: those specific and idiosyncratic actions and strategies that helped them succeed within their own indi-vidual environments.

Wanting to bring some order to my tales, I've grouped them by chapter according to broad categories that summarize a major theme of the plan. Categories include programs based on group support; pro-grams that ask you to balance carbs, fats, or calories; programs whose focus is faith-based; and programs that emphasize exercise. Because the underlying messages of many plans are similar, it's a somewhat arbitrary division—many plans could easily be categorized in another way. But I thought this method might help you more readily understand the plans.

Following each individual's story, I have included information about the particular plan he or she used. This information is readily available;

I gathered it from books, websites, press releases, and marketing brochures. What isn't easy is comparing the plans and settling on one that will work for you. That's the beauty of a book like this one. I've done some of the legwork for you.

In many cases, when a person has maintained weight loss for some time, the weight loss plan he or she used has since been updated. In these cases, I've noted updates to the plan, so that it is the most up-to-date information possible at the time of publication.

As you read about each weight loss plan, keep in mind that this book is a reference tool, and not a medical manual. People who shared their professional knowledge with me—experts in the fields of overweight and obesity, diet, nutrition, and fitness—plenty of insights to pass along. However, while the information is designed to help you learn about weight loss strategies and choices, and the success profiles are intended to be motivational, this book is not a substitute for seeking medical advice from a doctor.

Not surprisingly, I found that what's true about Americans in general is true about weight loss seekers in particular—we can be quite stubborn individualists. Many people followed a plan of their own making, used one plan and later switched to another, or picked out only what they wanted from a name-brand plan and mixed in their own elements. That adaptability was very rewarding to hear about. After all, it's what this book is about: not what *should* work but what *does* work.

My hope is that by reading these inspiring stories and comparing the weight loss plans, you'll find your way to the crucial inner motivation that will drive your success. That you'll go on to make your own stuttering call to Lands' End. For while William Faulkner once said that the only thing worth writing about is the human heart in conflict with itself, my desire for you is that you will know the joy of ending this one monstrous inner conflict once and for all.

Chapter Two

It's You and Me, Baby—Or Not

Choosing How Much Help You Want

When I thought about why I waited so long to do something about my weight, I came up with a lot of reasons. I worked full time. I had my own business. I was caring for our son and volunteering at his school, all while trying to remain viable in my profession. To keep up, I reasoned, I needed to read widely and write every day, not be checking in at the front desk for a spin class.

But, to be honest, my biggest hindrance was myself. I denied the truth; I didn't want to admit I looked and felt as bad as I did. For the longest time, the mirror lied to me. It lies to most of us, in fact. Very few people see themselves as others do. One Pew Research Center survey found that nine in ten people believe that most of their fellow Americans are overweight, but only four in ten see themselves as overweight.[1]

Even when faced with the truth, I firmly believed that I could take care of the situation, if and when I wanted to. After all, I was my own boss. Nobody was going to tell *me* what to do.

Ultimately, I was humbled to realize that I was guilty of one of those old-fashioned, outdated Seven Deadly Sins. No, not Gluttony, but Pride.

I didn't want anyone's help, even though it was obvious I wasn't helping myself. I was doing just fine by myself, thank you very much. It's nonsensical that just when I was feeling the worst about myself, I was the most prideful, but there it is. "The heart is deceitful above all things and beyond cure. Who can understand it?"[2]

I thought that people who paid money for gyms were frivolous, that people who bought prepared meals from weight loss programs were lazy. That these morally defective people were just going to give up anyway, so why were they even bothering? Inwardly, I scoffed at those hyper people who ran, biked, walked, or worked out at home. *Surely, I make better use of my time,* I crowed to myself.

When my day of reckoning came, it was a huge hurdle to admit that I needed help. For me, the solution was to join a gym. Still, I'm pretty much anonymous there. I go in, swim my laps, and leave. I like to go during the day with all the seniors, when all is calm, and they haven't yet cranked up the music for the after-work muscle crowd.

Anyone who decides to act will face the same question: How much personal attention do I want—or need—from others to succeed? It helps to know yourself well: Are you a person who will exercise only in a class setting? Or are you a private person who would rather die than show up in Spandex at a jock gym? Could meeting one-on-one with a personal trainer keep you motivated? Would you thrive with the encouragement of a support group?

One young man I talked with said he purposely chose a small, private gym. "If it had been one of those big, Gold's Gym type of places, I wouldn't have done it, because I was too self-conscious," he said. Another man joined a YMCA, feeling at home in the communal atmosphere. One woman used the workbook of a small-group plan, but she didn't choose to join the group.

Following are three people who involved the help of others in varying degrees, from the impersonal avenue of the Internet, to the one-on-one relationship of a personal trainer, and finally to the immersion approach of a residential weight loss center. And they've all succeeded.

Lynne Modranski

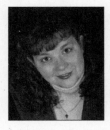 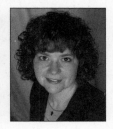

Steubenville, Ohio
Age: 48
Occupation: Web design
Accomplishment: Lost 30 pounds
How She Did It: SparkPeople

For Lynne Modranski, the old adage that knowledge is power is absolutely true. When she wants to know something, she looks it up—generally online.

"I'm at my computer all the time," she says. "I've got a crazy schedule, with my own website design business, composing music, and being the worship leader at my church, and I have my children and grandchildren nearby, but I'm always on the Internet."

So it was natural for Lynne to look online in 2007 when she got serious about losing weight.

Lynne was a yo-yo dieter. Over the years, she'd tried many programs—Free to Be Thin, the Carbohydrate Addict's Diet, and Naturally Thin, among other plans. She would enjoy a period of success, but then she'd just gain the pounds back, along with some bonus pounds.

Lynne traces her weight struggle back to her childhood. She grew up on a beef farm, where meat and potatoes—in large quantities—were on the dinner table nightly. Every evening, her family enjoyed big bowls of ice cream or popcorn before going to bed. As a child, these habits weren't a problem. Lynne more than worked off the meals helping her dad bale hay or working in the garden with her mom all day. The problem arose when her habits followed her into her adult life.

"By the time I was married, I could eat any guy under the table!" she says.

Many years, and three pregnancies, went by. Only 5 feet, 2 inches tall, Lynne gained 60 pounds during her first pregnancy. She managed to get back down to about 140 pounds, but after her third child, she found herself weighing in at about 170 pounds.

Lynne learned a lot from her forays into the various diet programs. From the book *How to Become Naturally Thin by Eating More* by Jean Antonello, she understood that by starving herself on diets, her body was reacting to the perception that it was facing a famine and simply storing up sustenance for lean times, hence the weight gain after a loss. She learned how to control portion size and make simple substitutions, like skim milk for whole milk.

In 1996, Lynne decided that she was going to stop fighting her weight and instead simply accept it. She figured that if she could learn how to maintain her weight, she would be happy with that.

But Lynne's new attitude of acceptance was jolted by a completely unexpected wake-up call. In 2007, at the age of 44, she suffered a transient ischemic attack, a sort of mini-stroke. Suddenly, Lynne was concerned about her health, not just her weight.

About that time, Lynne's sister told her she'd lost 25 pounds using an online program called SparkPeople. Lynne was intrigued.

"I was amazed at how much information is on the SparkPeople website, all entirely free," she says. "I loved the articles on health and fitness, and I began tracking my calories, meals, and exercise every day."

Although she'd tried counting calories before, Lynne said it was a laborious process of toting around a notebook, looking everything up, and writing everything down. With SparkPeople, she simply typed in what she ate and got back an analysis of the calories and the balance of protein, fat, and carbohydrates. She especially liked the feature that contrasted her actual balance of nutrients with how they should be balanced to achieve her goals.

"It was all the same information I'd known—eat fewer calories, less fat, and more protein—but I could see it all laid out in graphs. That visual information made it easy for me to make changes," she says.

Her first week on SparkPeople coincided with her church's Vacation Bible School, for which she was the music director. With kids, that's an active job. "It was like five days straight of two-hour aerobics," she says. She lost five pounds the first week.

Most of her weight came off gradually after that, anywhere from half a pound to a pound and a half a week. It took Lynne several months to lose 30 pounds. She was happy with her rate of progress, although some might consider it slow. "I figured when I got to 150 that it was OK to be there, because I used to be 170," she says. "I just took it a week at a time."

Some of Lynne's biggest changes have come in her restaurant habits. She and her husband eat out frequently, as she doesn't like to cook and feels she's not good at it. "We've literally had to throw meals into the garbage and go get a pizza," she says. She tracks components of restaurant meals using information on SparkPeople and the websites of individual chain restaurants.

Though many people like the support communities of SparkPeople, Lynne didn't get involved in them at first. "I'm the kind of person who likes to get to know people face-to-face," she says. Eventually, though, Lynne started an online SparkTeam with members of her church who wanted to connect but had no time to get together.

Today, at 137 pounds and wearing a size 6, Lynne is content, though she'd like to get down to 120 pounds. She enjoys shopping for clothes now. Where she used to dress in long blazers, layers, and bulky clothes, she now buys cropped jackets and other more formfitting clothes that she loves.

Though she dislikes exercise, Lynne makes sure to add activity into her day. She and her daughter, a Turbo Kick instructor, work out with a group at church twice a week, and she uses Wii Fit another two days a week. She golfs—and walks the course—when she and her husband have the time, and she swims when she has access to a pool. But she admits it's still something she forces herself to do. "I don't get that endorphin rush from exercise that other people talk about," she says.

Lynne draws a direct connection between her spiritual life and her physical well-being. "I find that on the days I spend time in Scripture, I have more success at resisting cravings and keeping on track," she says. "When I am faithful, he is faithful. I believe he sends the Holy Spirit to remind me, *You don't want that.*"

All in all, Lynne is a glass-half-full kind of person, and she encourages other people to be, too.

"I don't get discouraged or worried about my progress or lack of progress," she says. "Instead, I just think to myself, *Look at the good. Look at what I haven't gained.* I always encourage people to put things in perspective. I have grown by leaps and bounds, and I get better every day at incorporating changes into my life."

Thanks To

My sister, Brenda, who lost 25 pounds using SparkPeople.

My daughter, Julia: She's really into healthy living, and she encourages my husband and me to be, too.

SparkPeople: I am impressed by Chris Downie, the founder of SparkPeople, and everything that is available at absolutely no cost.

My Tips

The thought that helped me more than any other was that if I could learn to maintain my current weight, I could learn to maintain at a lower weight. I have made many small substitutes that anybody can make—pretzels instead of potato chips, skim milk instead of whole, and water and decaffeinated iced tea instead of carbonated drinks, which tend to make me draggy. At a restaurant, I'll either ask for something off-menu, like a grilled chicken breast and steamed veggies, or I'll order an entrée and ask the server to hold the sauce or the cheese, or whatever. I'll split a meal with my daughters or look for the low-calorie meals at places like Applebee's or Eat'n Park.

SparkPeople[3]

"Whether you want to fit into your 'skinny jeans,' improve your health and fitness levels, change your outlook and mood, or reach all new goals, The Spark can help you transform your body and your life. What are you waiting for? Spark your life today!"

—*The Spark: The 28-Day Breakthrough Plan for Losing Weight, Getting Fit, and Transforming Your Life* by Chris Downie (Carlsbad, CA: Hay House, 2011)

SparkPeople founder Chris Downie says he and his wife were early eBay employees whose windfall allowed them to do what they'd always wanted to do—help people get healthy. More than ten million people have joined SparkPeople since it started in 2000, with 175,000 joining each month.

SparkPeople is a free online program that combines informative articles and blogs with personal calorie, nutrient, and exercise trackers, meal plans, recipes, and online support communities. Its program is a four-stage diet plan that is personalized by users. Users enter their height, weight, and amount of intended daily exercise, as well as a target weight and date. These prompts result in recommendations for calorie, fat, and carbohydrate intake as well as a personalized fitness plan.

The four diet phases consist of the Fast Break, which gives users a simple goal to complete in the first few weeks as a springboard for other goals; Healthy Diet Habits, which addresses success strategies such as portion control, exercise, and hydration; Lifestyle Change, which stresses consistency and motivation; and Spread the Spark, which completes the diet with tips and goals for continued success.

Like Lynne, many people say they are interested primarily in the information available on the site. But for other users, the support of other weight loss seekers is the big draw. Users can connect by blogging on their member page and following others' blogs, commenting on message boards, or joining a SparkTeam. SparkTeams are groups of users united by common interests or goals; for example, there are teams of vegetarians, single parents, college students, and faith groups. In another interactive section, users share their weight loss and fitness "secrets."

The site offers many types of tools to encourage progress. The SparkPoints system is a motivational tool that allows users to earn awards and trophies for their progress. Progress can be tracked through charts and graphs and other means of feedback. There are apps for iPhones, Android devices, and BlackBerry phones. The site even breaks out information for the teen audience, those with health conditions, those wishing to manage their money, and those planning a healthy pregnancy.

This plan might work for me because...

- ☑ I'm at my computer all the time.
- ☑ Information is what I need to get going.
- ☑ I'm self-motivated and don't need a lot of hand-holding.
- ☑ Online communities of support are there if I want them.

Todd Peterson

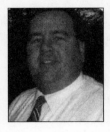 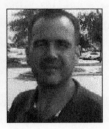

Memphis, Tennessee
Age: 41
Occupation: Sales professional
Accomplishment: Lost 105 pounds
How He Did It: Personal trainer at home

Todd Peterson played football in high school, so when as an adult he decided to do something about his weight, he realized that to succeed he needed a player-coach kind of relationship.

"I knew I hadn't done anything about it before because no one was making me do it," he says.

So in 2005, when his wife asked him what he wanted for Father's Day, Todd told her he didn't want a tie or another shirt—he wanted a coach. "Help me find somebody who can help me lose weight," he replied.

Although he was sincere, Todd, a salesman who works for an agent of United Van Lines, knew that even then he hadn't entirely bought into the deal.

"I asked my wife to do it for me because I was lazy," he says. "And I thought, *Now it's off my back and she can't blame me if it doesn't work out. . . . Oh, and hand me another hamburger.*"

Todd's wife called his bluff. She presented him with a list of three personal trainers. It was Todd's job to close the deal. He called each of them and met with Derek Curtice, the founder of SimpleFit in Memphis. Even then, Todd wasn't fully on board.

"At the time, I weighed about 280 pounds. Derek asked what my goal weight was, and I said I didn't have one. I just wanted to lose some weight. I thought I could buy into losing maybe 25 or 30 pounds," Todd recalls. "So Derek said, 'Great, 200 pounds it is.' And I'm thinking to myself, *Lose 80 pounds? This guy is crazy.*"

Yet, when Derek knocked on his door at 5 A.M. a few days later, exercise ball in hand, Todd let him in. Despite his initial reluctance, Todd says that at that moment he became committed to his weight loss "hook, line, and sinker."

The two worked out together for an hour three days a week, starting with simple squats and crunches and gradually adding in resistance bands and weights. Even after Derek left, Todd says he would work out another twenty to thirty minutes. On alternate days, Todd worked out on his own, following a forty-five-minute routine Derek created for him.

At the same time, Todd changed his eating habits, following guidelines Derek gave him. Making these changes was the harder job for him. Old habits die hard.

"I traveled a lot in my job and I never ate breakfast. I thought that was the way to lose weight," Todd says. "By lunchtime, I'd be starving, so I'd really pound that all-you-can-eat buffet. If I was home, I'd have a bag of Cheetos before dinner, fall asleep watching TV, and wake up at ten-thirty for a glass of whole milk and chocolate chip cookies."

It was also while traveling that Todd observed the habits of his coworkers and bosses and felt the stirrings of a desire to help himself.

"My bosses and I would plan to meet up at breakfast, and they'd get up early to work out in the fitness room. Meanwhile, I'm just wanting to sleep in," Todd recalls. "But sometimes these things were playing in my mind, and I'd go try out the treadmill—when no one was there—but after five minutes, I'd be thinking, *Forget this!*"

These habits and halfhearted attempts had their predictable effect. Todd gradually found maneuvering through life more difficult. After climbing up two or three flights of stairs to meet with a client, Todd says he would have to walk around in the hallway for a few minutes so he wasn't huffing and puffing when the client answered the door.

So Todd buckled down and gave it his all. He gives his wife a lot of the credit. "She'd call me at the office and ask whether I wanted chicken or fish for dinner, and it would be ready for me when I got home," he says. When he ate out, he consulted Derek's list of healthy restaurant choices. And even though he wasn't required to keep a food journal, Todd did, just to keep himself honest.

Incredibly, in just a little over ten months, Todd battled his weight down to 172 pounds—more than 25 pounds below the 200-pound goal weight Derek had set.

Today, maintaining at 175 pounds, Todd considers himself a fortunate man. His health is good, even though diabetes runs in his family. He's pleased with the fact that his life insurance carrier no longer considers him a high risk and has moved him into the "extremely preferred" category. But more importantly, he has a new outlook on the future.

"I want to be here to play with my son, and my son's children. Derek and I would talk about family, and he'd always say, 'Do you know what a tremendous gift you're giving to your wife and son? You're going to be around for them,'" Todd says. "Derek more than gave me back my life. He gave me a new life."

Thanks To

My wife, Carol, and my son, Parker: I am so blessed in my life.

Derek Curtice, personal trainer and SimpleFit founder.

My Tips

In the South, it's all about gravy, cheese, and dessert. You have to learn how to live! You can't have dessert every night, but you can have it maybe one Saturday night a month. Not everyone is going to support you. They'll say, "Go on, have a cupcake. It's Easter," or your niece's birthday, or whatever. But if you're going to lose weight, it has to be your only goal.

How to Choose a Personal Trainer

Like Todd Peterson, you might feel at a loss when it comes to finding a personal trainer. Yellow page listings are daunting, and if you belong to a gym, playing eenie, meenie, miney, moe with the photos on the staff board is a dicey game.

The biggest mistake people make when choosing a personal trainer is to go by looks, says Laura Kruskall, a registered dietitian who is chair of the Department of Nutrition Sciences at the University of Nevada, a fellow of the American College of Sports Medicine, and an ACSM-certified health and fitness instructor.

"A popular reason people choose a particular trainer is based on appearances. They pick someone who looks the way they want to look," Dr. Kruskall said in an interview. "That's not a good way to choose."

Instead, says Dr. Kruskall, check into the person's background for a degree in exercise science or a similar emphasis. Then check the trainer's certification. Don't be taken in by vague credentials touting a person as a "certified personal trainer," Dr. Kruskall warns.

"Anyone can say they're a personal trainer. It doesn't mean anything. Some gyms have their own certifying programs, and you can even buy your certification online," she says.

A number of organizations offer certifying exams for personal trainers. You'll need to wade through an alphabet soup of certifications and certifying groups. Your best bet, Dr. Kruskall believes, is to look for credentials from the American College of Sports Medicine (ACSM), the National Strength and Conditioning Association (NSCA), or the American Council on Exercise (ACE).

Ask friends and family for referrals, or use the phone book if you need to. Call a number of trainers and either chat on the phone or make an appointment to visit. Most trainers offer a free consultation at which you can determine whether he or she is a good fit given your goals and personality.

"Remember, you'll be sweating in front of this person, bending over, maybe wearing a low-cut top," says Dr. Kruskall. "Personality and comfort level are big factors."

Thinking about why you want a personal trainer might also lead you to the right person. Many people need the help of a professional to remain faithful to an exercise program, so look for someone you find motivating. You might also want the guidance of a trainer if you have not exercised or been active before; along with the help of your doctor, the trainer can provide an initial fitness assessment and lay out a safe and effective exercise plan. If you've been exercising but seeing little or no results, a trainer can lead you in a more effective workout. Or, if you have been injured, a personal trainer can work in conjunction with your physical therapist to suggest modified exercises that suit your limitations.

Many personal trainers offer meal plans as part of their package. Before you follow any dietetic advice, however, you'll want to talk with your doctor. Personal trainers are qualified to give general, nonmedical nutritional information, Dr. Kruskall says, but if you have a medical condition, it can be worsened by the wrong nutritional advice. For the specifics of a diet, you might want to seek the help of a dietitian, she suggests.

This plan might work for me because . . .
- ☑ I need one-on-one help.
- ☑ I'm willing to commit to regular exercise.
- ☑ I can find a personal trainer at my gym or arrange for sessions at home.

Susan Ray

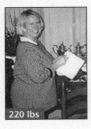 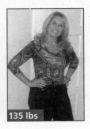

220 lbs   135 lbs

Urbanna, Virginia
Age: 51
Occupation: Residential design and renovation
Accomplishment: Lost 85 pounds
How She Did It: Duke Diet & Fitness Center

"You have such a beautiful face. If only . . ."

All too many people have heard this statement at some point in their lives. Susan Ray knew how to fill in that blank.

At 5 feet, 4½ inches and 225 pounds, Susan knew without anyone telling her that she was overweight. She hated how she looked. A woman highly attuned to fashion, she couldn't buy anything that looked good on her.

"I had a few pairs of black pants that worked, and that was it," she says. "I had four hundred pairs of shoes, because that's the only thing I could find to fit me!"

Susan hadn't always struggled with her weight. Unlike many people, she grew up in a home with healthy habits. Her mother made good, healthy meals, and the family rarely had desserts. Neither she, nor her parents, nor her three sisters had weight troubles.

But when Susan went off to college, her odyssey began. Separated from her home environment, she took to the habits of college students everywhere.

"I ate all the time. Cafeteria food, pizza, popcorn, desserts, late-night snacking. I had no idea of the damage junk food could do," Susan says.

"The salad bar, I never touched it. I put on those ubiquitous Freshman Fifteen—and all before Christmas break, too!"

From then on, Susan waged a constant war with her weight. She married and with her husband opened a string of restaurants along the East Coast from Florida to Maryland. At home, they cooked huge meals and ate at odd hours.

The final blow was the couple's opening of a gourmet deli. The chef they hired knew what their customers wanted.

"He made unbelievable breakfasts, cookies, pastries. I opened the deli every day, and I just picked all day long. At home, I'd make pasta with cream sauces, baked potatoes loaded with everything, steak salads smothered in full-fat Caesar dressing," Susan recalls.

Susan tried many times to get her weight under control—a low-carb diet, starvation, low-fat diets. She always had the best success with low-fat diets, at one point losing 40 pounds. But the pounds always seemed to come back.

In her early forties and approaching her highest weight, Susan wasn't experiencing any debilitating health effects yet. Her stamina was good. To exercise, she'd walk for miles. But emotionally, she was suffering.

"I felt terrible about myself," she says. "But the more unhappy I was, the more I turned to food for comfort."

Susan's breaking point came in 2003 when she took a trip to Italy with a group of girlfriends. Traveling had become increasingly hard for Susan, and this time was no exception.

"I was so uncomfortable on the plane," she says. "It was such a tight squeeze, I could barely fit into the seat. I was twice as big as any of my friends."

It was on that flight that Susan, despairing, thought: *How have I done this to myself?*

That question was a turning point for Susan. The restaurant business was taking a toll on her personal life, though, and soon her marriage ended. Alone, jobless, and unsure of what to do next, Susan took an honest assessment of her future.

"Truthfully, I asked myself, 'How marketable are you?'" she says. "And I had to say, not so marketable. Our society is not inclined to welcome obese people."

At about this time, a friend of Susan's told her about his experience at the Duke Diet & Fitness Center in Durham, North Carolina, and suggested she give it a try. She knew it would cost her plenty, and she knew it would be hard work, but she was excited about the prospect.

"I was so pumped!" she says. "I just knew it was going to work for me. I gave myself to it 100 percent."

For six weeks, Susan lived in an apartment across from the Duke Center on the campus of Duke University. She immersed herself in the experience—taking every nutritional and exercise class, attending every individual and group counseling session, swimming in the pool, eating healthy meals in the cafeteria, and nurturing friendships with her classmates.

"The best thing is that you're with other people who are struggling with weight, just like you are," she says. "The doctors, the nutritionist, the staff all make it the most comforting environment imaginable. No one judges you; you're all there for the same reason."

In her six weeks at Duke, Susan lost 20 pounds. At home, she continued to lose, and she went back to Duke for two weeks in the spring. In total, she lost 85 pounds within a year. Today, she weighs 145 and wears a size 8/10.

Susan's daily diet is rich with fruits, vegetables, and whole grains and low in fat, yet she enjoys eating out and doesn't consider any foods forbidden. She has remarried and lives next door to her best friend, who is her walking buddy six days a week. The two walk about five miles a day. In addition, Susan does a light weight training routine at home.

In August 2005, Susan appeared on NBC's *Today* show on a weight loss segment. Every other year or so, Susan returns to Duke to meet up with friends from the program. She will never lose her gratitude for the program that helped her gain control of her life.

"I went to Duke knowing that I was giving myself a gift of a new future," she says. "I came away with the knowledge that I deserve to be this healthy and this happy. I am worthy of being thin and feeling good, and I owe that to myself."

Thanks To

My family: My parents and my sisters were my biggest supporters. They'd send me cards while I was at Duke, saying, "We're proud of you! Go for it!" There's nothing better than getting a letter in the mail when you're away from home.

My Tips

I found it easier to succeed by breaking my goal into smaller increments. I'd say to myself, "I want to lose five pounds." Then, when I lost that five pounds, I'd reset and say the same thing, "I want to lose five pounds." If I had gone into this thinking, "I need to lose 100 pounds," it would have been too overwhelming. The thought that powers me on every single day is, *How good can I be to myself today?* And it's not just about the food—you have to learn how to deal with the emotional triggers that make you reach for food.

The Duke Diet & Fitness Center

"We are more likely to be successful with achieving long-term weight control if we outsmart the problem, rather than try to defeat it with brute force, or sheer willpower, alone."

—*The Duke Diet: The World-Renowned Program for Healthy and Lasting Weight Loss* by Howard J. Eisenson, MD and Martin Binks, PhD (New York: Ballantine Books, 2007)

The Duke Diet & Fitness Center is based in Durham, North Carolina, across from the campus of Duke University. It offers residential programs lasting from one to four weeks. Patients receive medical and fitness evaluations, take daily fitness classes, and engage in individual and small group sessions dealing with behavioral health and medical management, fitness, lifestyle choices, and nutrition, as well as menu planning, grocery shopping, cooking demonstrations, and guided restaurant outings. The patient has regular one-on-one check-ins with medical and behavioral staff.

During the patient's initial assessment, a registered dietitian helps plan a personal nutrition program, which includes three meals and a snack each day. For many years, Duke offered just the traditional low-fat, higher-carbohydrate meal plan, but today it offers moderate- and low-carbohydrate approaches. The plans are based on a daily calorie count that is adjusted to fit each individual's situation. Once the patient reaches goal weight, the daily calorie count of the maintenance plan increases.

After a person leaves the center, he or she has access to the center's Personal Coaching program, regular mailings, and weekly group phone calls. The center also sponsors tune-up visits and annual reunions for program graduates.

The center's online weight loss program, DukeDiet.com, is available to program participants and graduates, as well as those who cannot attend the program in person. The website provides up-to-date weight management information and tools including food logs, exercise trackers, weight trackers, and interactive message boards.

This plan might work for me because . . .

- ☑ I would like to be totally immersed in a weight loss program.
- ☑ To succeed, I think I need a support team of professionals.
- ☑ I would like to have healthy habits modeled for me.
- ☑ I can take time away from my job and life to achieve my goals.

Chapter Three

It's a Balancing Act

Tracking Carbs, Proteins, and Fats

We've all been warned not to mention politics or religion at the dinner table. You might want to add a caveat about bringing up Robert Atkins, too.

Atkins is, of course, the famous doctor and author whose diet advice turned conventional wisdom on its head with the publication of *Dr. Atkins' Diet Revolution* in the 1970s. At the time, almost every doctor, dietitian, and government researcher preached, "Eat less sugar. Eat less fat. Bread and potatoes are where it's at."[1]

Dr. Atkins's revolutionary thought was that refined carbohydrates and starches, not fat, make us fat. Most experts of the time—and still today—consider that fats, being calorie-dense, lead to obesity, and the name of the game is to cut calories.

Instead, Dr. Atkins believed that carbohydrates are more directly linked to obesity because they stimulate the body's production of insulin and cause it to store fat tissue. Dr. Atkins also pooh-poohed the idea that the fats and cholesterol of his low-carb diet damaged the heart or led to other health problems.

I think that even before I knew about the Atkins diet, I tried it. One summer I had a job slinging hash on a steam line at a GM parts factory, hair net, scratchy uniform, and all. I rebuffed the pressure from my fellow cafeteria workers to have a smoke, but when they talked up a diet that supposedly allowed me to eat all the bacon, cheese, eggs, and fried chicken we were serving up, I couldn't resist.

Apparently, I didn't get the full Atkins memo, because the idea of lean sources of protein never occurred to me. And while I happily filled my plate with proteins, I somehow didn't get the part about cutting out the carbs. I came back for seconds on the french fries, bread, and pieces of pie. Needless to say, my so-called diet didn't work.

Today, the carbs versus calories debate rages on, particularly in the media, with experts weighing in on either side.[2] Yet despite the acrimonious debate, it's probably fair to say that without Dr. Atkins, we would not look at the nutrients in our food the way we do today. Virtually every diet coming into existence today suggests limiting your intake of refined sugars and flours. And low-carb diets are here to stay.

Here are three people who found success on diets that either limit carbohydrates, stress the "right" carbs, or balance them in particular percentages with proteins and fats.

Jimmy Moore

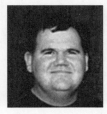 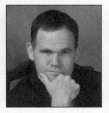

Spartanburg, South Carolina
Age: 39
Occupation: Health blogger, author, and podcaster
Accomplishment: Lost 180 pounds
How He Did It: Atkins Diet

Jimmy Moore is livin' la vida low-carb. That's the theme of his life—and his books, his blog, his podcast, and his online videos.

At age 32, Jimmy weighed 410 pounds. He was on medications to treat high cholesterol, high blood pressure, and labored breathing. He had no hope that his life could be any different.

"I believed this was just the way I was supposed to be," he says. "My family was fat, and I had been fat my whole life. My mom was a single mom who had to feed three growing kids, so she bought what she could afford, which was pretty much all carbohydrates and sugar-laden junk food."

It didn't help that Jimmy lived in the South most of his life, a part of the country notorious for its high-carb comfort foods like grits, cornbread, and biscuits, and his jobs only worsened his dilemma. "I worked at places like Shoney's, Taco Bell, and Domino's Pizza while I was in college, and my dad owned three restaurants," he recalls.

Over the years, Jimmy had tried many diets, all of them essentially low-fat. But even when he dieted, he never once gave a thought to his sugar consumption.

"I was addicted to Twizzlers—a naturally fat-free food after all!" he says. "Every diet I tried, I was eating a lot of sugar. Everything I knew was predicated on low-fat eating, because it was the way I was told you had to eat to lose weight."

At times, he did lose weight, a lot of it. In 1999, he lost 170 pounds in nine months on a virtually zero-fat diet of his own making. But he was grumpy and "psychologically messed up," he remembers. And, ultimately, he wasn't able to stick with it.

"One day, my wife asked me to get her a Big Mac meal, supersized, with a Coke, and I said to her, 'I'm just going to get one for myself, too,'" he remembers. "That was it. In four months, I gained back all 170 pounds. I was just rebelling, thinking that this was the way I'd have to eat for the rest of my life."

But in 2003, at age 31, Jimmy was forced to face himself. His brother Kevin, just four years older, had suffered a series of heart attacks, and he wondered whether he would be next. He was a substitute teacher and had come in for some hurtful comments from students.

Ultimately, though, it wasn't an external voice but an internal one that broke through. That year, he attended a church festival that featured a climbing wall. Jimmy thought that at 6 feet, 3 inches tall he should be able to reach the top easily. So with kids all around him zipping up the wall, he went for his first foothold.

"I started up and on the first step, my foot slipped, and I fell," he says. "I tried again, and again I fell. The people behind me weren't laughing or anything—my church family was very supportive. But I was determined. On the third try, I slipped again, and this time, I twisted my foot and sprained my ankle."

At that moment, the defeated climber thought to himself, *Jimmy, you are out of control!*

Jimmy vowed to take on his weight again. He wasn't up for another low-fat attempt, but he knew two people who had succeeded on the Atkins diet. For Christmas, he received *Dr. Atkins' New Diet Revolution,* and he read it cover to cover. On January 1, 2004, he resolved to begin his low-carb lifestyle. But right off, he ran into trouble.

"That first day, I thought I was going to die. I had the worst headache, my body ached. I was sprawled out on the couch, and I pleaded with my wife to just kill me now," he says. Nevertheless, he persevered and within a few days the symptoms subsided.

In the first month, Jimmy lost 30 pounds. The second month, 40 more pounds were gone. Within 100 days, he lost 100 pounds. He had joined a gym and was running on a treadmill, but obviously Jimmy was thriving on a diet that worked out to about 60 to 70 percent fat, but with just 20 grams of carbohydrates a day, including two cups of low-carb vegetables.

For breakfast, Jimmy would have three to four eggs with cheese; for lunch, some kind of meat with cheese and mayonnaise; and for dinner, steak or chicken over spinach leaves with full-fat ranch dressing. He snacked on almonds or macadamia nuts, sugar-free chocolates, and Atkins bars.

Within a month of starting, Jimmy entered a weight loss contest sponsored by a local radio station—a disc jockey challenged volunteers to lose a literal ton of weight. Four other people joined him.

Despite his early bolt out of the box, Jimmy hit a wall at 300 pounds. For ten full weeks, he didn't lose a single pound. He wavered but didn't turn back. "I focused on why I was doing this and just pushed through," he says. To his surprise, he lost eight inches off his waist during that time, despite the stalled scale.

At the end of the year, Jimmy was the only contestant left. He had lost 180 pounds on the Atkins diet. Among other prizes donated by local sponsors, he won a particularly apt one—a year's worth of weekly steak dinners.

Jimmy attributes part of his success to his exercise routines, which include resistance and interval training along with competitive volleyball, pickup basketball, and volunteering as a referee for youth sports at his church. He takes a variety of vitamin supplements and holds his carbohydrate level to around 30 grams a day.

Succeeding at the Atkins diet has literally changed Jimmy Moore's life. In 2005, he published a book, *Livin' La Vida Low-Carb: My Journey from Flabby Fat to Sensationally Skinny in One Year*. A second book followed, *21 Life Lessons from Livin' La Vida Low-Carb: How the Healthy Low-Carb Lifestyle Changed Everything I Thought I Knew*. He blogs at *Livin' La Vida Low-Carb*, writes for nutrition- and health-related websites, records podcasts with diet and fitness experts, and produces online videos. He is tireless in urging others to take control of their lives, no matter what weight loss plan they choose.

"Don't feel like you have to eat a certain way, because many roads will take you there," he says. "It's not about willpower but rather a steadfast resolve to make better choices. Commit to do it, even when it hurts, because it is so worth it in the end."

Thanks To

My faith: God is at the center of my life. I give him all the glory for blessing me in weight loss and life.

Dr. Robert Atkins: Without him, the world wouldn't even know what a carbohydrate is.

The author Gary Taubes: He continues to be at the forefront of the low-carb revolution.

My wife, Christine: She has stood by me whether I was 410 or 230 pounds. I love that woman to pieces!

My Tips

Sugar is rat poison. Read labels—if you see double-digit sugars, run like the wind. Don't be afraid of fats, especially saturated fat. Avoid grains, vegetable oils, and anything labeled low-fat. Choose fresh foods from a local farmer like grass-fed beef, pastured eggs, and non-starchy vegetables. Enjoy nourishing foods that keep your blood sugar levels steady.

The Atkins Diet

"The Atkins diet isn't a peculiar, exotic diet. It's the human diet raised to its healthiest pitch and stripped of the 20th century food inventions that are so economically delightful and so physiologically disastrous."

—*Dr. Atkins' New Diet Revolution* by Robert C. Atkins, MD (New York: M. Evans and Company, 1992)

The Atkins diet has been around since 1972, when cardiologist Dr. Robert Atkins decided the way to eat was low-carbohydrate rather than low-fat. Atkins rejected the long-held view that eating fats makes you fat, and he believed there is no need to count calories. The biggest culprits in weight gain, he said, are the refined sugars and flours of today's processed foods.

The Atkins diet is a four-stage, high-protein, high-fat plan that severely restricts carbohydrate intake. By restricting carbohydrates, Dr. Atkins believes you ingest fewer of the kind of calories that are typically converted into body fat, and the body is forced into burning stored fat.

During the two-week induction phase, only 20 grams of carbohydrates a day are allowed, and 15 grams come from low-carb vegetables. In the second phase, you are allowed a gradually increasing amount of daily carbs, as long as you keep losing one to three pounds a week. This phase continues until you're within five to ten pounds of your ideal weight. The third phase adds even more carbs each week as long as you're losing about a pound a week and continues until you reach your target weight. The final phase is a maintenance plan that allows the carbohydrate level of the third phase. If you gain five or more pounds above your goal weight, you return to the first phase. In time, Dr. Atkins believes the dieter discovers his or her tolerance for carbohydrates and can adjust daily allowances to maintain a desired weight.

In all phases, grains, fruits, and dairy products are restricted, but proteins like red meat, eggs, and cheese and fats like butter and cream are perfectly acceptable. From proteins, the body absorbs amino acids, and from fats, the body absorbs glycerol and fatty acids. But Atkins believed the simple sugars absorbed from carbohydrates overwhelm the system with excess glucose. His diet is intended to put the body into "ketosis," a state in which the body is burning fat placed in storage by insulin, the hormone that converts excess carbohydrates into stored body fat.

The plan has been updated several times, most recently as *The New Atkins for a New You: The Ultimate Diet for Shedding Weight and Feeling Great*, which includes vegan and vegetarian options.[3]

This plan might work for me because . . .

- ☑ Low-fat, low-calorie plans haven't worked for me.
- ☑ I like the idea of eating foods that are restricted on other plans.
- ☑ I am OK with eating a lot of protein and severely cutting back on carbohydrates.

Vickie Silcox

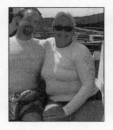 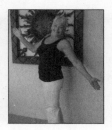

Palmdale, California
Age: 53
Occupation: Artist
Accomplishment: Lost 77 pounds
How She Did It: South Beach Diet

As a young girl, Vickie Silcox personified the California life—she was the quintessential bikini-clad beach babe.

As an adult, Vickie took on another persona, this one no less dramatic. After many years in construction adminstration, she followed her dream and took up glass painting full-time. She donned the artist's cloak, literally.

"As an artist, you can have a certain flair. You're almost expected to have an artsy look," she says. "I had this burgundy velvet cloak that I'd wear—it gave me a sort of Stevie Nicks look. It was gigantic!"

Vickie isn't exaggerating—the cloak literally was gigantic. At the time, Vickie weighed 248 pounds and wore a size 18/20. It's not that Vickie imagined herself the starving artist, but despite the numbers, she didn't really see herself as a large woman.

"You know how they blur the photos of celebrities to make them look perfect?" she says. "That's how I saw myself, with softened edges. I saw a thinner person in the mirror."

Although we all imagine California as the land of the toned and tanned, even there you can make the wrong health decisions. Vickie's career in construction meant a stressful, "new nightmare every day" kind of life.

"I dealt with the stress through alcohol and food," she says. "I overcame the drinking, but I was a stress eater, big-time. I had crazy, weird hours and got my meals off lunch trucks—hamburgers, fries, burritos, fried chicken, potato chips—everything greasy and cooked in oil."

Vickie gained weight with each of her three pregnancies, one time gaining 80 pounds. Though she managed to lose most of the weight each time, a few pounds would stick around. Later, menopause didn't help her cause. Waking up with night sweats, she'd head to the kitchen for a snack, even if just a bowl of cereal, hoping it might help her get back to sleep.

Over the years, Vickie tried several times to lose weight. She tried a 10,000-steps-a-day walking program and bought an elliptical trainer and a recumbent bicycle for her home. At one point, she hired a trainer and managed to lose 10 or 15 pounds, but they eventually came back.

When Vickie transitioned to the artist's life, her food choices didn't improve much. She worked twelve to eighteen hours a day, having pasta or sandwiches on white bread and chocolate chip cookies for lunch, and she traveled on the weekends. On the road, she traded the lunch truck for the food available at the art shows where she sold her work. Always on the run, she stopped at fast food places for the convenience.

Over the years, this kind of eating had its effect, and the pounds gradually added up on her 5-foot, 6-inch frame. Then in 2010, at age 52, some vacation photos brought her up short.

"We'd gone to Hawaii and when I saw the photos, I was devastated," Vickie says. "I didn't see myself in soft focus any longer—this time the edges were sharp and it was awful."

More than the photos, it was her husband's concern that finally got through to Vickie. "It doesn't matter what I weighed, my husband was never harsh with me. He never criticized me or made me feel fat," she says. "But when we saw the photos, he said to me, 'I'm concerned about you.' I knew then that I had to do something."

Vickie considered a lot of weight loss plans, but the food didn't appeal to her, particularly on the delivered meal programs. And she had one nonnegotiable—whatever plan she chose, it had to include milk. "If I couldn't have milk, it was a deal breaker for me," she said. "One day, I googled 'diet and milk' and up popped South Beach."

Vickie went out and bought three South Beach books: the diet book, a cookbook, and a guide for grocery shopping. She liked the looks of the recipes, especially the side dishes that rounded out a meal's protein. "The sides are beautiful," she says, "zucchini cheese bake, mashed cauliflower with sour cream and chives, brown rice, a dipping sauce for bread."

The next day, February 25, 2011, Vickie started the South Beach Diet. Within two weeks, she'd lost 20 pounds. "This is the easiest thing I've ever done," she says. "I just started dropping down through the sizes—I had to give away clothes I'd bought for a new size before I even took the tags off."

Thinking it was going too smoothly to be true, she went to her doctor's office one day and asked to use their scale, just to be sure she was getting an accurate reading. It was true; she had lost 42 pounds. Over five months, Vickie lost 77 pounds, and today she's aiming for another few pounds. From a size 18/20, she's dropped to a size 10. Incredibly, she lost her weight without any deliberate exercise.

In each phase of the South Beach Diet, Vickie has found recipes she loves. "I'm just not going to sacrifice taste, so I had to find recipes that I would like," she says. "My go-to recipe in the first phase was an espresso custard topped with mini dark chocolate chips. The chips were the size of lint, but they did the job for me!"

Besides enjoying her new recipes and habits, Vickie feels she's gotten a handle on what to do after "indiscretions." "I just go back to Phase 1 for a day and get the sugar or whatever out of my system," she says. "I've learned to stop myself, because I don't want to keep creating cravings for myself. I ask myself, 'Do I really want to begin all this again?' and the answer is no, just no."

Although Vickie has stopped going to art shows, she has a plan for the velvet cape she used to wear to them.

"I'm going to build a wooden frame and stretch the cape out on it just to remind myself how much material it took to cover me," she says. "I did not believe that I would ever feel like myself again. I keep asking myself, 'Have I really lost this weight?' And the answer is, 'Yes! I really have lost the weight!'"

Thanks To

My husband, Scott: For looking at me lovingly, no matter what I weighed.

My weight loss soul sister, Cynthia Callahan: She and I are administrators of Facebook's South Beach Intermediate Support Board. She is a joy, my mentor. She validates everything; she reminds me that what I'm doing means something.

My Tips

You have to decide that this is a lifestyle, not a diet. A diet is temporary. It expires. You can't be on a diet for the rest of your life. Read the *South Beach Diet* book cover to cover, so you understand it completely. It's not complicated. It's work, yes, but joyous work. You'll find recipes that you love: steak au poivre, sweet potato fries, egg "muffins," melon-and-blackberry salad, pork tenderloin with peach salsa, whole wheat pancakes—and of course the Chilled Espresso Custard, a recipe you can find on the South Beach Diet website.

The South Beach Diet

"The South Beach Diet teaches you to rely on the right carbs and the right fats—the good ones—and enables you to live quite happily without the bad carbs and bad fats."

—*The South Beach Diet: The Delicious, Doctor-Designed, Foolproof Plan for Fast and Healthy Weight Loss* by Arthur Agatston, MD (Emmaus, PA: Rodale, 2003)

Miami cardiologist Arthur Agatston developed the South Beach Diet for overweight heart patients. In the first two weeks of this three-phase diet, food choices are severely limited: no starches, no fruit, no alcohol, and no sugar. The second phase allows a little of the foods you enjoy, whether it's pasta, chocolate, or a glass of wine. The third phase is the lifelong stage that allows you to eat "normal size" portions of "normal" foods, even rich desserts, if you can manage to eat just three bites. Two snacks a day are allowed in all phases.

The diet is based on the glycemic index, a measure of how rapidly blood glucose levels (and, therefore, insulin levels) rise after eating a carbohydrate. In its final two phases, the diet allows low-glycemic carbs like whole grain breads, pasta and cereal, vegetables and fruit, some fats, lean meats, and low-fat dairy products. But by avoiding the highly processed, high-glycemic carbohydrates, such as the ones found in white breads and white rice, baked goods, snacks, and other convenience foods, Agatston says the body can overcome its insulin resistance and properly process fats and sugars, leading to weight loss. And, he says, the body's cravings for sweets and bad carbs will disappear.

While Agatston believes that exercise is an essential part of a cardiac health plan, he created the diet to be effective regardless of the dieter's exercise habits. Yet he notes that physical activity will speed weight loss.

The plan has been updated through the years, most recently as *The South Beach Diet Supercharged: Faster Weight Loss and Better Health for Life.*[4]

This plan might work for me because . . .

- ☑ I need a total break from my current eating habits.
- ☑ I like the idea of a phased plan that adds foods back in gradually.
- ☑ After my success, I want to be able to enjoy some of my favorites again.

Nancy Inglehart

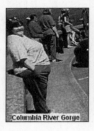
Columbia River Gorge

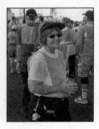

Portland, Oregon
Age: 59
Occupation: Special education paraeducator and nutritionist
Achievement: Lost 165 pounds
How She Did It: Zone Diet

Nancy Inglehart used to zone out on fast food. Now she's in the Zone, where she's 165 pounds lighter and 100 percent more energetic.

Nancy's upbringing in Connecticut, in the embrace of a family with both Italian and German roots, put her on an early track to unhealthy eating habits. Her dad, while a hardworking man, had a temper and was strict about the family's schedule and habits. When her mother was incapacitated by illness, Nancy was packed off to her grandmother's house, where she sometimes spent long periods of time.

"*Manga!* That was the mantra I grew up with," she recalls. "For my grandmother, eating was comfort. Cooking was the answer to everything—for when you were happy, for when you were sad, for indulging after church, or to get yourself a man."

The years dealt Nancy some crushing blows. Her mother was ill throughout Nancy's entire early life, and her dad took on the responsibility of keeping the family together. Her husband was diagnosed with lupus at the age of 37, and their daughter died of heart disease at age 11. The couple raised their two other children, who were only ten-and-a-half months apart in age. Nancy eventually cared for her parents during their final illnesses.

All the while, Nancy led a busy and often stressful working life, with her own medical transcription business, working in doctors' offices and eventually making a career change to education. She was a stress eater, big-time.

"When my son was a teen, I'd ask him to go to Taco Bell and get me a dozen tacos," she said. "I promised him I wouldn't eat them all at once, that I would save some for tomorrow. But then I would sit down to watch TV and devour all twelve of them."

For dinner, Nancy admits, she would cook pasta and eat the entire one-pound package herself. She was in despair over her eating habits, but seemingly powerless to stop herself. Over the years, she tried a wide range of diets and exercise plans—Richard Simmons, Free to Be Thin, the grapefruit diet—but eventually she would fail.

In her early fifties, Nancy's weight peaked at 350 pounds. The time to act had come. Although she had endured some rude comments from schoolchildren, and she knew her health was suffering, what really got her attention was being unable to find clothes that fit.

"My back hurt; I couldn't walk. I couldn't get any clothes to fit me. Even Wal-Mart didn't carry stretchy pants large enough for me," she says.

Nancy had simply had enough, and she knew she had to make a decision. One day in March 2003, she was flipping through channels and came across Barry Sears talking about his Zone weight loss plan. She was intrigued enough to buy the book. And then she went to work. "The first thing I did was clean out my refrigerator," she says. When she started, she weighed in at 325 pounds.

Used to doing her own cooking, Nancy liked the idea of being in control of her meals. She prepared meals and snacks using the Zone's 40-30-30 formula—40 percent carbs, 30 percent proteins, 30 percent fats—and began to lose weight, but she soon found herself bored with the recipes in the book.

Heading to the Internet this time, she found FormulaZone, a website of Zone-friendly meal plans, recipes, and advice. Not only did she find recipes there, but she submitted her own to the thousands in the database. She was such a devotee of the site that she became close friends with the owners, Cale and Karen Bergh. Cale even started getting some mysterious packages from Nancy.

"My comfort foods are crunchy ones, like Kettle chips or soy crisps. If I can't control myself, I do what I call a ritual cleansing, and I mail the bag to Cale," she says.

Surprisingly, Nancy found the weight just dropping off. "I liked the food, because it was real food, it was my food," she says. "I began feeling better, and I was not as hungry. I was losing the cravings and I had more energy."

Fifteen months later, Nancy had lost 165 pounds. Although she could barely get up and down stairs when she began, she started walking as soon as she could, incorporating more steps into her daily routine and building up to benefit events, like the annual Susan G. Komen Race for the Cure and Portland's Providence Hospital Annual Bridge Pedal and Stride.

When she thinks about her journey, Nancy is amazed but saddened by the realization that society treats overweight people as outcasts. Her experience bears it out.

"One day, when I was over 300 pounds, I was in the parking lot at Costco, trying to fit all my stuff into my car. People were driving by and laughing at the fat woman," she remembers. "The other day, I was doing the same thing, and a man stopped his car, got out, and said, 'Let me help you with that.' I'm not a different person, but people perceive you differently."

Today, energetic is the only word to use when you talk about Nancy. During the day, she works in special education for a public school district and serves on two state-level special education committees, and in her off hours, she is a home health care and hospice worker. She is working on her business degree, starting up a nutritional counseling and in-home catering business called Bridgecity Nutrition, and consulting on the FormulaZone website.

"I used to be crabby and irritable. I'd just come home from work and crash," she says. "Now I have so much energy, when my feet hit the floor in the morning, I'm ready to go. This has literally changed the whole course of my life."

Thanks To——————

Cale and Karen Bergh, founders of FormulaZone.com.

Author Bob Schwartz, *Diets Don't Work.*

Author Geneen Roth, *When Food Is Love.*

My Tips

If you can get past the first ten minutes of a craving, you can beat it. Divert your attention—walk the dog. I'll pick up ice cream at the grocery store, then head over to the produce section. After a while, I can put the ice cream back. Don't reward yourself with food. Get a jar, and every time you go to the store and put the ice cream back, or whatever, put a dollar in the jar. At the end of the week, or the month, go to a movie or buy some new clothes.

The Zone Diet

"The Zone is a real metabolic state that can be reached by everyone, and maintained indefinitely on a lifelong basis. . . . In the Zone you'll enjoy . . . freedom from hunger, greater energy and physical performance, as well as improved mental focus and productivity. . . . Every time you open your mouth to eat, you're applying for a passport to the Zone."

—*The Zone* by Barry Sears, PhD, and Bill Lawren (New York: HarperCollins, 1995)

Seeking to avoid the fate of the men in his family who all died of heart attacks, biochemist Barry Sears created this diet that aims to achieve stable blood sugar levels and hormonal balance, so that the body draws on stored body fat for energy. According to Sears, the body functions best when every meal you eat contains a ratio of 40 percent carbohydrates, 30 percent protein, and 30 percent fat.

While it looks like a high carbohydrate diet, in reality the Zone allows only carbohydrates from "good," low-glycemic sources. "Bad" carbs are found in the usual suspects—bread, pasta, and rice—along with some vegetables and fruits you wouldn't suspect, like carrots and cranberries. Sears believes many people are insulin resistant, which makes the high-density, high-glycemic carbohydrates of the standard—and now out-dated—food pyramid ineffective, and even unhealthy, for many people.[5]

The 40-30-30 ratio is calculated by first determining your daily protein requirement with a formula that estimates your lean body mass and level of physical activity. Maintaining this constant ratio helps the body stabilize its hormones, Sears says, placing your body in what he calls "the Zone." By balancing out your hormones, he believes, the body releases less insulin into its bloodstream, contributing to weight loss. Sears also claims that eating this way lowers your risk of developing other chronic diseases.

The tricky part of the diet is balancing every meal using Sears's "block" method. In later books, such as *Mastering the Zone*, *Zone Perfect Meals in Minutes*, *What to Eat in the Zone*, and *Zone Meals in Seconds*, Sears provides meal plans and recipes in which the blocks are calculated for you.[6] Helping the Zone dieter figure it all out is also the mission and business of FormulaZone.com founders Cale and Karen Bergh of Broomfield, Colorado.

This plan might work for me because . . .

- ☑ The idea of balancing, rather than restricting, foods appeals to me.
- ☑ I am willing to track the nutrients in my meals and even in my snacks.
- ☑ I don't want to eliminate carbohydrates, but I would like to choose healthy carbs.

Chapter Four

You Can Count On It

Limiting Calories One Way or Another

Jerry B. Jenkins, the wildly prolific author and speaker, has maintained a weight loss of 135 pounds for many years. He does it by counting calories. Using DietPower.com, he has taken the mystery—and the imprecision—out of calorie counting. After all this time, and even when he doesn't have online access, he does the hard work of counting.

"It remains an obsession. When I'm not near the computer, I'm constantly jotting down what I've eaten and how many calories I have left," he said to me.

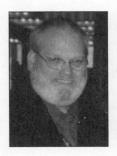 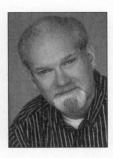

"It's a worth-it war."

—Jerry B. Jenkins, author

Many people feel the way Jerry does, whether they're actually counting calories or simply eating in a way that limits them. Many weight loss plans rely on low-calorie intake or on low-fat intake, which necessarily results in a low-calorie plan. "You just can't eat a bowl of broccoli big enough to take in too many calories," as one person put it to me.

But what are calories? And why should we keep track of them? The definition of a calorie doesn't make much sense at first glance—it's hard to see how it relates to food. A calorie is a unit of energy. So far, so good. This much we all learned in science class.

Of course, we associate calories with food, but they actually apply to anything containing energy. For example, a gallon of gas contains about 31 million calories. Now there's an entrée for you!

Specifically, a calorie measures the amount of energy, or heat, that it takes to raise the temperature of 1 gram of water 1 degree Celsius (1.8 degrees Fahrenheit). Does that help any? No, I didn't think so. (It does explain, though, why we burn a few calories when we drink iced beverages—your body has to work to heat them up. Bring on the iced tea!)

You might be confused, too, if you've ever heard the word *kilocalorie*. When we say, "This bag of chips has 400 calories," what we're really talking about is kilocalories—1,000 calories equals 1 kilocalorie. So, a bag of chips containing 400 food calories contains 400,000 regular calories, or 400 kilocalories. The same applies to exercise—when a fitness chart says you burn about 100 calories for every mile you walk, it means 100 kilocalories.

But let's not quibble. Let's just talk about the word *calorie* that we all know and hate.

We humans need energy to breathe, move, and pump blood, and we acquire this energy from food. The number of calories in a food is a measure of how much potential energy that food has. A gram of carbohydrates (including sugar) has four calories, a gram of protein has four calories, and a gram of fat has nine calories. Foods are comprised of these three elements. So, if you know how many carbohydrates, fats, and proteins are in your food, you know how many calories, or how much energy, you are taking in.

Armed with this knowledge, the person wanting to lose weight must make a second calculation of an appropriate daily calorie limit, given how many calories he or she "burns" throughout the day, in order to create a consistent calorie deficit and achieve weight loss.

That's the logic behind lowering or tracking your calorie count. For some people, like Jerry Jenkins, calorie counting is an exact science. Many weight loss plans keep track of calories directly or through a point system that simplifies the tracking of calories. Other plans, by their very nature, limit calories without you having to actively track them.

You can count me in as one of those people who isn't very exact about things. The meandering rows of my vegetable garden are quite artistic, I think. And balance a checkbook? Even given my history as a financial journalist and my role as the family banker, tax preparer, and investment manager, I can't get excited about that little chore.

I make meals that combine proteins, carbs, and fats. I estimate the caloric content of my snacks. I eyeball portion sizes. Despite an upbringing that forbade card games, I can tell you when a piece of chicken is the size of a pack of cards. I watch the clock when I exercise, but I don't own a heart rate monitor. My blood pressure looks good at the doctor's office, but I don't know from day to day how it's doing. Nothing about the numbers has been exact.

But the truth is that by simply keeping a minimally attentive eye on my intake and expenditure of calories, I brought my daily total down. I couldn't tell you exactly how much of a calorie deficit I created, but the numbers speak for themselves. At any given time in my quest to lose 30 pounds, I knew I was succeeding when the scale was trending downward.

If I had kept a closer eye on calories, it might not have taken me three long years, and thousands of laps, to drop three dress sizes. Many people already know this. Here are two people who lowered their calorie intake—whether deliberately or simply by their new food choices—and succeeded.

Lori Kimble

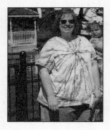 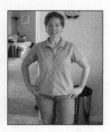

Fort Edward, New York
Age: 42
Occupation: Medical transcriptionist
Accomplishment: Lost 105 pounds
How She Did It: Calorie counting

Remember the *Looney Tunes* character Wile E. Coyote? Over and over, he'd rig up a contraption to drop an anvil on the lightning-fast Road Runner. That cartoon image is embedded in Lori Kimble's mind.

"At my heaviest, I weighed 250 pounds," says Lori. "I saw that number on the scale, and I could see in my mind a Wile E. Coyote anvil marked '250 lbs.' It dawned on me then—250 pounds is halfway to 500 pounds, and I could see myself weighing that much if I kept going the way I was."

But having that realization and acting on it were two different things for Lori.

"I was frustrated because I thought, *I'm going to weigh 500 pounds because I don't know what to do about it,*" she says.

Lori recalls always being heavy—or at least chubby. She has no memories of ever being a healthy weight. From an early age, she was drawn to comfort foods like macaroni and cheese, pasta, white rice, bagels, and spaghetti. Hamburger Helper was a dinner staple at her house. The only vegetables she liked were broccoli and corn. She and her sister snacked at home, and they liked their sweets.

Like many people frustrated with their weight, Lori was always trying one diet or another, but she failed every time. "I had in my head that I only had to put up with this diet for awhile, and then I could go back to eating the way I always had," she says. "It was an all-or-nothing attitude that just wasn't working for me."

In 2003, Lori read *The Sugar Addict's Total Recovery Program* by Kathleen DesMaisons. The book made her realize that her previous weight loss attempts may have failed because she was simply replacing high-fat foods with seemingly healthy low-fat foods that were instead loaded with sugar. By weaning off of processed foods, refined carbohydrates, sugars, and what she calls "white things" and replacing them with proteins and whole grains like brown rice, she lost 20 pounds in one year.

This success spurred Lori on to address other problems with her diet, like portion sizes. She joined Weight Watchers and lost another 60 pounds but then hit a frustrating plateau.

"I was eating very little point-wise, exercising hard, and seeing no progress," she says. "I cried every week weighing in. This went on for six months."

At the time, living in temporary housing without a kitchen, Lori and her husband began picking up food from a Mexican takeout place, and her weight started coming back on.

"I tried eating right again, and I tried going back on Weight Watchers and several other things, like eDiets and the low-glycemic plan GI Impact," she says.

But by this time, Lori was exhausted.

"I was so tired of thinking about food all the time. I just wanted someone to tell me what to eat," she says.

Lori found relief by joining Nutrisystem and ordering their packaged meals for a few months. She found it to be helpful in once again training her to recognize an appropriate portion size. She liked the balance of fats, proteins, and carbs—the meals included more protein than she was used to having, and that helped her stay full longer.

When she felt ready, Lori transitioned from Nutrisystem to cooking her own meals. She combined some elements of Nutrisystem and the

Zone Diet to come up with meals that combined nutrients in a way that kept her from feeling hungry.

Exercise also figured into Lori's success. She and her husband are avid bike riders. They generally take one long bike ride each weekend—at least when the weather in upstate New York cooperates—usually about 40 miles. She is training for a 100-mile bike ride and has participated in her first triathlon.

Gradually, Lori began to see success again. "It was a slow process, but that just made my weight loss feel more permanent to me," she says. Within a few years, Lori's total weight loss came to 105 pounds. At 5 feet, 2 inches, she wears a size 8 today, where once she wore a size 24.

Although Lori's success came from several different programs, one thing remained constant—calorie counting. Throughout her weight loss journey, Lori logged the caloric value of her foods. She used the system provided by the plan, like Weight Watchers Points or Nutrisystem's calorie counter, and when she was on her own, she sought help from an online calorie counting program, LiveStrong's MyPlate.

Determining her ideal daily caloric intake was a process of trial and error, Lori says. She eventually settled on about 1,500 calories a day for weight loss. "Anything lower than 1,400 and I get cranky," she says. When she is in a maintenance mode and on days when exercise has her body crying out for sustenance, she might up the calorie count to 2,000 a day.

Logging calories and exercise choices isn't a chore for Lori. "I'm a bit dorky that way," she says. "I like seeing the numbers."

Another motivator for Lori has been tracking her progress on her blog *Finding Radiance*. Her blog is filled with photo after photo of her colorful and appetizing meals.

"Once I began arranging meals on a plate to take photos, my food looked more appealing to me, and I began to get excited about food again," she says. "I'm not afraid of food anymore. Cupcakes aren't evil. If I really want something, I can make room for it and really, really enjoy it."

Today, Lori continues to track her calories, food choices, and exercise. For her, it's the key to success.

"Now I have the complete puzzle put together! I feel like I can live this way for the rest of my life," Lori says.

Thanks To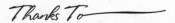

My husband, John Vaughn: He's my rock, the best support I have. He's lost 40 pounds along with me, and we've enjoyed getting fit together.

My blog readers: This community has been invaluable to me. I always have support when I need it, and I enjoy supporting others when they're struggling. It makes you realize that you're not alone after all.

My Tips

You can't have an all-or-nothing attitude. Don't think you're going to run five miles if you've never taken a step. If you eat something you shouldn't have, don't think, *Well, I can just go ahead and eat what I want. The day is shot anyway.* But don't beat yourself up. It's OK to be a little imperfect. Most of all, don't give up!

Here is a recipe I love for protein-rich pancakes.

Recipe for: **Protein Pancakes**

1/3 cup 1% fat cottage cheese

1/3 cup rolled oats

1/3 cup egg substitute, or 1 egg plus one white

1/8 teaspoon baking powder

dash of vanilla

dash of cinnamon

Splenda to taste (optional)

Blend all ingredients in a blender; the batter should be smooth. Make them like regular pancakes. Makes three big pancakes. You can also make waffles with this batter. Top with your favorite fruit topping. Here is one of mine:

Recipe for: **Banana Maple Topping**

1 small ripe banana

1 tablespoon real maple syrup

In a small bowl, mash the banana well until it is liquidy. Stir in the maple syrup. Heat in the microwave for about 20 seconds.

Losing Weight by Counting Calories

As Lori discovered, losing weight by counting calories requires that you create a calorie deficit—taking in fewer calories than you expend over time.

To lose one pound per week, for example, you need to create a calorie deficit of 500 calories per day, or 3,500 a week. You can do this by consuming 250 fewer calories a day and burning an extra 250 calories through physical activity, or through some other combination of these two measures.

In order to create a consistent calorie deficit, you first need to know what amount of calories will sustain your current weight. This formula depends on several factors: age, gender, height, weight, and activity level. Numerous websites can take you through the calculation.

The formula generally begins by calculating your basal metabolic rate (BMR), or the rate at which your body burns calories while at total rest. For example, using the calculator on the website www.bmi-calculator.net, a woman who is 5 feet, 4 inches tall, weighs 160 pounds, and is 50 years old would have a BMR of about 1,417 calories per day.

Next, factor in your level of daily activity. You burn calories over and above your BMR, even if you have a desk job or engage in no purposeful exercise. Here is the Harris Benedict Equation for determining daily caloric needs:

Sedentary (little or no exercise): BMR x 1.2

Lightly active (light exercise/sports 1–3 days/week): BMR x 1.375

Moderately active (moderate exercise/sports 3–5 days/week):
  BMR x 1.55
Very active (hard exercise/sports 6–7 days/week): BMR x 1.725
Extra active (very hard exercise/sports and physical job): BMR x 1.9

If the woman in the example considers herself sedentary, she would multiply 1,417 by 1.2 to arrive at 1,700 calories per day for weight maintenance. To lose weight, this woman would have to decrease her caloric intake or increase her activity level or both.

Determining how many calories you take in daily can be accomplished fairly easily using an online calorie counting program. These programs can be highly specific, listing the caloric value of everything from an apple to a meal at a chain restaurant. FitDay, SparkPeople, DietPower, MyPlate, and CalorieKing are five popular programs mentioned by people in this book. Keeping a food log over time will help you get a handle on how many calories you generally consume per day.[1]

The caloric value of what you eat in a typical day may shock you. If asked to guess, most people underestimate their daily caloric intake. But often, you can make simple changes that add up over time. For example, I replaced butter on my toast with a heart-healthy butter substitute, which has half the calories of butter—50 calories per tablespoon instead of 100 calories. I began making my own salad dressings when I found that commercial dressings often contain sugar, which has 16 calories per teaspoon. I use a mix of half sugar and half sugar substitute in my coffee. Now, if I could only replace the half 'n half with skim milk, I'd have it made! But some measures are just too drastic, if you ask me.

Ken Romeo

Reno, Nevada
Age: 53
Occupation: Geriatric and sports doctor
Accomplishment: Lost 115 pounds
How He Did It: Atkins Diet[2] and the Pritikin Program

Sports doctor Ken Romeo was opining about matters of health to the ball players of the Astros one day when he was stopped short by the team's catcher.

"Why should we listen to you, doc? You're fat," the catcher said.

That word *fat* struck Ken Romeo with all the force of a major league fastball.

As a doctor, Ken had seen plenty of overweight patients. In fact, just from looking at the statistics and lab results on a patient's chart, he could visualize with almost one 100 percent accuracy what that patient looked like before the exam even began. Yet it seems he couldn't visualize himself with any accuracy.

Ken weighed 315 pounds—of course, he knew that—but he, like so many of us, didn't really see his weight for what it was.

"You realize you're overweight, because maybe you waddle or you wear out easily, but you look in the mirror and the only thing you see is the feature you think defines you," Ken says. "You say to yourself, *I have great hair* or *I have a beautiful smile*. It's almost impossible to take a cold, hard look at yourself when your mind can so effectively block out the negative."

Something about the ball player's words got through to Ken, though, and he decided on a dramatic test. He took a brown paper grocery bag, cut two holes for his eyes, and put the bag over his head. Thus attired, he stood in front of a full-length mirror and took a good, long look at himself.

"Boy, was that a rude awakening! By eliminating all the features I thought were compensating for my weight, I saw my body for what it was. And I had to conclude that the catcher was right. I was fat," he says.

At 6 feet, 1 inch tall, Ken wore a size 4X shirt and had a 54-inch waist. It was unquestionably time to act.

But it wasn't so easy for Ken to decide what to do. While he knew plenty about healthy food, the reality was that it wasn't always available to him. He traveled frequently, both with the Astros and in his role as a team physician to the U.S. Olympic boxing team, and he found himself hanging around stadiums full of nachos and cheese but bereft of fresh produce. Not only that, but Ken had some things firmly in mind that he wasn't going to do.

"I love food and I hate to exercise. Odd for a sports doc, I know," Ken says. "Going on a diet that was based on starvation or calorie counting wasn't an option for me. I didn't have the patience for that. I was kind of left with the alternative of 'eating away' my fat."

Ken was drawn to the Atkins diet, one that is high in protein and low in carbohydrates. He thought metabolically it had merit, but he asked a few of his cardiologist friends what they thought. "They said they didn't care what I did as long as I took off the weight," he says.

The thought of eating traditionally forbidden foods like steak, eggs, butter, and cheese appealed to Ken. He felt good enough about his decision to act that he even started walking for exercise. Even so, sticking to the regime could be a challenge at times.

"I'd enter the cafeteria at an Olympic Training Center in Colorado Springs, and I'd ask the cooks for some mayonnaise for my two or three cheeseburgers—no buns—and every eye would be on me. The chefs actually had to go into the back of the kitchen to get the mayo," he says. "I could feel the athletes looking at me and thinking, *Dude, go on a diet!*"

Ken found to his surprise that the diet worked. In about thirty days, his weight plummeted by 35 pounds to 280 pounds. Within a year, he lost 40 more pounds. Still, he dreaded his annual physical, fearing what all the proteins and fats in his diet would mean for his health. "I was never so scared in my life, waiting for my blood work," he says. "But everything looked great. Good cholesterol was up, bad cholesterol down, triglyceride numbers were great. My doctor told me, 'Whatever you're doing, keep it up!'"

Yet although Atkins was working for him, Ken had some regrets.

"It was summer and the grocery stores were filled with colorful fruits and melons, foods that you know are high in fiber and antioxidants, and I couldn't have them in the quantity that I wanted them," he says. "I'd see them and think, *There has to be more to life than cheeseburgers and steaks*."

To continue his weight loss success, Ken turned to the Pritikin Program, a low-fat, low-protein diet that is essentially the antithesis of the Atkins diet. "I looked at the athletes I was spending my days with and saw that high performance went hand in hand with a Pritikin-like diet," he says.

But because the Pritikin Program was formulated in the late 1970s, Ken thought it was high time for a few modifications.

"The Pritikin plan demonized virtually all fats and oils, yet today we know so much more about good fats versus bad fats," he says. "I tempered out some of the radical parts of the Pritikin plan to make it livable for me. If I want an olive oil dressing on my salad, I'll put it on."

Initially, Ken found himself gaining a few pounds of what he knew was water weight, but soon the scale started dropping down again. Another 40 pounds came off. At his lowest weight, Ken's scale read 200 pounds. His second healthy decision—to quit a pack-and-a-half-a-day smoking habit—put a few pounds back on, though, and today his weight hovers between 215 and 220. "I'd rather have an extra 15 pounds than still be smoking," he says.

Ken has adopted his Pritikin way of eating for good. It's not so radically different to cook this way, he found. For example, making a chef salad might simply mean substituting chicken for red meat and eliminating the egg yolks. He doesn't think too closely about portion sizes or food quantities. "I eat until I am full and then I stop," he says.

Ken would like to lose a few more pounds. His days are busy—in addition to his advisory role for the U.S. Olympics, he specializes in treating Alzheimer's patients in their homes. He walks and does yard work for exercise. By eating in a way that works for him, he knows that he will be able to meet his goal, so he's not worried about it.

"There's no hurry. I know it will happen," he says. "That's the good part. As long as I eat the right things, I am confident that I will continue to lose weight."

Thanks To

Google: All that information is out there!

My Tips

Your mind is your own worst enemy. Don't think that you're going to lose 10 pounds for a wedding or to wear a bikini. There are no quick fixes. You don't find the solution at a pharmacy; you find it at the grocery store. You have to keep pounding away at it. Your life depends on it.

The Pritikin Program

"Not only is the Pritikin Diet safe and healthy, but it maintains your ideal weight—without any restrictions on food quantity. You can eat as much as you like of many of the permissible foods. All day long, if you wish."

—The Pritikin Program for Diet and Exercise by Nathan Pritikin with Patrick M. McGrady; recipes by June Roth (New York: Bantam, 1984)

Nathan Pritikin was diagnosed with heart disease in his early forties. It was the late 1950s, and cholesterol was barely understood at the time. Pritikin wasn't a doctor—he was an engineer and an inventor—but he knew from studying the groundbreaking work of a California doctor that his cholesterol level, at close to 300, was dangerously high.

Pritikin didn't follow the advice of the day, though, which was to stop exercising, take it easy, and nap often. No one said anything about eliminating the pervasive foods of his daily diet: eggs, bacon, beef, butter, and ice cream. Instead, Pritikin undertook an eating plan that was rich in fruits, vegetables, whole grains, and beans. He switched to lean meat, seafood, and nonfat dairy foods in moderation and began to exercise. His cholesterol level dropped to 120.

The focus of Pritikin's program is on unprocessed, or minimally processed, high-fiber foods and is dramatically low in fat. The original Pritikin plan suggests fewer than 10 percent of your daily calories come from fats. Because of the lack of fats and the emphasis on fruits and vegetables, the plan is naturally low in calories.

Pritikin's son, Robert, updated his father's plan several times, to add more flexibility into his father's plan. In *The Pritikin Principle: The Calorie Density Solution* he modified the plan around the concept of calorie density.[3] Foods that are calorie-dense pack a lot of calories into a small amount of food, he says, and by avoiding calorie-dense foods like baked goods, cheese, fried foods, and ice cream and focusing on low-calorie-dense, high-fiber fruits and vegetables, a person can eat more and feel full longer. The plan suggests eating five or six small meals throughout the day to further avoid hunger.

Specifically, the plan suggests a daily diet of at least five half-cup servings of whole grains and starchy vegetables like beans and potatoes; four one-cup servings of raw vegetables or four half-cup servings of cooked vegetables; no more than three and a half ounces of lean meat; two servings of nonfat dairy; and no more than a quarter cup of nuts. Refined foods, such as white flour, pasta, and white rice, ideally are eliminated. Other foods, such as condiments, sweeteners, and unsaturated fats, are "caution" foods.

The updated plan suggests at least forty-five minutes of daily aerobic exercise like brisk walking, weight training two to three times weekly, and stretching every day.

The Pritikin Longevity Center & Spa in Miami, Florida, is a residential facility that incorporates the Pritikin Program into programs of one or more weeks. Pritikin meals can also be mail-ordered from the center. The Pritikin Center's chief medical director, Robert A. Vogel, MD, and the president of the Pritikin Organization, Paul Tager Lehr, published an updated version of the plan, titled *The Pritikin Edge: 10 Essential Ingredients for a Long and Delicious Life.*[4]

This plan might work for me because...

☑ I want to improve my health as well as lose weight.
☑ I like the idea of having no restrictions on certain healthy foods.
☑ I think I can adapt to a radically different way of eating.
☑ I am willing to exercise regularly.

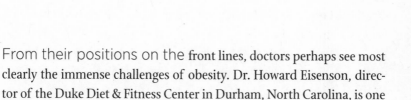

Chapter Five

Get with My Group

Seeking Strength in Numbers

From their positions on the front lines, doctors perhaps see most clearly the immense challenges of obesity. Dr. Howard Eisenson, director of the Duke Diet & Fitness Center in Durham, North Carolina, is one eyewitness to the devastation of this heartbreaking battle.

"We often see people at their most desperate," Dr. Eisenson said to me. "They're hopeless, depressed, and some are nearly bedbound from physical limitations. They're thinking, *How can I go another day like this?*"

Many people I interviewed expressed this same thought. At their lowest point, many considered suicide. It seemed the only way to end the pain of their existence. Yet their story did not end.

"Through our program, many people tell us they have gotten their lives back," Dr. Eisenson says. "We've seen them come back from the abyss."

Dr. Eisenson attributes much of the success of the Duke program to the extensive system of support the staff builds around its participants, as well as the support that program participants provide for each other.

"We try to give them everything we can think of to give them a success experience here," he says. "We give them strategies and messages of encouragement. People leave here feeling hopeful. But we give them a dose of reality, too. We let them know that their continued success rests in the ability to create support systems at home."

For many people, support systems—whether in a residential facility or in their everyday environment—become the key to success. It's why so many weight loss plans are grounded in the practice of weekly meetings. And chances are, at your local Curves you get a little cheerleading along with your workout. Even web-based plans have their message boards and blogs.

Many people told me that they depended on the support of others for a rush that would keep them going. "Nothing felt better than the applause I got each week when our group leader announced my weight loss," one man said to me.

For some people, just the presence of another person in their lives or in their thoughts is a huge motivator. A friend of mine had her husband in mind when she joined Weight Watchers.

"George is an Air Force chaplain, and he was deployed in Kuwait for four months. My gift to him was going to be my weight loss," says Roxanne, who weighed 147 at the time and wore a size 14. "So I took the whole plan on board and planned my meals around the point system. It was an easy way to track what I was eating, and it caused me to be conscious about my choices."

By monitoring her food intake and increasing her exercise and activity level, Roxanne dropped 15 pounds in time for her husband's return. Since then, she has adopted the Weight Watchers plan as her lifestyle. In further evidence of the power of a group, she took up ballet, a childhood passion, joining a class at a local studio. "It wasn't pretty, but I swallowed my pride and I went twice a week," she says.

Through the lives of three other people, let's look at the power of a group in gaining control of your weight.

Veronica "Roni" Noone

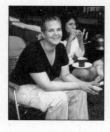 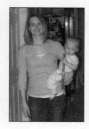

Joppa, Maryland
Age: 35
Occupation: Web publisher and business owner
Accomplishment: Lost 66 pounds
How She Did It: Weight Watchers

Most women plan for a healthy pregnancy. Roni Noone had a plan for *after* her pregnancy.

Two weeks after giving birth to her son Ryan, Roni walked into her local Weight Watchers meeting for her second attempt at the program, baby in tow. She weighed in at 210 pounds, but she wasn't discouraged.

"I knew what to do. Everything was in my corner. I was confident, even looking forward to it," she says. "I knew I could do it."

From her teen years on, Roni remembers being heavy. She considered herself a "chunky" girl, and she didn't like it. One childhood moment in particular haunts Roni.

"I was 12 and I weighed about 150 pounds," she recounts. "One time a friend of my mom's, a man, said to me, 'We weigh the same.' He really didn't mean it negatively, but still it was a devastating comment."

Roni began skipping meals, lying to her mother about having eaten, and hiding food to eat later by herself. At age 14, she took a job at McDonald's, where she made her own concoctions, grilling huge burgers in sausage grease and constructing sundaes smothered in strawberry and chocolate toppings.

Alternating this kind of eating with bouts of sporadic dieting, Roni's weight fluctuated over the years. She graduated from high school a size 12. But college—with its social life and carefree lifestyle—did major damage.

"I came home from my first semester at college and, during a holiday meal, a relative said something at the table about the weight I'd put on. It just about made me cry," she says.

Roni made continued efforts to lose a few pounds, each time settling in a higher weight range. Graduating from college, she weighed in the 180s, and in the year she attended graduate school, she shot up to 210. She wore a size 16 suit to her graduation and a size 18 while interviewing for jobs.

Depressed and angry with herself, Roni decided in January 2000 to try again. She tried zero-calorie diets, a weight loss clinic, even diet pills. She had the most success with a low-carb diet, managing to get down to 155 pounds, but she was miserable. "I was obsessed. I dreaded eating out; I agonized over every decision," she says. "I just couldn't eat that way long-term."

In 2004, Roni and her husband began to talk about starting a family. Roni knew she had to find a healthy way to lose weight. Weight Watchers fit the bill.

"I fell in love with the plan. I just thought, *This is logical*," she remembers. "For someone like me, a little OCD, it's perfect. I love keeping statistics, plotting my progress, going to meetings, and weighing in. The meetings added a layer of accountability that I needed."

In fact, Roni found she loved the supportive atmosphere of the meetings. "I was glad to have people to ask questions of, somewhere I could go for reputable answers. I found a lot of friends there," she says. "Before, it was always me just popping pills by myself, just me trying to make it work."

At her first meeting, Roni weighed in at about 230 pounds. By following the plan, she lost 11 pounds over the next four weeks. But then she discovered she was pregnant, and the deal was off.

"I did eat healthy foods throughout my pregnancy, but I ate excessively," Roni admits. "I ate entire cantaloupes, banana smoothies, fried foods, burgers. I ate for eating's sake. I felt it was my last hurrah."

Not surprisingly, Roni gained 70 pounds in her pregnancy. Coming home from the hospital in June 2004, she weighed 210 pounds. But this time she knew what to do, and back she went to her meetings.

Adopting the Weight Watchers plan for nursing mothers, Roni began to steadily lose weight, most often just two pounds a week. By January 2005, she had reached her goal weight of 149 pounds.

Roni found keeping within her point range a welcome challenge.

"The plan appealed to my creative side. I was excited about figuring out how to eat the biggest portions possible for the lowest amount of points and still eat foods I enjoyed," she says. "I make the best burger ever, on an English muffin, with spinach and pickles, and it has only four points!"

Gradually, Roni lost her aversion to exercise. She began walking with Ryan on her back, dancing around the house with him. She turned off the television and enacted a "five story" rule for herself—in any building up to that height, she has to take the stairs. In 2007, she joined the Y and began walking on a treadmill and biking on a reclining bike. She graduated to cardio, cycling, and step classes and, eventually, started entering 5K races.

Today, at 5 feet, 9 inches tall, Roni weighs 144 pounds and wears a size 6. Although she doesn't consciously count points, she finds her eating habits ingrained. She'll make meatballs with ground turkey, weigh the cheese she puts into baked ziti, and divide her meals and snacks into rough point estimates. She is grateful for her success, and she wants to keep it that way.

"When I joined Weight Watchers, I had a list of goals I wanted to meet. I wanted to have something to celebrate every week. I wanted to be the one to raise my hand in the meeting and share my accomplishment. I wanted to be a success story," she says.

Roni's weight loss journey has transformed her life. Under the umbrella of Skinny Minny Media, Roni has been blogging for several years about weight loss and healthy living. She recently compiled recipes from her websites into a book, *GreenLiteBites: Favorites from the First 3*

Years, and she founded FitBloggin', an annual conference for health and wellness bloggers.

Roni says her blogging and social media business keep her on track. Ultimately, though, she gives her children—in 2011, another son followed her first—all the credit for her success.

"I didn't want to be an afraid-to-have-fun mom, a mom who sits out, a mom who won't put on a bathing suit because she's ashamed of her body," she says. "My sons gave me all the motivation I needed. They have given me a renewed sense of life and purpose."

Thanks To

My sons Ryan and Evan, my husband Bill, and my mom Gerri.

My Weight Watchers leader, Wendy: She showed me it is possible.

My Tips

Rearrange your fridge and put fresh produce, veggies, yogurts, and healthy foods on the shelves. Put the other stuff in the drawers, so you won't see it first. Bring food with you—I always look like I'm going on a trip, packing my apples, yogurt, half sandwiches, and granola bars. Trick yourself into thinking you're eating more than you are—bulk up burgers with lettuce, tomatoes, pickles, and green pepper slices, or add veggies to homemade pizza. Don't stress about parties or special occasions—just make good choices after you get home.

Weight Watchers

"In order to overcome the powerful myth that it is not possible to sustain weight loss, you need to have all four components in place: making wise food choices, being physically active, making positive lifestyle changes, and creating a supportive atmosphere."

— *Weight Watchers Weight Loss That Lasts: Break Through the 10 Big Diet Myths* by James M. Rippe, MD, and Weight Watchers (Hoboken, NJ: John Wiley & Sons, 2005).

Weight Watchers began in the early 1960s when Jean Nidetch, a woman who had lost weight at the New York City Obesity Clinic, began inviting friends to her home in Queens to discuss weight loss techinques. As the meetings developed into a formal program, the weekly meeting became its cornerstone.

Until recently, the traditional Weight Watchers Points plan assigned points to foods according to their caloric value, and the dieter made food choices to remain within a daily point limit. In 2010, Weight Watchers overhauled its plan, and today it is called Points Plus. It is still focused on counting calories, but it now assigns points to foods based on their nutritional value.

The new plan emphasizes using points wisely by eating foods rich in fiber and protein. Previously, for example, a 100-calorie apple was treated the same as a 100-calorie cookie. Now, the plan allows unlimited quantities of fresh fruits and non-starchy vegetables, and assigns more points to calorie-dense foods that have more fat and simple carbs. No foods are off-limits, but foods that are high in calories and low in nutritional value are now limited.

The goal of creating a calorie deficit through food and exercise choices remains the same. As before, daily point allowances are based on body weight and weight loss goal. You earn extra points for exercise and can apply them to your daily diet or speed weight loss by not using them.

To become a member and attend meetings, you are charged a one-time membership fee and weekly meeting fees; you must pay the weekly fee even for missed meetings. Meetings begin with a confidential weigh-in. After reaching and maintaining your goal weight for six weeks, you become a lifetime member and may attend meetings at no charge, if you weigh in once a month and are no more than two pounds above your goal weight. Group leaders speak on and lead discussions of topics relevant to weight loss.

If you don't wish to attend meetings, Weight Watchers also offers an online program at WeightWatchers.com, including various tools and message boards. You can buy a Points Plus pocket guide listing popular foods, a mobile phone app, or a Points Plus calculator. You also can access the online database of 40,000 foods. The program's prepackaged food can be found at most major grocery store chains.

This plan might work for me because . . .

- ☑ I would like specific guidelines in making food choices.
- ☑ I think I would enjoy the support of others in my situation.
- ☑ Weekly meetings would encourage me to be faithful to my plan.

Marie M.[1]

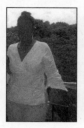 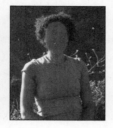

Raleigh, North Carolina
Age: 39
Occupation: Attorney
Accomplishment: Maintaining a 72-pound loss
How She Did It: Overeaters Anonymous

When Marie started practicing law, she spent big bucks on new clothes for her court appearances. Although she weighed 240 pounds, she thought that she had finally made peace with herself and accepted her weight.

But her peace was short-lived. It always was. As a child, Marie remembers that her busy parents—her father in the construction business and her mother an architect—used food to engender momentary good feelings.

"I was showered with a lot of attention, but my parents used food to calm me, quiet me, and reward me," she says.

Growing up in New York City, Marie remembers shopping in New Jersey with her mother. On the way home, they'd stop at Dairy Queen or a candy shop. When her sister was born, she was promised a jelly doughnut to ease her anxieties about the new baby. She remembers bingeing for the first time at age 7, after her parents separated. At age 10, she and her sister lived with an aunt in Nigeria for a year, an experience she recalls as wonderful but that increased her feelings of anxiety and insecurity.

As early as kindergarten, Marie's parents were concerned about her weight. One day, she passed out in her kindergarten classroom because her mother had restricted her food so severely. By the time she turned 14, when her father died after a battle with lymphoma, Marie's emotional upheaval and eating habits began to take their toll. Within four months, she gained 70 pounds. At 5 feet, 10 inches, she weighed 220 pounds. Even then, she knew that her eating habits were tied to her emotions.

"I was longing for intimacy and love. I went to a weight loss camp the following summer, and I loved it," she remembers. "It hurt me that smaller kids could be picked up or given piggy back rides. I had one memorable moment at camp when a girlfriend said to me, 'It's OK. You can sit on my lap,' and she didn't tease me about being too heavy."

Yet it was also a friend who later introduced Marie to purging.

"When I was 17, a friend and I went out to lunch. Afterward, she said she knew how to get rid of the food," Marie says. "It was like manna from heaven! I thought, *Why didn't I think of that?*"

Marie tried undereating, too. Wanting to shape up for her senior prom, she cut back to 500 calories a day, exercised, and smoked. Within a month, she lost 30 pounds. She considers this her first of two anorexic episodes, although bulimia became a long-term condition.

Over the years, Marie's weight fluctuated in response to the emotional turbulence of her life. Her mother contracted Lyme disease and eventually could not walk. Marie bounced from one relationship to another, gaining and losing weight. She'd go through periods of intense exercise, what she calls "exercise bulimia." Her bulimia waxed and waned, and although she was depressed about it, she resisted seeking help.

"I didn't want people to think I was crazy," she says.

In her late twenties, Marie stopped exercising for six weeks while she studied for the bar exam. Her weight shot up from about 230 to 260 pounds. Joining a "pay and weigh" program again a few years later, Marie lost 63 pounds, but she never attained her goal weight range of 160 to 175 pounds. Two years and another destructive relationship later, she regained the weight and then some. She no longer suffered from bulimia, but she continued a pattern of binge eating.

By the time Marie moved to another city and was outfitting herself for the courtroom, she became embroiled in a family crisis that brought her to her knees.

"I confronted my sister and her husband about some of their personal issues, and it turned into a big blowout, complete with yelling, screaming, and crying," she recalls. "It made me realize that I was a big hypocrite because my own life was out of control, and I was the one who needed help. It was my first step toward surrender."

Searching the Internet, Marie happened on Overeaters Anonymous (OA). "Something just clicked," she says. "It was the start of God doing for me what I couldn't do for myself." She made a phone call and attended her first meeting.

"I heard one woman share her story. She talked about things I had done in secret that I had never shared with anyone," she says. "That night I knew that I was home."

By the time she attended her third meeting, though, Marie was in agony. "I cried through that whole meeting," she says. "I realized then that food had always been my best friend and constant companion, and I knew I'd have to surrender it."

The next morning, December 7, 2006, Marie called the local OA contact, who agreed to sponsor her, and they began working the twelve steps together.

From that day, Marie has followed her own eating plan, abstaining from her addictive foods, including sugar. Adhering to OA's tradition of allowing members to choose their own eating plan, and to avoid dwelling on food, she prefers not to talk about her specific food habits, even at meetings. She will say that she hasn't found it difficult to adopt new eating patterns.

"Initially, I never wrote down a list of what to eat or not eat. Once I surrendered, I instinctively knew what to eat," she says. At one point, however, she did consult a dietitian, one of the avenues that OA suggests for gaining dietary information.

Over the course of 18 months, Marie lost 72 pounds. "I am now a size 10, which I can barely comprehend, but the biggest joy is the freedom I have from food obsession," she says. "Not only have I not eaten my binge foods for four years, but the true miracle is that I haven't wanted to eat them."

Marie is in daily contact with her sponsor, does her twelve-step work every day, keeps a daily food journal, and uses what OA calls "tools," such as writing, sponsoring, and service to others. She starts each morning with prayer and meditation. Combining these activities with her involvement in a supportive church community, Marie feels happy and free for the first time in her life.

"I no longer pick up food in response to emotions or life circumstances," she says. "Every morning I wake up with the beautiful gift of abstinence and for that I am grateful."

Thanks To

The founders of Overeaters Anonymous.

My Tips

Surrender is the first step to freedom. Keep coming back until the miracle happens for you!

Overeaters Anonymous

"We admitted we were powerless over food—that our lives had become unmanageable."

—Step 1, The Twelve Steps of Overeaters Anonymous

Overeaters Anonymous was founded in January 1960 by Rozanne S. and two other women in Los Angeles to help people who consider themselves "powerless over food." It is now based in Rio Rancho, New Mexico, but meetings can be found worldwide.

OA offers a program of recovery from compulsive overeating and other forms of eating disorders, including binge eating, bulimia, and anorexia. It uses the Twelve Steps and Twelve Traditions of OA, which are based on the steps and traditions of Alcoholics Anonymous. Members are meant to gain recovery through the peer support of meetings and other means, such as establishing a plan of eating, sponsorship, telephone contact, writing, and service to others. OA is self-supporting through member contributions.

OA addresses not only weight loss but also physical, emotional, and spiritual well-being. It does not promote any particular religion or diet. OA members are encouraged to develop a food plan with the help of a health care professional and a sponsor. The emphasis on anonymity is meant to encourage people to honestly share their experience, knowing that what they say will be held in confidence.

Meeting formats vary, but many open with the Serenity Prayer, the Twelve Steps, and a reading that describes compulsive overeating. A speaker may talk about his or her life, or someone might read from OA or AA literature. Other members share their experiences, and new attendees have the opportunity to introduce themselves and speak if they like. Members can both be sponsored and sponsor others.

This plan might work for me because . . .

- ☑ I want the structure, support, and motivation of a regular meeting.
- ☑ I don't mind having to find my own eating and exercise plan.
- ☑ I need to deal with the emotional underpinnings of overeating.
- ☑ I am open to a spiritual dimension in my weight loss journey.

Stacy Merriman[2]

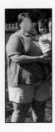 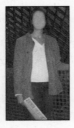

Lancaster, Pennsylvania
Age: 42
Occupation: Software trainer for a public library system
Accomplishment: Lost 200 pounds
How She Did It: Recovery from Food Addiction

When Stacy Merriman attended her first meeting of the twelve-step group Recovery from Food Addiction, she was confronted with an eating plan that banned just about everything she could imagine—sugar, flour, wheat, cheese, nuts, butter, caffeine, alcohol—and weighed and measured everything else.

These people are insane! she remembers thinking.

But in her heart, Stacy knew it was her own lifestyle that was truly insane. In 2000, at the age of 30, she weighed about 370 pounds, although that's just her estimate. "Scales stop at 350 pounds, and I wasn't about to go to a truck stop to weigh myself!" she says.

Many days, Stacy called in sick to her job as a social worker. Her legs and feet were always swollen and her skin was stretched so tightly she thought it might rip. Every evening, she would fill a shopping cart with binge foods. Having recently married, she would hide food around the house or binge in the car. In one sitting, Stacy would typically eat two McDonald's meals or a large pizza, a bag of cookies, a bag of chips, a dozen doughnuts, a pint of ice cream, and a big bag of M&M's.

"I was totally insane at this point. I was ready to die. I just didn't have the guts to kill myself," she says.

Years of out-of-control eating had gotten Stacy to this point. In fact, her earliest memory is from about age two, when she would wake before the rest of her family. In the kitchen, she'd stir spoonfuls of sugar into a glass of water, making a syrupy drink that she would polish off. Although not a binge eater then, she was a grazer, eating whatever and whenever she wanted. At school, she was popular and played sports, but by fifth grade she weighed 185 pounds and could no longer participate. By her senior year, she was close to 6 feet tall, weighed 240 pounds, and wore a size 24.

At a friend's suggestion, she started following the Weight Watchers program on her own, and within five months she lost 60 pounds. But once in college, she began overeating and binge drinking, gaining and losing weight through her college years, usually settling at about 240 pounds.

Between Stacy's junior and senior year at college, she began a crash diet and adopted a triathlon exercise routine, each day running three miles, swimming one mile, and biking one mile. Yet still she was bingeing at night. Working an office job at the college, she stole money from co-workers' desks and emptied out the candy machine at night. Eventually she was caught.

"I was the straight-A perfect good girl. No one would think it was me. But it was my cry for help," Stacy says.

Stacy was forced into counseling and began attending Overeaters Anonymous meetings, where she found immediate help. "It was such a relief to know I wasn't alone," she says.

For seven years, Stacy went to OA meetings and worked its Twelve Steps, but still she struggled. She returned sporadically to the Weight Watchers plan but repeatedly lost and regained the same 80 pounds. In 1996, she just gave up.

"Everywhere I went, people always told me that moderation was the key—you need to learn to have just one," she says. "To myself, I would think, *Maybe if I just don't pick it up, that's what would work.*"

On August 20, 2000, Stacy found someone who agreed with her. A friend contacted Stacy about joining a band—in her teens and early twenties, Stacy had been an R & B singer. The woman invited her to a meeting of Recovery from Food Addiction (RFA), where Stacy first heard that it is possible to be addicted to food. The message rang true for her.

"I've got the genes for addiction," she says. "My father was an alcoholic who left us and eventually shot himself. Both of my grandfathers were alcoholic, as well as a host of uncles, aunts, and cousins. And those in my family who aren't alcoholic are food addicts."

Although Stacy's first thought was that the RFA folks were insane, she adopted the entire plan, following it to the letter. Within a week, she says, she became "totally clean," losing even her cravings. And by following the Twelve Steps, reflecting and praying, journaling and clinging to her RFA sponsor, walking on a treadmill and weight training, she began her journey downward. "It truly is one day at a time," she says.

Today, Stacy weighs 165 pounds and wears a size 10/12. She has returned to the Catholic church, the faith of her youth, where she sings in a worship band. She and her husband have two beautiful girls, ages 4 and 2, that she calls gifts of recovery, as she was previously infertile. She stays in touch with her sponsor and is herself a sponsor. Every day, Stacy wakes up grateful for her recovery.

"By the grace of God, I now have eleven years of unconditional abstinence," she says. "It's an unreal feeling, and my brain has to catch up to being a thin person. I wish this blessing for all food addicts."

Thanks To

Kay Sheppard, author, mental health counselor, and eating disorders specialist.

My fellow singer, soul mate, and RFA sponsor, "Terry."

My husband: He always saw the real me, even when I tried to push him away.

My Tips

I weigh and measure everything. Even when I travel for business, I am always whipping out my scale. Early in my recovery, if I couldn't make it to an RFA meeting, I'd go to an Alcoholics Anonymous meeting.

Recovery from Food Addiction

"Members of Recovery from Food Addiction believe that abstinence from sugar, flour, and wheat is the most important thing in our lives; for without abstinence we do not have a life."

—Recovery from Food Addiction,
www.recoveryfromfoodaddiction.org

Based in Houston, Texas, Recovery from Food Addiction is one of several twelve-step groups, including Food Addicts in Recovery and Recoveries Anonymous, that target food as an addictive substance. RFA asserts that people can be genetically disposed to food addiction, not simply driven to compulsive overeating.

RFA members remain abstinent from all forms of sugar, flour, and wheat. Weight loss is not the primary goal, but it is an expected outcome of abstinence. Members are not required to adhere to a particular diet; however, its approved eating plan is outlined in *Food Addiction: The Body Knows* by Kay Sheppard.[3]

Sheppard's plan includes daily portions of fruit, protein, dairy, grains, and vegetables. Fat is limited to one portion of an approved type a day, and limits are placed on condiments, sweeteners, broths, and spices. Portion sizes differ for men and women. Food is weighed and measured, and portions can be adjusted to prevent too rapid a weight loss.

In addition to its total ban on sugar, flour, and wheat, the food plan also prohibits cheese, butter, sour cream, and other fats; alcohol and caffeine; nuts, seeds, rice cakes, and popcorn; many fruits; and some grains and cereals. The plan's motto is: "When in doubt, leave it out!"[4] Exercise is suggested but is limited to forty-five minutes a day.

RFA meetings are shaped around the Twelve Steps and Twelve Traditions originally set down by Alcoholics Anonymous. A group leader is a member in recovery with at least thirty days of abstinence; members rely heavily on their sponsors. The group also endorses other books by Kay Sheppard, including *From the First Bite: A Complete Guide to Recovery from Food Addiction.*[5]

This plan might work for me because . . .

- ☑ I believe I may be addicted to certain foods.
- ☑ I want the structure, support, and motivation of a regular meeting.
- ☑ I am open to a spiritual dimension in my weight loss journey.
- ☑ To succeed, I need a finely detailed and restrictive eating plan.

Chapter Six

Heaven Help Me

Choosing a Faith-Based Focus

"Faith takes over when willpower fails."

When my husband and I facilitated a support group for addictions recovery at our church some years ago, we often heard this sentiment from people in recovery from addictions to alcohol, drugs, smoking, or eating disorders. The same can be true for weight loss seekers. A spiritual outlook on the road to weight loss can be a powerful motivator.

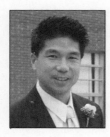

"I live in L.A., a place of vanity where it's all about looks. But I take a spiritual approach that integrates the inner self with the outer self. God made us with mind, body, soul and spirit, and He said, 'Be transformed.'"

—Erik Akutagawa, founder of Competitive Spirit performance coaching, whose clients include elite athletes and people seeking weight control

As early as the 1950s, Presbyterian minister Charlie Shedd published *Pray Your Weight Away*, a bestseller that rebuked gluttony as a sin. "When God first dreamed you into creation, there weren't 100 pounds of excess avoirdupois hanging around your belt," he wrote.[1] He suggested doing karate moves and sit-ups while reciting Scripture. He preached his message well into the 1970s, when he published *The Fat Is in Your Head*.

About that time, Carol Showalter, a Presbyterian pastor's wife in Texas, founded 3D (diet, discipline, and discipleship), the first nationwide church-based weight loss program. Other programs followed: Free to Be Thin, Overeaters Victorious, Thin Within, Lose It for Life. Some programs piggybacked on national crazes, such as the Believercise aerobics program of the 1980s. Today, Christians can choose Christian yoga, Christian Zumba, and Christian Pilates, among other faith-based diet and exercise regimens.

If churches are turning to weight control programs, it may be because churchgoers struggle mightily with weight. In several studies, Dr. Kenneth Ferraro, a professor of sociology at Purdue University, found that religious people are more likely than nonreligious people to be overweight.[2] The findings surprised him.

"In the 1990s, all the evidence showed that being in a faith community was good for your health," Dr. Ferraro said to me. "In terms of smoking, alcohol, and high-risk sexual activity, religion seemed to promote health. But weight is a different story."

Food, Dr. Ferraro suggests, is often the only acceptable vice left to an otherwise teetotaling and smoke-free congregation. In addition, he guesses, faith communities are welcoming groups in which everyone finds acceptance. And the culture and traditions of some denominations may also play a part—Southern Baptists, he finds, lead the way in obesity (church suppers! prayer breakfasts! fellowship breaks!), while Jewish and non-Christian religious groups are the leanest.

Even more alarming, a study by researchers at Northwestern University's Feinberg School of Medicine suggests that young people who frequently attend religious activities are more likely to be obese in adulthood. In fact, they were 50 percent more likely to be obese by middle age than those who did not participate in religious activities in young adulthood.[3]

Getting the message, some churches are literally breaking new ground. In Raytown, Missouri, for example, First Baptist Church has built a $14 million community and fitness center and staffed it with personal trainers and volunteers who organize sports leagues with an enrollment of five hundred participants at any given time.

In Davenport, Iowa, St. Mark Evangelical Lutheran Church has an active Wellness Committee, started ten years ago by a parish nurse. Its outreach programs include blood pressure screenings, flu clinics, exercise and weight loss groups, classes for caregivers and new mothers, healing services, and newsletter articles addressing health issues.

For his part, Dr. Ferraro plans to study the role of pastors in modeling fitness. If ministers are fit and incorporate fitness opportunities into their ministry, he wonders, will congregants follow their lead? He might want to start with Dr. David Ireland, pastor of the 5,000-member Christ Church in Montclair, New Jersey, who, after losing 65 pounds himself, challenged his congregation to lose 10,000 pounds. (While the church didn't hit that mark, they did shed 3,000 pounds.)[4]

For now, weight loss seekers continue to flock to church-based weight loss programs. Here are three people who found not only spiritual sustenance but success there.

Heidi Bylsma

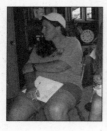 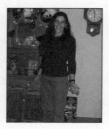

Cool, California
Age: 49
Occupation: Homeschooling mom, writer
Accomplishment: Lost 100 pounds
How She Did It: Thin Within

Many people claim they wrote the book on weight loss, but Heidi Bylsma actually did.

An experienced dieter, Heidi once lost 100 pounds using Weight Watchers. Gratified, she applied to be a group leader, but she was turned down. Although her ending weight of 175 pounds was fine for her 5-foot, 7-inch height and represented muscle tone hard-earned from strength training and running marathons, her Body Mass Index (BMI)—a calculation of body fat using a person's height and weight—wasn't acceptable. To qualify, Heidi estimated she'd have to be technically anorexic.

The injustice of the rejection stung. After the birth of her children, Heidi had become obsessed with losing those 100 pounds. Her diet and exercise routine was intense, and her desire for fitness crowded out everything else in her life.

"I missed a lot of the early years of my children's lives because I was out running and training for marathons," she admits. Although she won her war with weight, her heart was heavy.

When a local church in Sacramento, California, began offering a Christian weight loss workshop that linked eating behaviors with earning

God's favor, she attended, even though she was at her goal weight of 175 pounds.

"At the first meeting, the other women thought I was crazy to be there, but they didn't know how wrong they were," Heidi says. "I had every bit the problem with food they did. My husband calls this my 'bulimic period,' as I would eat and then exercise all the more to be sure not to gain weight. Everything I did was out of fear."

Sidelined by an overuse injury, Heidi's routine came to a sudden halt. In no time, she gained back 70 pounds. Disheartened, she returned to the workshop and began offering classes at her church in Granite Bay, California. Again she suffered an accident, breaking a leg and dislocating an ankle in a rollerblading accident. At that time, a friend told her about a book titled *Thin Again*.

Heidi was excited about the book, whose program was based on an earlier plan called Thin Within. It teaches a hunger and satisfaction approach to eating and encourages people not to fill the heart's void for God with food. In daily devotions, she began to talk about her weight control journey using Thin Within on an e-mail distribution list she had started called "Bread of Life."

Late in 2001, the devotions came to the attention of Thin Within's founders, Arthur and Judy Halliday. Judy invited Heidi to work on a new version of the *Thin Within* book, along with curriculum for an online program. It was a seminal time in her life.

"What a delight it was to work on these projects," she says. "I was tutored and mentored by the Hallidays to embrace the truths that God wanted to work in my life inside and out."

But, as many people say, "God isn't finished with me yet," and Heidi would probably second that.

Over the next few years, Heidi faced many challenges. She was working through issues of childhood abuse, parenting an autistic son, and homeschooling her two children. The family moved to the foothills of the Sierra Nevadas in 2002, and within four years she gained back her weight and more. The scale now read 250 pounds.

"We had moved to the country so we could have horses, and now I was afraid to ride them for fear of hurting them," she says.

Ever the driven writer, Heidi began participating in an online group of Christian horse enthusiasts. One woman looked into Heidi's background and asked her to lead them in a Thin Within study. Although she had managed to drop back to 230 pounds, she was humbled. "These precious ladies had never seen me and had no idea I wasn't living the truths that I had helped put in a book," she says.

As Heidi puts it, once again God got hold of her heart.

"I knew I had to work on some issues, like forgiveness of others and my own rebelliousness," Heidi says. "Many of my eating habits stemmed from my anger toward God. People are shocked when I say that, but I truly think we sometimes feel ripped off by God. And my response to him was, 'I can *too* eat that.'"

Once again, Heidi began listening to her body's cues of hunger and satisfaction, and once again the weight began to come off.

"There is such freedom in not worrying about which foods are 'good' or 'bad' or what their point value or fat gram content is. I was free to just listen to my body," Heidi says.

This time, Heidi tried some new strategies that allowed her to "release" her weight, as Thin Within terms it. She began to listen to the words of Christian musicians, whose songs helped her turn over her circumstances to God.

"When I am reminded of Christ's sacrifices for me, I think, *I have a Savior who laid down his life for me. Will I not lay down some food if he calls me to?*" Heidi says.

"Sometimes when I think I am hungry, my soul is calling out for food. Rather than feed a spiritual or emotional need with physical food, I can feast on the 'right' kind of food for my mind and heart," she adds. "Praying, reading Scriptures, or calling a friend to encourage her may be what I really need."

Heidi also began to exercise using Dance Praise, a video game similar to Dance Dance Revolution. To her delight, her teen children, Michaela and Daniel, joined in. Within a year, she dropped down to 150 pounds. Once a size 24, she was now a size 10. She was itching to get back on her horse.

"In May of 2007, I rode my horse Harley for the first time in three years! He is the horse I always dreamed of having," Heidi says. "Riding him bareback with a halter—gosh, riding him at all—was a lifelong dream come true. I was free! Free from all the extra weight, free from fear of my horses, free from the fear of dying young."

And, in a bit of perfect justice, Judy Halliday again contacted Heidi, knowing nothing of her journey and struggles. Heidi put her writing skills to work for the book *Raising Fit Kids in a Fat World*. And she's led groups of women through the *Thin Within* book at her church.

"God has freed me of 100 pounds by the simple method of listening to hunger and satisfaction and running to him for everything else I need," she says. "No obsessions! No gimmicks! Just a solid biblical approach that changed my life."

Thanks To————

Arthur Halliday, MD, and Judy Halliday, RN, authors of *Thin Again* and *Thin Within*.

My Tips

I like frequent small meals. It trades the mentality of *How much can I get away with?* for *How little does it take to sustain my body?* If I take four times as long to eat half as much, I feel like I have had twice as much food. At McDonald's, I love the grilled chicken chipotle snack wrap. My favorite breakfast is one slice of Orowheat Winter Wheat bread with peanut butter and honey-almond granola with a half cup of milk, and I usually don't eat all of it.

Thin Within

"When you allow the Lord to meet your needs, you will find a fulfillment that you never knew existed. You will begin to need less

food as you realize that much of your eating has been triggered by something that food really can't satisfy. You will begin to see that you can become authentically thin within, from your heart and soul outward."

—*Thin Within: A Grace-Oriented Approach to Lasting Weight Loss* by Judy Halliday, RN, and Arthur Halliday, MD (Nashville, TN: Thomas Nelson, 2005)

Judy Wardell Halliday and Joy Imboden Overstreet began offering Thin Within workshops in 1975. The program began as a secular organization, but following Halliday's spiritual conversion in 1982, it took on a spiritual focus. In 2002, the Hallidays launched Thin Within as a national faith-based weight loss and wellness program. The book *Thin Within* was republished that year as a grace-oriented approach to lasting weight loss. [5]

The three-phased plan is based on the biblical verse, "'Everything is permissible for me'—but not everything is beneficial. 'Everything is permissible for me'—but I will not be mastered by anything" (1 Cor. 6:12). Progressing through the three phases is a journey intended to allow you to break free from a strict reliance on food laws, and embrace a freedom that is grounded in a growing discernment of what is healthy for your body.

This "grace-based" approach contrasts with programs that emphasize food rules and prohibitions, and with faith-based programs, that treat eating habits as signs of spiritual obedience or disobedience. Food and nutrients are not weighed, counted, or tracked, though Thin Within does encourage eating healthy and balanced meals.

A guiding principle of Thin Within is that you can trust the God-given signals of hunger and fullness. Using this principle, a person eats only when hungry and stops before becoming full. A "hunger scale" is used to gauge the need for food: at 0, a person is truly hungry and should eat. However, the body is physically satisfied at 5, which is when eating should cease. Continuing to eat past 5 causes overeating, and leads to being uncomfortably full.

The Hallidays acknowledge that it is difficult to stop at 5 on the hunger scale. We eat, they say, when we're upset, excited, anxious, depressed, or lonely. This kind of eating creates a relationship with food that has nothing to do with physical nourishment. Instead of nurturing this relationship, they urge pursuing a relationship with God. By reordering this relationship, we come to rely less on food to meet emotional and spiritual needs.

The 48-week program is broken into a series of 12-week sessions. Meetings include video testimonies, discussion, and prayer time. An online program is also available. The Hallidays encourage finding forms of exercise that you will enjoy and be able to incorporate into your life on a regular basis.

Over the years, the Hallidays have written many books that address what they call "disordered eating." In them, they tackle a wide spectrum of eating-related issues, including anorexia, bulimia, and obsessive focus on food. These books include *Get Thin, Stay Thin, Raising Fit Kids in a Fat World*, and *HEAL: Healthy Eating and Abundant Living: Your Diet-Free, Faith-Filled Guide to a Fabulous Life*, a book that is intended for young women.[6]

This plan might work for me because . . .

- ☑ I don't like heavily regulated eating programs.
- ☑ Grace and freedom sound like good concepts to me.
- ☑ I think I can rely on my body's signals of hunger and fullness.
- ☑ I'd like the support of a faith-based group.

Sandy Ward

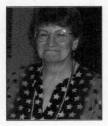

Berwyn, Maryland
Age: 68
Occupation: Retired co-owner of a sporting goods store
Accomplishment: Lost 37 pounds
How She Did It: First Place 4 Health

Can there be anything more disheartening than to have to quit as the leader of a weight loss group because you've gained too much weight? Sandy Ward was determined it wasn't going to happen to her.

Sandy had struggled with weight most of her life. She enjoyed those blissful early years of childhood without a thought about weight, but in her teens, she began a cycle of gaining weight and then thinning out as she grew taller. At 17, she took her first job at a life insurance agency on Louisiana Avenue in downtown Washington, DC. It was a time of life she cherishes.

"I remember going into work with my father, who also had a job in the city," Sandy recalls. "Streetcars were still running then, and I'd take them to shop at the department stores downtown."

After a few years, marriage followed, along with a move to the suburbs and the birth of her son, Danny. But Sandy's weight continued to plague her. At her highest weight, she reached 234 pounds. She tried many times to get it under control. In 1968, she joined Weight Watchers and lost 40 pounds, a full 10 pounds under her goal weight of 150. Yet that wasn't the end of the story.

Sandy was enjoying success in her professional life. A friend had started a sporting goods store in College Park, and Sandy began helping him out with administrative tasks. When her son entered school, she became a partner in the business, and they thrived in the niche market of skating and skateboard equipment. Along the way, however, Sandy quit going to Weight Watchers, because it was becoming costly for her to attend.

Over the years, the weight crept back on, although Sandy says she never hit her high weight again. Eight years ago, after having sold the business and retiring, she still wanted to do something to help herself. One Sunday, she found her opportunity.

"I was sitting in church waiting for the service to begin when I saw an ad for a First Place group that was starting up at my church," she says. "The ad just clicked with me somehow. I guess I was just ready for it, and I was determined this time."

Sandy went to the first meeting and liked both the people and the program of Bible study and group prayer, as well as the nutritional program of dietetic exchanges. Over the course of the 13-week program, she lost 40 pounds. But when it came time for the second session to begin, the leader had moved away, and the group had dwindled to just three women. They decided to continue anyway. And Sandy made another decision.

"I'm not the kind of woman who gets up in front of everyone and speaks," she says. "But I thought that becoming the leader of this group might be a good ministry for me." After a trip to Texas for a leaders' conference, she did just that.

But her success story doesn't end there, either. Eventually, even as a First Place leader, she began to put on extra pounds. In January 2007, she had another decision to make.

"The First Place people told me that often when leaders gain weight, they just quit, and I didn't want to do that," Sandy says. "I made a vow to God that I was going to take that weight off. I set a date for me to start and when that date came, that was it. Vows to God are serious!"

Returning to the First Place plan, Sandy cut back to a 1,200-calorie daily diet. She switched to mostly organic foods, and her menu became fairly simple. Gone were the extras she had been heedlessly enjoying.

"No more desserts and no more fancy Starbucks coffees," she notes. She walked and exercised to a DVD included in the First Place member kit.

Sandy's decision was a brave one. This time, her weight loss quest wasn't a matter of a silent vow. She was still a First Place leader. "I had to do it in front of everyone," she says. "It's hard to face your own demons and the people who have seen you fail." Yet, in six months' time, Sandy lost 37 pounds.

Today, the First Place program is thriving at Berwyn Baptist Church. Sandy says that usually around twenty people are signed up for the ongoing sessions. The meetings start with half an hour of socializing and a weigh-in: those who have lost weight are given First Place "money" to spend on prizes at the banquet they hold after each 13-week session. Sandy hands out written material about weight loss topics and recipes, which the group discusses.

The group is often large enough that they break up into smaller groups for the Bible study and prayer time, and Sandy often organizes groups for specific concerns, like diabetes.

To Sandy, First Place is more than a weight loss group. The members of her group make a commitment to God and to each other to deal with anything in their life that is out of balance. During one session, three people successfully quit smoking, an addiction some feel is harder to break than any other. And Sandy feels that as a leader she benefits even more than the group's members.

"I know I am getting my direction from God," she says. "He knew I would be a leader, and he has given me such a love and compassion for people with weight problems. When I see them, I just think, *Oh, bless your heart*, because I know the humiliation of it all."

Thanks To

The First Place group at Berwyn Baptist Church: Because we make the commitment to attend meetings, I see the same people from week to week, which makes this a very supportive group.

My Tips

At church functions, we set up a First Place table and invite people with special diet requirements to sit with us. We usually have a fruit tray. And, for those who can eat sweets, we like to serve Diet Cola Cake.

Recipe for: **Diet Cola Cake**
(equals 1 bread exchange)

| 1 chocolate cake mix, with pudding in the mix |
| 1 can Diet Cola |

Mix ingredients and bake according to directions in a 9 x 13 pan. Serve 1½ inch square pieces with fruit or fat-free whipped topping. (This recipe omits the eggs and oil usually called for in a cake mix.)

First Place 4 Health

"It is only when we give Christ first place in every area of our lives that He can reveal His plans for us and make us into His image."

— *First Place: Lose Weight and Keep It Off Forever* by Carole Lewis with W. Terry Whalin (Ventura, CA: Regal Books, 2001)

First Place began in 1981 as a ministry of First Baptist Church of Houston by a group of women including Carole Lewis, the woman who later became its national director. Today, renamed *First Place 4 Health*, it operates in partnership with the Southern Baptist Convention and claims half a million members in 12,000 groups across the country. It is a program of balanced living that aims to encourage members to put Christ first in their lives. The program has been updated as *First Place 4 Health: Discover a New Way to Healthy Living.*[7]

The program runs in 11- to 13-week segments during which members are asked to make nine commitments: group attendance, Bible study, group support, accountability, a nutrition plan, regular exercise, keeping a "commitment record," daily prayer, and Scripture memorization.

The food plan, which the founder calls a "live-It" instead of a "die-It," is an exchange plan similar to that of the American Diabetic Association. It is a balanced nutrition plan that breaks out to about 50–55 percent carbohydrate, 15–20 percent protein, and 25–30 percent fat. It outlines a daily diet of 1,200 calories or more that includes meat, bread, vegetables, fruit, milk, fat, and "free foods" that are low in calories. The number of allowable exchanges is based on the calorie level chosen. Members are asked to cut down on salt, sugar, and caffeine and to exercise at least three times a week.

Members purchase a First Place kit and Bible study materials. The kit includes commitment records, motivational tapes, a prayer journal, and Scripture memory verses. The book includes the entire exchange plan, sample commitment logs, exercise guidance, sample exercise logs, and a sample Bible study.

This plan might work for me because . . .

- ☑ I want to make a commitment to a group and can attend weekly.
- ☑ A food-tracking exchange plan would help me stay on track.
- ☑ I think cutting calories and fats would lead to weight loss for me.
- ☑ Putting Christ first in every aspect of my life is important to me.

Candy Nagel_____

Davenport, Iowa
Age: 57
Occupation: Medical records technician
Accomplishment: Lost 50 pounds
How She Did It: 3D (Diet, Discipline, and Discipleship)

There's something unnerving about the thought of sitting around in close quarters studying the Bible with a group of people you barely know. But Candy Nagel thought the discomfort worthwhile if it would help her lose weight.

For forty-six years, Candy had attended St. Mark Evangelical Lutheran Church in Davenport, Iowa, when the parish nurse started a 3D group. At 5 feet, 7 inches, Candy weighed 188 pounds and wore a size 16. She wasn't happy about it. "I had never weighed that much, even when I was nine months pregnant," Candy says.

With her daughters now grown and their weddings approaching, Candy decided it was time to act. "I didn't want to be the fat mother of the bride," she says.

Candy joined the group in September 2000. The class was small, ten people at most, and at first, the experience was daunting.

"I was apprehensive when I found out it was a Bible study, too. I had never attended a Bible study and felt rather inadequate about my faith," she recalls. "I had seen these people in church but had never spoken more than a 'good morning' to them."

The first meeting began with a weigh-in, which Candy found "painful," but her fears dissipated quickly. "The moment we started our lesson my uneasiness left me," she says.

Following the 3D plan, the group shared spiritual lessons using the book *Devotions for a New Beginning* and boned up on the American Diabetic Association's nutritional exchange plan. For Candy, adjusting to new portion sizes was the hardest part.

"My stomach growled for at least three weeks," she admits. "But I grew to like my eating pattern. My husband Rick joined me, and we would count out ten peanuts each for a snack or have a fat-free pudding instead of moose tracks ice cream."

On top of her new eating pattern, Candy got moving on a treadmill. "I started with a 20-minute mile and just about died," she says. But she kept at it, and eventually she could walk a 15-minute mile.

Within two months, Candy lost 20 pounds. At Thanksgiving, the group arranged to bring in provisions for their food pantry equaling their weight loss. Candy was proud to drag in two 10-pound bags of potatoes. After six months, Candy had lost 50 pounds. In October 2003, she wore a size 8 dress to her daughter's wedding.

To this day, Candy tracks her portion sizes and exercises every day, walking four miles and doing two hundred crunches. Ten pounds have returned, but at 148 pounds, Candy is comfortable and happy. Her blood pressure is under control without the use of medicine, and her husband's cholesterol levels have come down to an acceptable range without medication. She is grateful for the success she's had.

"I am thankful for the opportunity of attending a 3D program. I could never have done this on my own," Candy says. "Becoming friends with fellow church members and talking to them every Sunday like family, sharing recipes and information, was the best part of it. I feel extremely blessed."

Thanks To

Linda Litt, 3D leader at St. Mark Evangelical Lutheran Church.

Carol Curry, parish nurse.

My Tips

Casseroles are a thing of the past. I have also given up my Pepsi completely. I drink diet green tea and lots of water. I eat six small meals a day and believe portions are just as important as the food we eat. You don't

realize how much you eat until you write it all down. Writing down everything I ate and sharing that with the group kept me focused.

The 3D Diet

*"Food, like everything else, needs to come under the Lordship of
Christ. . . . The whole area of food brings out rebellion, fear, and
anxiousness, and it reveals a lot about who we are inside."*

—*3D: Diet, Discipline & Discipleship* by Carol Showalter (Orleans,
 MA: Paraclete Press, 2002)

The 3D program has its roots in a church group started on Cape Cod in
the early 1970s to help its members deal with problems like finances,
drinking, dieting, and even housework. Carol Showalter, a pastor's wife,
took the germ of that program—the idea that all problems come down
to diet, discipline, and discipleship—and expanded it into a nationwide
program. The program has recently been updated in the book *Your Whole
Life: The 3D Plan for Eating Right, Living Well, Loving God*.[8]

Billed as a holistic approach to integrating health and spirituality,
3D seeks to bring weight struggles into balance; for example, Showalter
stresses the concept of eating right, rather than dieting. The 12-week program includes Bible study, devotional readings, prayer, scripture memorization, and journal-keeping.

The 3D eating plan is based on the Dietary Guidelines for Americans
and the American Diabetic Association food plan, a calorie-counting
exchange plan of low-fat, high-fiber foods. You make choices based on
knowledge of the basic food groups and how to exchange foods within
groups. The caloric intake necessary for weight loss and weight maintenance is determined by equation. High-fat meats are not included in
the dietary plan, so if eaten, their added grams of fat must be taken into
account. A vegetarian diet and dietary plan is available.

Showalter de-emphasizes the term *exercise*, finding that people resist
the concept. The more realistic goal, she believes, is to strive for thirty
minutes of natural movement a day for weight maintenance and sixty

minutes for weight loss. This kind of movement includes walking on your lunch hour, taking the stairs instead of the elevator, parking further from the door, and walking around your house. Structured exercise can be added for weight loss. The 3D member kit also comes with a pedometer.

This plan might work for me because . . .

- ☑ I am as interested in spiritual growth as in weight loss.
- ☑ I like the idea of natural exercise, like walking.
- ☑ A food-tracking exchange plan would help me stay on track.
- ☑ I think cutting calories and fats will lead to weight loss for me.

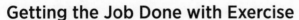

Chapter Seven

Do the Reps

Getting the Job Done with Exercise

"Stop fidgeting and sit still!"

How often did you hear this admonition when you were a child? Well, our parents could have saved their breath.

Researchers at the Mayo Clinic have found that people who fidget burn more calories than people who don't and, therefore, lose weight faster. The difference on average is about 350 calories a day, which amounts to a possible weight loss of 30 to 40 pounds a year.[1] That's quite a reward for the kind of annoying restlessness that used to get you in trouble.

How do you feel about movement? Almost everyone in the weight loss business says our bodies love exercise, crave it even. One founder of a weight loss plan chides that it isn't exercise but sitting still that is the unnatural act.

I beg to differ. I don't know about you, but I for one am perfectly happy sitting curled, catlike and unmoving, for hours at a time. It calms my mind, it quiets my heart. If my soul is ever to be still, I have to come to a complete halt.

Movement makes me feel unsettled and purposeless. When I settle down to read a book or watch a movie, I don't exhibit even the tiniest tics of movement. I don't twirl my hair, I don't drum my fingers, I don't pick at the polish on my fingernails, nothing. I don't fidget, in other words.

Thankfully, not everyone feels the way I do. While interviewing people, I was constantly amazed at how obsessive—how cheerful!—most weight loss seekers are about exercise. No matter how many hours they spent at the gym or pounding the pavement, they wanted more. They told me of how energetic it made them feel, how powerful, how in control.

This seems particularly true of runners. Running seems to be an almost addictive activity for some people. These folks don't just run a mile at a time. They get up at the crack of dawn and run marathons, *and* they get back in time for breakfast. My good friend Yolanda lost 66 pounds one year, most of it while summering at the Jersey Shore, where she got up every morning and ran, jogged, and walked for two and a half hours.

Exercise is good not only because it expends calories, but also because it boosts your metabolism and builds muscle, which cause you to burn calories faster. No one I talked with, and nothing I read, suggested anything less than 30 minutes of exercise a day, three times a week. Walking was the most recommended form of natural movement, while a daily rotation of aerobic and strength-training exercise was a frequently recommended fitness routine. Even though my soul protests, I am well aware that it is regular lap swimming, more than any change in my eating habits, that keeps my weight under control.

When you read the stories of the people in this chapter, you'll see how dramatically exercise can contribute to your success. After talking with these amazing people, I became more committed to my swimming, and I threw in some treadmill and elliptical work for good measure. These days, I'm even trying to wiggle my fingers and jiggle my legs a little while I read!

Christina Chapan

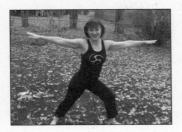

Oak Forest, Illinois
Age: 40
Occupation: Special education teacher
Accomplishment: Lost 30 pounds
How She Did It: Body-*for*-LIFE

"I'm a little obsessed about fitness," Christina Chapan admits.

That's putting it mildly. In addition to her teaching career, Chris is a certified personal trainer and teaches people to train for half and full marathons. She leads fitness programs at a special recreation facility and works with special needs clients at her gym. She incorporates fitness into her classes and is the high school boy's track coach for her district's charter school.

Chris arrives at her gym most days at 5:30 A.M., and some days she runs 20 miles with her running buddies. In 2007, when extreme heat forced a midrace shutdown of the Chicago Marathon after one runner died and hundreds of others were taken to local hospitals, Chris had reached the 18-mile mark and was disappointed she wasn't allowed to finish.

Chris says that as a child she hated physical activity. "I wasn't coordinated at all," she says. She always loved to eat, a passion she allowed to flourish when she went off to college. At 5 feet, 4 inches, and at her

111

heaviest weight of 156 pounds, she wore a size 16. Her moment of truth came when her younger sister announced she was getting married.

"I didn't want to be a fat bridesmaid," Chris recalls, "especially as the older, spinster sister!"

On the advice of a friend, she began a low-fat diet, a program she found easier to follow than other "counting" programs. "Counting calories is hard," she says. "Counting fat grams, you just stop at 20, and you're done for the day." In six months, she lost 30 pounds and fit into a size 6 dress, although not a bridesmaid dress, as her sister ultimately canceled the wedding.

After college, Chris took a job teaching second grade at Stone Church Christian Academy in Palos Heights, Illinois, and in 1997 had her own wedding, marrying her husband, Mike, a computer technician. Within a year, she went back up three dress sizes. "I was married and I had my dream job, but I wasn't happy with myself," she says. Over the years, the stresses of the job resulted in some bad habits that led to more weight gain.

"When you're working until seven or eight o'clock at night, and you're tired, those M&M's look awfully good," she notes.

In 2002, the youth pastor at her church mentioned Bill Phillips's Body-for-LIFE program. The structured program of 12-week exercise and nutrition challenges appealed to Chris. She relished the discipline of writing down the details of what she ate, her exercise regime, and her progress. Over the course of a year, she completed four challenges, losing 20 pounds and toning up her body in a way she had never experienced before.

Chris credits her commitment to fitness for saving her from serious harm in an accident that totaled her car. On her way to work one wintry Chicago day, her car skidded on an icy street, spinning and crashing into the car in front of her.

"I was sore, but I went to work for a half day anyway," she recalls. "I'm certain God protected me in that accident, and the doctors said my state of health and positive attitude had a lot to do with my outcome."

Yet Chris cautions that fitness can become a too-consuming passion. She admits she ultimately lost her second teaching job, in part, because her obsession with fitness caused her to stop focusing on her job. But she revels in her new job as a special education teacher at a public school, and she maintains her conviction that a person has to carve out time for her passions.

"You have to say, 'This is my time, and this is my way of dealing with stress,'" she says. Running a 31-mile ultramarathon recently helped her over the hump of turning 40. In fact, she believes her passion for fitness has helped her cope with the most heartbreaking disappointment of her life, her inability to have a child.

While she is a disciplined person, Chris appreciated that the Body-*for*-LIFE program allows for a little cheating. "You eat in a very healthy way for six days, and then you can have one day, or three meals, that are not what you'd call healthy," she says. For her, that means that on Friday mornings when the teachers and staff at her school host breakfasts, she can enjoy herself. She uses the book as a guide for her weight training, although she says she's "kicked it up a notch."

Chris remained on the Body-*for*-LIFE program even after it became her way of life, and she's lost and kept off 30 pounds with the program. For a while, she says, she joined a 24-hour, "muscle-head" gym, just for a kick. "I love new experiences and trying new things," she says. "It was neat to be around bodybuilders and people who were so into fitness."

Today, at 122 pounds, Chris is down to a size 4. She has incorporated Bill Phillips's new program, Transformation, into her daily routine, a program of 18-week challenges that stress internal as well as external change. She recently received recognition in the Transformation community for her volunteer work, which includes working at her gym with a special needs client and helping with the youth group and music program at her church.

"I think it's important to be involved with other people," she says. "You can be fit, but if you have no relationships, what good does it do?"

Thanks To

Pamela Smith, RD, nutritionist, author of *Food for Life*; *Eat Well, Live Well*; and *The Diet Trap*.

Doug Harris, youth pastor at Stone Church Assembly of God, Palos Heights, Illinois.

Bill Phillips, author of *Body-for-LIFE: 12 Weeks to Mental and Physical Strength* and *Transformation: The Mindset You Need. The Body You Want. The Life You Deserve.*

My Tips

Plan ahead! I make up several meals at a time so I have healthy meals ready to go. When we go out to eat, we choose places that have healthy entrées on the menu. Panera Bread has great soups and salads, and Applebee's has a good selection of Weight Watchers entrées.

Body-for-LIFE

"When you gain control of your body, you will gain control of your life. . . . No matter who you are, no matter what you do, you absolutely, positively do have the power to change."

—*Body-for-LIFE: 12 Weeks to Mental and Physical Strength* by Bill Phillips (New York: HarperCollins, 1999)

Bill Phillips founded and was editor-in-chief of a bodybuilding magazine, *Muscle Media*. In addition to the Body-*for*-LIFE program, Phillips was the creator of EAS (Experimental and Applied Sciences), a line of nutritional supplements now owned by Abbott Laboratories.

The Body-*for*-LIFE program is divided into two components, the Eating-for-LIFE Method and the Training-for-LIFE Experience, which together make up a series of 12-week personal challenges. Participants keep daily logs on what they eat, their exercise routines, and how they feel each day.

The Eating-for-LIFE segment of Phillips's book is brief. It contains a list of "authorized" nutrient-rich foods, from which the participant chooses a combination of quality proteins and carbohydrates and healthy fats. He encourages the use of nutritional supplements like his. The program's greater emphasis is on the exercise component, Training-for-LIFE.

The program gets more than twice as much attention in the book, with detailed photos of the exercises, and is divided between aerobic exercise and weight training. The inside covers of the book are plastered with before-and-after shots in the bodybuilding tradition. The rest of the book consists of Q & A, sample log sheets, and personal testimonies.

The program was tweaked in a subsequent book, *Body-for-LIFE for Women* by Pamela Peeke, MD.[2] It divides a woman's life according to four "hormonal milestones" and customizes the plan for each period. Dr. Peeke targets what she calls "toxic fat," the abdominal fat that compromises a person's health and suggests weight management to attain a goal of eradicating fat for health, rather than cosmetic, reasons. Phillips also wrote *Eating for Life* to expand his nutritional philosophy and include recipes.[3]

Bill Phillips has since sold his interest in EAS and Body-*for*-LIFE, but his new book, *Transformation: The Mindset You Need. The Body You Want. The Life You Deserve* is a similar program of 18-week challenges that are less taxing physically, but incorporate methods for shaping a healthy body, mind, and spirit.[4]

This plan might work for me because . . .

- ☑ I am a goal-oriented person who loves a challenge.
- ☑ Setting short-term deadlines keeps me motivated.
- ☑ I have plenty of time to exercise and weight train.
- ☑ General guidelines are all I need for meal planning.

Nancy Sebastian Meyer

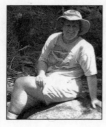 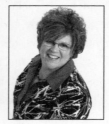

Lancaster, Pennsylvania
Age: 50
Occupation: Speaker, author, and singer
Accomplishment: Lost 30 pounds and 3 dress sizes
How She Did It: Curves, First Place 4 Health, and Personal Trainer[5]

It can be hard to see the good—let alone God—in the circumstances of our lives, particularly when they aren't all that wonderful. But speaker and author Nancy Sebastian Meyer manages to do just that.

Nancy married a pastor, just as she had always hoped to do, and they had a daughter. A singer, she made recordings of Christian music and started a women's ministry called Hope4Hearts. But a few years into her life with her husband, Rich, he quit the pastorate and declared himself to be an agnostic, a person who believes it is not possible to know whether God exists. He took a number of jobs and endured periods of discouragement, while Nancy picked up the pieces of her life.

Eventually, Rich landed a good job in the human resources department of a large dairy producer. The couple worked on their differences, and she continued recording, writing, and speaking to women about finding hope and seeing God's hand in difficult situations. With Rich's blessing, she even wrote about their "spiritually divided" marriage.

In May of 2007, Nancy abruptly faced another stark reality. One weekend, Rich let her know that he wanted her to start sharing in the family's financial responsibilities—paying for her own car, her own clothing, and a third of the household expenses. "You're just playing at your ministry 'quote' work," he told her bluntly.

"God used Rich to push me to get serious about the business part of ministry," she says. "He upped the ante for me and made me realize I needed to get smart about my ministry and business."

Part of her awakening was to meet with her publicist. Again, she was confronted with a person whose brutal honesty would change the course of her life.

"We were planning a photo shoot, and my publicist said, 'Nancy, I guarantee you, you will get more calls if you lose 20 to 40 pounds,'" she recalls.

Nancy almost crumpled at that. "I just wanted to bawl," she says. Instead, Nancy made an immediate commitment.

"I heard the voice of the Spirit saying very gently to me, *This is the moment, honey,*" Nancy says. "I said to my publicist, 'You're absolutely right. I am going to do it.'"

Nancy says she had dieted at least every two years for as long as she could remember. In college, she dieted so rigorously that she got down to 117, but although she was just 5 feet, 2 inches tall, she looked so emaciated that even her doctor was concerned. When she married, she weighed 130, and by the end of the first year, she had gained 20 more pounds. At her highest weight, following her pregnancy with her daughter, Becky, Nancy weighed 195.

Over the years, Nancy had her best success with Weight Watchers, but she always gained the weight back. This time, Nancy used the aerobics video and workbook of the faith-based First Place 4 Health program to outline an exercise and eating plan. Already a member of Curves, she intentionally fulfilled the three-times-a-week, thirty-minute circuit-training program. But she was discouraged about her slow progress and went to see her doctor.

"He asked me whether I was really working out at Curves or just socializing," she says. "I decided I was probably socializing too much, so I began to push myself harder—*much* harder."

Nancy faithfully worked out at Curves three days a week, stopped chatting and started working between circuits, and used her aerobics video the other four days of each week. She wrote down everything she ate, got rid of things like white flour and sugar, added dark greens to her salads, and snacked on Kashi bars. She asked a close personal friend, a woman with a degree in physical education, to serve as her trainer.

Nancy has 20 to 25 pounds to go, and she works hard at it. When she travels, she either uses the hotel's fitness center and swimming pool or gets a travel pass for a nearby Curves. She avoids large meals and brings single-serving baggies of her own homemade protein shake to mix with water. "I often break through weight barriers on a trip," she says.

Despite her progress, Nancy continues to come in for lashings of brutal honesty. After she began losing weight, Nancy's daughter wasn't too sure she liked her new mom.

"Becky told me, 'You look too good, too put-together, too unapproachable. I think people need to see you as an ordinary, fun-loving, chubby person,'" Nancy says. After a mother-daughter talk, though, it seems the girl's objections had more to do with herself than with Nancy. "I think she objected to the fact that we resembled each other more, and she wanted to be her own person," she concludes.

In her books and her speaking engagements, Nancy continues to have a passion for storytelling and finding good in the eye-opening encounters of life.

"I've learned to value the distinct gifts God has given me," she says. "I'm so thankful that I've gotten to this point in my life."

Thanks To

My publicist, Beth Fisher, president of Masterpiece Marketing.

My physician, Dr. Charles Mershon of Cornerstone Family Health Associates.

My friend and health coach, Gwen Diller.

Linda, at Leola Curves.

Carole Lewis, director of First Place 4 Health.

My Tips

I won't do anything just because it's healthy for me. It has to be a "me" thing—I have to make it fun, as well as practical, or I won't do it. I need to make my own plan, but I play with it. I keep a written log, but I do it on the computer and make it colorful.

Curves

"Successful fitness and weight management requires a 'three-legged stool' approach.... By following a comprehensive approach of exercise and weight management combined with the third leg of embracing change, you will dramatically improve your chances for long-term success."

— *Curves Fitness & Weight Management Plan* by Gary Heavin, Nadia Rodman, RD, and Cassie Findley, MS, Ed. (Waco, TX: Curves International, 2008)

A nutritional counselor and fitness instructor, Gary Heavin started the Curves franchise in Harlingen, Texas, in 1992. Since then it has grown to 8,000 women-only outlets. Currently, Curves is rolling out its new program, Curves Complete, a three-pronged program that includes exercise, diet, and motivational components.

The Curves workout is a 30-minute machine circuit interspersed with cardio activity between machines that is recommended three to four times a week. The circuit is a complete workout that includes strength and cardio training, along with stretching. Curves also has recently added a Zumba option that combines the Curves workout with the Latin dance craze.

The Curves nutritional plan is a three-phase plan that addresses two of the concerns weight loss seekers often have: convenience and portion control. In Curves Complete, each participant has online access to a customized meal plan, which is based on an assessment of food preferences, dietary needs, and other individual factors. New to the plan is a Heat & Eat option, which allows you to include healthy frozen meals.

In the new program, participants will meet weekly with their motivational coach to review their meal plan and their daily exercise habits to determine what is working and what needs to be tweaked. The one-on-one coaching is geared toward enabling participants to continue with successful strategies once they complete the program. Each week, participants will receive a review sheet that outlines their food choices, exercise goals, and water and vitamin goals. Daily videos, made possible through a partnering with the Cleveland Clinic, will be available for informational and motivational support. Online message boards and a Facebook page provide means of sharing support with other participants.

Gary Heavin believes that the weight loss battle is won not by willpower, but by embracing a conscious change, which is a gradual process of setting goals, overcoming obstacles, planning for emergencies, and finding the motivation you need.

This plan might work for me because . . .

- ☑ I would like some support and cheerleading.
- ☑ I'm pressed for time, so thirty minutes three to four times a week sounds good.
- ☑ I want to go to a gym, but I would rather work out with other women.
- ☑ I like the idea of making a conscious change rather than white-knuckling it with willpower alone.

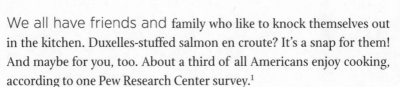

Chapter Eight

Special Delivery

Letting Others Do the Work

We all have friends and family who like to knock themselves out in the kitchen. Duxelles-stuffed salmon en croute? It's a snap for them! And maybe for you, too. About a third of all Americans enjoy cooking, according to one Pew Research Center survey.[1]

Yet today we spend 49 percent—virtually half—of our food budget in restaurants and ordering takeout, according to the National Restaurant Association. And we don't want to stop there—more than two out of five people say they would like to eat out or order in even more often.[2] This is an odd dichotomy. We say we like to cook, yet we choose not to much of the time.

When it comes to losing weight, our aversion to cooking may become even stronger. Taking the time to shop for healthy ingredients, read labels, balance nutritional components, control portion sizes, and master healthy cooking methods can all combine to make us throw up our whisks in defeat.

That's why many people just pick up the phone. The diet food home delivery market is huge and growing ever larger. Today, it's estimated that people spend about $924 million a year on home-delivered diet foods from about thirty companies like Nutrisystem, Jenny Direct, Medifast, and Seattle Sutton's Healthy Eating.[3]

The convenience factor couldn't be higher. You place your order and it comes to your doorstep. You put the boxes, bags, and packages in your cupboards and take out what you need when you need it. Foods are ready-to-eat, microwavable, or prepared with minimal effort, like boiling a package in a pot of water.

One couple I know chose Medifast's Take Shape for Life program, which entails eating five small, 100-calorie "meal replacements" throughout the day, using the company's snack bars and foods, plus an evening meal. The couple's "lean and green" dinners, as Medifast calls them, consisted of one serving of a lean meat and three servings of low-carb vegetables. "Even before we started, we knew we'd succeed," they told me. And they did—together they lost 245 pounds in a year's time.

On top of the convenience, delivered food programs take the guesswork out of what, and how much, to eat. Everyone I talked with said that eating packaged meals reset their idea of a proper portion size, and they got an idea of what to eat once they stopped the deliveries. Many people said that having a set menu removed the possibility of forbidden foods calling out to them when they opened the refrigerator. One woman said ordering prepared meals relieved her of the burden of working her husband's program for him. "I didn't have to do all the shopping, meal planning, and food preparation, and then have to persuade him to eat it," she said.

All of these factors add up to a recipe for success for many people, including the following people who dialed their way to weight loss.

Robert Hartwell

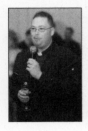 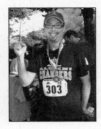

Bronxville, New York
Age: 43
Occupation: Pastor
Accomplishment: Lost 100 pounds
How He Did It: Nutrisystem

Most people make their weight loss resolution only after the annual holiday binge. But it was on New Year's Eve 2007 that the Rev. Robert Hartwell's weight loss odyssey came to a dramatic close.

That morning, he stepped on a scale on NBC's *Today* show in front of 10 million people.

The journey of this pastor of Village Lutheran Church began at Thanksgiving the previous year. Robert's church had started a campaign to pay down an $8 million mortgage it had assumed for a building project.

One day, Robert got a baffling call. A former parishioner, someone who kept close ties with the church, offered to make a substantial donation. But there was a catch.

"This donor asked me how committed I was to the project, and I started to tell him what I planned to give," he says. "The donor brushed that off and said instead that he wanted me to commit to losing 70 pounds, and if I did so, he would donate $5,000 for each pound lost."

It was both an intriguing and a heartbreaking offer.

"I was crushed—mortified—that someone had discovered that I was overweight, although of course everyone saw it when I stepped into the pulpit each week," Robert says. "But this donor said he wanted to know that I was as committed to the project as he was."

Given the unusual nature of the pledge, Robert talked with church leaders to make sure that accepting the offer wouldn't cheapen the image or mission of the church. Although the other pastors and deacons found the offer "wacky," they saw no reason to reject it. So was born "The Skinny on Sacrifice" campaign.

Although up this point Robert hadn't acknowledged his weight problem, he certainly understood how it had happened.

"My life is so hectic. I was always eating on the run. I'd grab a muffin between hospital visits, get home from council meetings at 10:30 at night, exhausted and ravenous, and grab a couple of sandwiches and chips," he says. "And I was a volume eater—I could eat a half a pizza by myself or eight White Castle burgers at a time."

By the time the sly donor came into the picture, the 6-foot-tall pastor weighed about 270 pounds. After consulting with his parish nurse, Robert took up the challenge. Robert chose Nutrisystem, and he followed it to the letter.

On a food plan of about 1,500 calories a day, Robert lost ten pounds almost immediately and continued to lose two to three pounds a week. He and his wife, Sue, had always walked for pleasure, and Robert made sure he got in his two to three miles a day.

After six months, Robert ramped up his exercise routine in the gym at next-door Concordia College, where he is an adjunct professor. A congregant who is a personal trainer showed him how to use the machines for both cardio workouts and strength training. The college atmosphere was stimulating.

"I was there with the 19- and 20-year-old baseball players, and they motivated me to keep going," he says. He began going to the gym five days a week, on top of his family walks.

Meanwhile, an employee at the church's school who happened to be a lighting director for the *Today* show brought the pastor's challenge to the attention of a producer. Wanting a religious-themed holiday feature, the producer asked whether Robert would be willing to weigh in on the show the morning of December 31, 2007.

"I had already told the donor that I wouldn't weigh in during a church service, and here I was agreeing to do it in front of a live audience on national television," he laughs. "Barring Jesus projecting it in the sky over the earth, it couldn't get any bigger than that!"

Robert agreed to do the show, but he had a few conditions: he wanted to be fully clothed, but he didn't want to wear shoes, and he wanted to bring his own scale. So far, so good. But just before he stepped out onto the stage, someone clipped a microphone to the back of his shirt. "This thing must weigh five pounds!" he protested.

No matter. Robert made the donor's 70-pound goal, with eight pounds to spare. Keeping his end of the bargain, the donor wrote a check for $390,000, which church members augmented with their own funds for an even $400,000.

Since then, Robert's goal has changed—while he originally targeted 200 as his goal weight, he is maintaining his weight at 180 pounds and is working on strength training and toning. "Age is no friend to loose skin," he says. He still uses Nutrisystem—he orders a box now and then because he enjoys the food and finds it helpful in maintaining his weight. But he has also made his diet rich in omega-3s, healthy grains, and low-glycemic carbs and protein.

And the newly svelte pastor made a deal of his own. On Ash Wednesday a few years ago, "when everyone is thinking of mortality, ashes to ashes, dust to dust," Robert asked parishioners to join in a challenge cooked up with Nutrisystem to see how many pounds the church community could lose in a year's time. The congregation lost thousands of pounds, and many more community members picked up lifelong healthy lifestyles.

Ultimately, a change in lifestyle is what Robert believes makes a difference. "We have even changed the way we plan our fellowship events. In addition to the high-sugar foods that people love and often bring, we try to make sure there are healthy options," he says.

Robert has become an avid runner. In November 2011, he and four others ran the New York City Marathon to raise funds for the church's Christian school. "Running is such a great way to stay healthy and to find balance and harmony in the middle of a hectic life," he says. "I often find myself praying or praising God in my morning runs and thank God that my new healthy lifestyle allows this righteous pleasure."

With new insight, Robert says he now believes that weight loss is not only an individual pursuit yielding personal satisfaction, but it's also a goal with wide-ranging possibilities for strengthening family and community ties.

"Food is a shortcut. We use food to show love, to reward our children for their accomplishments. It's ridiculous," he says. "Food is really a substitute for spending time with each other. We've decided we're not going to do that anymore."

Thanks To

The anonymous donor to Village Lutheran Church.

My wife, Sue: She never made me feel guilty about not eating her food.

Parish nurse Joy Elwell and parishioner Rich Foster, my personal trainer.

God, for his grace and motivation to reach new goals.

My Tips

For our church coffee hours, I've encouraged everyone to bring in fruits and vegetables. It costs more, but we feel good about it. I don't go to donut shops, and I'm not buying that stuff for my kids anymore.

Nutrisystem

Nutrisystem began more than thirty years ago, morphing from a liquid protein diet provider into today's meal-based program. The meal plan offers foods low on the glycemic index, so that blood glucose levels rise slowly over a long period of time, with the goal of maintaining constant blood glucose levels and reducing hunger.

Nutrisystem's 28-day Basic program provides a choice of more than 130 menu items, including entrées, desserts, and snacks. You can choose either a favorites package or design your own menu. The food comes in shelf-stable packaging and does not need to be refrigerated or frozen. To the meal items, you add fresh fruit, vegetables, and dairy items. The Nutrisystem Select program offers more than 150 menu items, including fresh-frozen menus and ready-to-go foods.

The program can be tailored to men or women, diabetics, vegetarians, or seniors. The difference lies in how many of the items on offer fit the requirements for each category, while the senior plan includes a multivitamin. The packaged food includes snacks, so you eat five or six times a day, depending on your program.

With this program, you have no visits to brick-and-mortar stores. For nutrition and weight loss counseling, you call or seek online help. Your initial package comes with a "Results Kit" that includes an exercise video, behavior modification guide, meal plan, daily diary pages, and online access to message boards, articles, forums, and counseling.

This plan might work for me because . . .

- ☑ I like the convenience of prepackaged meals.
- ☑ I need a program that removes much of the decision making surrounding food.
- ☑ I don't need a lot of hand-holding.
- ☑ I need to allow for snacking throughout the day.

The Freberg Family

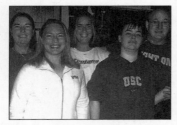

L-R: Laura, Kristin, Karen, Karla, Roger

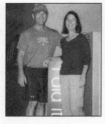

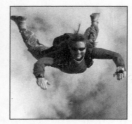

Laura and Roger   Kristin

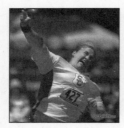

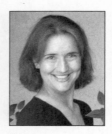

Karen   Karen

San Luis Obispo, California
Ages: 59, 58, 31, 28
Occupations: Two professors, a retired food products manager, and an Army captain
Accomplishment: Lost 263 pounds
How They Did It: Jenny Craig

Question: What do these four people have in common?

- A former pro football player and retired Nestlé product manager
- A psychology professor and textbook author
- An Army captain and West Point instructor
- A former Olympic-caliber shot-putter and strategic communications educator

Answer: A weight loss story.

Together, Roger and Laura Freberg and their daughters Kristen and Karen lost 263 pounds using Jenny Craig. Daughter Karen was the catalyst.

"Karen was a four-time All-American shot-putter and a finalist in the 2004 Olympic Trials. She holds four national power lifting records," says mom Laura, 58, a professor at California Polytechnic State University and a textbook writer.

On graduating from the University of Southern California with a master's degree in public relations, Karen weighed 285 pounds and wore size 26 pants. Even though she is 6 feet tall, this was not an unusual weight for a woman of her sport and athleticism. But after her track and field career ended, she wanted to lose her "thrower's weight."

"To be a good shot-putter, you have to do heavy weight lifting," says Karen, 28. "But, since I was retired, I knew that I had to lose the weight. The habits I had after ten years of eating with the football players just weren't working."

One day in October 2006, Karen decided to drop in at her local Jenny Craig office. Her dad, Roger, 59, remembers saying to her, "Don't leave without signing your mother up!"

Laura did, in fact, tag along, wanting to gain control over her 5-foot, 9-inch, 210-pound, size 16 frame. Mother and daughter signed up. After she and Karen received their first shipment of meals, they discovered that portion control would be a challenge, even with healthy food on their table.

"California is all about fresh fruit—bananas, grapes, you name it. We ate good food, just way too much of it. We'd sit down to eat a bowl of cherries that was about four times what we should be having," Laura says.

Controlling portions and calories with the delivered meals, the women's weight loss was almost immediate. Karen lost 15 pounds in the first week alone, while Laura lost six. From then on, one to two pounds a week was standard.

Meanwhile, dad Roger, 6 feet, 4 inches tall and 325 pounds, was approaching his date with destiny. He carried over his own habits from his days as a UCLA athlete and later as a defensive lineman for the Los Angeles Rams, who drafted him in 1974. During his playing days, he estimates he consumed about 10,000 calories a day.

A love of food ran in Roger's family. His grandmother ran test kitchens for several manufacturing companies, including Swift & Company in Chicago.

"My grandmother taught me everything about the love of baking and cooking. She was one of those outstanding women of the 1920s and '30s who had no boundaries in achievement," says Roger. "She went to wonderful restaurants and occasionally took me with her. I had the opportunity to see commercial kitchens and experience really good food."

Roger's later career as a product manager for Nestlé and Mars, and then his retirement hobby as the family chef, furthered his predicament. By 1999, he weighed over 400 pounds and was diagnosed with diabetes. Even though he brought his weight down to 325 pounds on an exchange plan, his diabetes still wasn't completely under control.

One day in December 2006, he happened past the kitchen table, where Laura and Karen were having Jenny Craig cupcakes. "I said, 'What's that?' I didn't realize I could have something like a cupcake and still lose weight," Roger says. He became the third family member to sign up.

The family's oldest daughter, Kristin Graham, 31, wasn't home to witness the family transformation. A graduate of West Point, she is a demolitions expert and a major in the U.S. Army, now teaching systems engineering at West Point after serving two tours in Iraq. But she began to wonder whether Jenny Craig could help with her own struggles.

"In the Army, you can be kicked out for not making weight," Kristin says. "We did a lot of running, seven to ten miles a day, and I was really tired at the end of the day. I needed something that would keep me from stopping for chicken nuggets, fries, and a coffee."

Not only that, but Kristin says that in the Army, some social activities are almost mandatory: when your commanding officer suggests an evening out, you go out. Kristin needed a way to compensate for the extra calories of the outings.

In May 2007, Kristin hopped on the bandwagon. At the time, she weighed 170 pounds. Although that sounds reasonable for her 5-foot, 7-inch height, she was actually at the top of the military's required weight range. To lose a few pounds and maintain her weight, she began having one or two Jenny Craig meals a day.

For all of the Frebergs, the decision to use a delivered meal program made weight loss almost automatic. Laura recalls reading Brian Wansink's book, *Mindless Eating: Why We Eat More Than We Think*, and being struck by research showing that, on average, people make more than two hundred decisions about food each day. To her, that meant more than two hundred opportunities to make the wrong choice.

"What I like most about the Jenny Craig system is that no decisions have to be made," Laura says. "I prefer to use my time, energy, and neural activity on my work and hobbies, not thinking about food."

Karen likes the simplicity of the system and believes that it is particularly suitable for athletes in transition. "It's easy and simple, and I would recommend Jenny Craig to athletes who have finished their athletic career," she says. Karen remained on Jenny Craig as she earned her doctorate degree and went on to teach strategic communications at the University of Louisville in Kentucky.

It's ironic that one of the Frebergs' most passionate shared hobbies is cooking. On the weekends, the Freberg kitchen turns out the likes of seafood gumbo, crab quiche, prime rib dinners, raisin-blueberry cinnamon rolls, raspberry chocolate truffle cake, and strawberry-amarula cheesecake.

To counterbalance the damage their hobby could inflict, the Frebergs package leftovers in appropriate meal-sized portions and store them in a chest freezer. "We have about a thousand freezer containers," Laura says.

The Frebergs' system seems to be working. Laura has reached her goal weight of 131 pounds—down 79 pounds—and wears size 4 "Barbie doll" suits.

Roger is holding at 235 pounds—a 100-pound loss—and wears size 31/32 jeans, down from a size 44/46.

Karen has lost 85 pounds and wears a size 8/10. She is working toward losing another 30 to 40 pounds. She takes spin and kickboxing classes and has competed in a 5K—a feat she finds amazing because, she says, for a thrower, one lap around the track is considered a long-distance run.

And at 155 pounds and size 4/6, Kristin has lost 15 pounds and is at the low end of her approved weight range.

The Frebergs' youngest daughter Karla, 26, is autistic and follows her own nutritional plan, but Laura says she's been more careful now that weight control is a family affair. All maintain an active lifestyle and continue to use Jenny Craig meals for weight maintenance.

"For me, it's peace of mind," concludes Laura. "It's worth all the money in the world."

Thanks To

Health issues motivated the Frebergs. Laura's blood pressure was borderline high, Roger is diabetic, although it's being controlled without medicine, and all were mindful of their family history of colon cancer.

My Tips

"Seize the day. Put no trust in the morrow!" (Horace). Never go more than two or three hours without eating; have something to take the edge off your hunger. Set a comfortable window of a few pounds, and if you go over, get strict with yourself. Give all your "fat clothes" to Goodwill. Choose your treats wisely and indulge at lunch, not dinner. Enjoy all the time you have that you used to spend worrying about your weight!

Jenny Craig

One of Nutrisystem's former employees, Genevieve Guidroz, started the competing Jenny Craig program in the mid-1980s. The Jenny Craig philosophy centers squarely on the intangibles of weight loss: managing stress and emotions, increasing your enjoyment of healthful eating and exercise, and learning to differentiate between physical and emotional hunger.

The program comes with a six-week membership fee. You can call or stop in at a Jenny Craig center for a free informational visit. If you join, you receive a personal profile that will determine your daily calorie level and individual meal plan.

The program is based on the U.S. government's Dietary Guidelines for Americans and is a low-fat, low-cholesterol diet. On the program, you choose calorie levels ranging from 1,200 to 2,300 calories a day. The program is intended to help participants lose 1 percent of their body weight per week, with a minimum goal of a 5- to 10-percent loss.

The program consists of frozen and dry packaged foods, with a two-week minimum order. You supplement the program with fruits, vegetables, grains, and dairy items. Included in the plan are Jenny Craig-branded vitamin and mineral supplements, bars, and shakes. When ordering, you can choose a favorites package or customize your own meals. Plans can be customized for seniors, vegetarians, and diabetics, but vegans or those who desire kosher meals may not be able to participate in this plan.

Membership includes one-on-one weekly consultations with a Jenny Craig representative, either by phone—called Jenny Craig at Home—or in person. Membership comes with a "Success Manual" that has tips on such topics as dining out, exercising, dealing with lapses, and motivational messages. In addition, the website offers online support components, such as forums, newsletters, an interactive online journal, a weight tracker, and menu planners. The program includes a transitional plan that can help you learn to prepare healthy food on your own.

This plan might work for me because . . .

- ☑ I like the convenience of prepackaged meals.
- ☑ I need a program that removes much of the decision making surrounding food.
- ☑ I have room in my freezer to store my meals.
- ☑ I would benefit from having a personal consultant to educate and motivate me.

Chapter Nine

I Did It
My Way

Independent Souls Just Forge Ahead

Americans have a reputation as highly independent souls who like to do things their own way. It's a notion that is certainly borne out in the realm of weight loss.

In 1994, two researchers—James O. Hill, PhD, professor of pediatrics and medicine at the University of Colorado Health Sciences Center and director of the National Institutes of Health's Center for Human Nutrition, and Rena R. Wing, PhD, a professor in the department of psychiatry and human behavior at Brown University's medical school—founded the National Weight Control Registry to track people who have lost weight and kept it off over time.[1]

To date, about 7,000 people have logged their weight loss stories into the database. To qualify, a person must be at least 18 years old, have lost at least 30 pounds, and have kept it off for one year or more. Participants have reported losing up to 300 pounds and keeping it off for as long as 66 years.

Among other findings, the study turned up data showing that almost half of successful registry members—45 percent—designed and followed their own weight loss program. I can certainly believe this. In looking for people to interview, it was far easier to find people who went solo, or who took from a program what they wanted and ignored the rest. When I asked why someone would go it alone, more than once I heard, "I'm just not a joiner."

While people in the NWCR study may have struck out on their own, their avenues to success have been pretty much the same. Ninety-eight percent of participants modified their eating habits, and most people report continuing to eat a low-calorie, low-fat diet in order to maintain their weight loss.

Similarly, 94 percent of people said they increased their level of physical activity, with the most frequently reported form of activity being walking. On average, people report exercising one hour a day. And where do they find the time, you might ask? Sixty-two percent report watching fewer than ten hours of television a week.

Here are two people who found and fashioned their own way to weight loss, mixing and matching among weight loss plans and coming up with their own way to success.

David Ireland

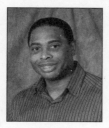

West Orange, New Jersey
Age: 50
Occupation: Pastor, ministry leader, author, and speaker
Accomplishment: Lost 65 pounds
How He Did It: "Lose the Snickers"

Usually, when you say grace before a meal, it's a one-way street. You sit down, you give thanks, you begin. One day at the table, however, Dr. David Ireland got an answer.

"I was ministering in Trinidad about fifteen years ago, sitting down to eat lunch. I don't remember what I was having, probably something fatty and high in carbohydrates," David says. "I began to say grace, 'Lord, bless this food. . . .' Right then, I heard the Spirit say to me, *David, how can I bless that?*"

Growing up in New York City, David had been an active young man, walking everywhere and playing baseball. He led a demanding and active life, pursuing undergraduate and graduate degrees, marrying his wife Marlinda, raising two daughters, and founding Christ Church in West Orange, New Jersey.

Over the years, without really noticing, he gradually put on weight. "It's one of the ways we deceive ourselves. You just don't see yourself in the mirror," he says.

By the time he turned 42 in 2004, David found himself at 248 pounds. Even after his experience in Trinidad, he had managed to ignore divine promptings. As with anyone, particular foods found their way into his hands more often than they should have.

"I was in love with Snickers bars. Those and peanut M&M's. They were my addictions," he says. "I convinced myself that I couldn't live without them."

Unlike many people, though, David had no resounding epiphany about his weight.

"Mine was no New Year's resolution. I had no illness, no threat to my health. I just woke up one day and realized I had done this to myself," David recalls. "Overeating is a choice. You can't blame McDonald's, you can't blame TV commercials or society. You can't blame Mom for cooking or Dad for taking you to Chuck E. Cheese. They are not the culprits."

Given his academic inclinations, David started reading up on nutrition. He adjusted his eating habits. Instead of fruit juices, he drank water. Instead of fried food and fast food, he grilled salmon and steamed vegetables. David's Snicker-bar days were over.

Exercise began to figure into David's schedule, too. He started to walk, although to begin with, he could barely manage a block. In time, he was walking a mile, then two miles, five miles and then ten, and then he was jogging, then running. His efforts were not without the occasional hitch.

"One morning, about 5 A.M., I was out jogging. I'd gone about ten miles, and my knee started acting up. I had no cell phone, no way to get home," he says. "I prayed, 'In Jesus' name, wake Marlinda up! Come pick me up! I'm in South Orange!' In the end, I had no choice but to hobble ten miles home."

After a year, he hired a personal trainer, a member of his congregation, and began meeting with him three times a week. David gradually upped the ante for himself. One day, he read about an Army Ranger competition that required participants to do 80 sit-ups in two minutes, 80 push-ups in two minutes, and 12 pull-ups, then run two miles in 13 minutes. He took the idea to his trainer and enlisted three other men to join him. He worked at it until he could meet all four requirements.

After losing 60 pounds, David set his sights on the New York City Marathon. In 2005, he registered for and won a spot. He trained for five months, running 40 miles a week. The day dawned, and David took his place among 37,597 runners.

"I was just trying to finish. That was my goal," David says. "At about mile 17, I did think to myself, *Why am I doing this?* But I did complete the race."

In fact, David crossed the finish line in 5 hours, 9 minutes, and 18 seconds, coming in ahead of about 10,000 other finishers. Since then, he has run in a number of full and half marathons and continues his work at the gym.

David was so inspired by his newfound fitness that he took it to the pulpit. He felt it was high time. "In my twenty-five years in ministry, I can honestly say I had heard only one sermon on the topic of stewardship of the body," he says.

Dr. Ireland spoke for five weeks on the spiritual motivations and physical means of healthy living. He challenged his 5,000-member congregation to lose 10,000 pounds over a 12-week period and assembled a team of doctors, dietitians, and trainers to assist them. At the final weigh-in, the congregants stacked up 3,000 lost pounds.

As with any testimony, it is David's own personal experience that speaks volumes.

"There's hope! There's hope!" he says. "I am a living witness. If I can do it, you can do it."

Thanks To

The prompting of the Holy Spirit.

"'Everything is permissible for me'—but not everything is beneficial. 'Everything is permissible for me'—but I will not be mastered by anything" (1 Cor. 6:12).

My Tips

You can't microwave success—make a lifestyle change for a lifetime. I cook meals ahead of time and put them in containers in the refrigerator, so everything's ready for me. I take snacks out with me: pears, apples, hard-boiled eggs. My favorite snack is organic peanut butter on crisp-bread crackers.

How Many Calories Did That Burn?

Runners do burn up a lot of calories. But determining how many calories you burn with any given activity is not an exact science. Many factors come into play—your gender, how much you weigh, and how vigorously you go at it, for example. At the gym, the calories you burn on a machine can vary according to whether you're gripping the handles or swinging your arms and even whether you're listening to music.

In fact, when asked, people generally overestimate the amount of calories they're burning. So consider this one fact. Say you eat a Big Mac meal with medium fries. (Let's assume a diet drink, just to be virtuous.) According to McDonald's nutritional information, a Big Mac has 540 calories, while the medium order of fries has 380 calories; the entire meal totals 1,480 calories.[2]

How long do you think you'd have to exercise to burn off those calories? An hour? Two hours? According to the most recent data, a 154-pound person would need to walk briskly for more than three hours to account for this meal! A more sedate pace would require more than five hours of hoofing.

The Department of Health and Human Services regularly publishes and updates its Physical Activity Guidelines for Americans, a document that along with the Dietary Guidelines for Americans is considered the best information available on the topic of health and weight control. The latest data suggests that the average person should engage in two and a half hours of moderate physical activity a week to reduce the risk of chronic disease. For weight control, the ante is upped to five hours a week, in addition to keeping caloric intake within certain limits, although a doctor's permission is suggested for this level of activity.[3]

Check out these government statistics for an idea of the number of calories per hour various exercises and activities burn.[4] These figures are approximate numbers based on a person who weighs about 154 pounds. Calories burned per hour will be higher for persons who weigh more than 154 pounds and lower for persons who weigh less.

Moderate Physical Activity	Calories Burned Per Hour
Hiking	370
Light gardening/yard work	330
Dancing	330
Golf (walking and carrying clubs)	330
Bicycling (less than 10 mph)	290
Walking (3.5 mph)	280
Weight lifting (general light workout)	220
Stretching	180
Vigorous Physical Activity	Calories Burned Per Hour
Running/jogging (5 mph)	590
Bicycling (greater than 10 mph)	590
Swimming (slow freestyle laps)	510
Aerobics	480
Walking (4.5 mph)	460
Heavy yard work (chopping wood)	440
Weight lifting (vigorous effort)	440
Basketball (vigorous)	440

This plan might work for me because . . .

- ☑ I am self-motivated and don't need a lot of hand-holding.
- ☑ I know what changes I need to make to my diet.
- ☑ I'm willing to commit to regular exercise.
- ☑ I can figure out an exercise plan on my own.

Sandee Kuprel

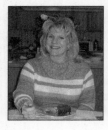 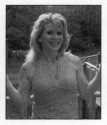

Holt, Michigan
Age: 44
Occupation: Wife and mother, nutritional consultant
Accomplishment: Lost 70 pounds
How She Did It: Flour-free, sugar-free diet, exercise, and a twelve-step program[5]

During the Christmas holidays in 2004, Sandee Kuprel stepped on a scale and saw a number she couldn't believe: 205.

"I panicked, and then I told myself it was just water weight," Sandee recalls. "I sucked in real hard, looked in the mirror, twisted and tilted just right so I could look smaller, and I thought, *Yes, it's just water. I'm sure I don't weigh that much.*"

Yet Sandee couldn't will away the thought that she did indeed weigh that much. Just under 5 feet, 3 inches and wearing a size 18, Sandee had nowhere to hide the pounds. She tried fasting and drinking only green drinks, but after a few days, she broke her fast at Wendy's. This started a cycle of fasting and bingeing that made her feel worthless.

"I felt like a stuffed pig," she says. "I found myself sitting in my closet crying, asking God, 'What's wrong with me?'"

In reality, Sandee was a strong woman who had already quit smoking and drinking. These were habits she had seen decimate her family: her grandmother and grandfather, mother, father, and aunt all died within a few years of each other. Her grandmother made it into her seventies and her grandfather into his eighties, but the last years of their lives were miserable. The others died in their fifties and sixties, their health ruined by alcohol, diabetes, lung cancer, and other debilitating diseases.

Alcoholics Anonymous helped Sandee become alcohol-free at age 25.

"After my son was born, I realized I had a problem with alcohol," she says. "I wouldn't drink when he was awake, but I became determined to break the cycle for the next generation."

Cutting out the cigarettes was harder—it took about ten years to cut out the smokes and taper off the nicotine gum at age 38.

But lifelong eating habits can be even more difficult to break than smoking or drinking—after all, you have to eat. And the habits instilled by Sandee's family were deeply ingrained.

"Gramma Lu was so much fun, so full of life. Add Gramma, shake, and have an instant party," Sandee recalls. "She always had lots of food around. Chips, candy, nuts, fried chicken, her dumplings that we called sliders, and dough gods—deep-fried homemade bread dough made with lard that we slathered with butter and honey. We made pasta salads with Miracle Whip and drank lots of soda."

"My dad's idea of a vegetable was to open a can of corn, take out a spoon, and you're good for the week," she says. "I really didn't know that there was anything wrong with this way of living. It was just how we ate. It was how we bonded, and we all enjoyed it."

Sandee says she was about 20 pounds overweight for most of her adult life, an amount that didn't bother her. Though she didn't have the same diet as when she was a child, she clung to her favorite foods. "I didn't want to give up ice cream," she says.

Yet the deaths in her family left her bereft and emotionally fragile, and she began to put on the pounds.

"There's no way to describe how this all felt. The rug was pulled out from under me. I was devastated, and I felt abandoned," she recalls. "It was a very dark world, very dark."

When fasting failed to give Sandee the results she wanted, she tried a diet that allowed five or six small meals and snacks a day. But the snacks included small bites of candy bars and snack cakes, and soon she'd find herself eating more and more of the sugary treats, and then she'd find herself at a fast-food place for dinner. "I figured I'd already blown it, so I might as well," she says.

Sandee was starting to suspect that sugar was a problem for her. About that time, she came across a twelve-step program for overeaters that confirmed her suspicions.

"I heard how sugar and flour were highly addictive, that once you eat any amount, your body goes into overdrive trying to get the next fix," she says. "It excited me to know what was wrong with me. I knew deep down that the description fit me to a tee, that I was an addict, strange as that may sound."

Although she was terrified to say she would never eat sugar or flour again, Sandee said she was willing to give it a try—one day at a time.

"I needed to face a lot of the fears I had. I ate to deal with everything I was stuffing," she says. "I said to God, 'You're going to have to give me the willingness to be willing,' because I didn't have it in myself."

A deeply spiritual person, Sandee combined her new way of eating with prayer and meditation. In all of her journeys through addiction, the Old Testament prayer of Jabez was one that she claimed for herself: "Oh, that You would bless me indeed and enlarge my territory, that Your hand would be with me, that You would keep me from evil, that I may not cause pain."[6]

Her group meetings became a support system as Sandee worked through the emotional turmoil of her life. And as she became adept at cooking without sugar and flour, she began to see dramatic results. Her weight started to come off at a rate of about ten pounds a month. Within 11 months, she had reached her goal weight of 130—a size 2 on her muscular frame.

Today, Sandee maintains her weight at 133 pounds and wears a size 4—a concession to her husband. "When I get down to a size 2, he says I look drawn," she says. She commits her daily food intake to her sponsor by e-mail, is increasing the raw foods in her diet, and has cut down on meats. For protein, she relies on chicken, legumes, yogurt, soy, and a protein powder. And although she didn't use exercise to lose her weight, she loves to walk now, and she uses aerobics, weight training, and yoga DVDs at home.

Sandee worked hard to escape the destructive habits of her past, and today she looks to the future to maintain her healthy self.

"Everything I used to do was based in fear," she says. "Now I don't look at the moment. I look at the big picture. The things that I want to do in the future—travel, enjoy my son and daughter—I want to do in a healthy way. I want to leave a new legacy for my children."

Thanks To

My faith: It is all definitely God. I just do the next right thing.

My sponsor and the fellowship.

The Twelve Steps.

My Tips

One of the biggest challenges of a no sugar, no flour diet is how to cook. I started compiling recipes, and people would ask me for them, so I've posted them on my website, www.happy2beme.com. I weigh and measure foods, although I don't take a scale out to restaurants. My favorite restaurant is Mongolian BBQ, where you choose your meats, vegetables, and sauces and they grill it for you, but now I use only soy sauce and dry spices. I've continued to make transformations in my life. I stopped drinking coffee two years ago, and I drink green tea now. I'm still working on getting PepsiMax out of my life.

Dr. Gott's No Flour, No Sugar Diet

"The key to weight loss is simply to burn more calories than you take in. . . . I have found, and my patients' successes have verified, that eliminating flour and sugar from your diet is a simple way to cut calories instantly."

—*Dr. Gott's No Flour, No Sugar Diet* by Peter H. Gott, MD, with Robin Donovan (New York: Wellness Central, 2008)

The flour- and sugar-free diet that Sandee Kuprel adopted for herself, but did not want to reveal, is similar to Dr. Peter H. Gott's No Flour, No Sugar diet. Dr. Gott is a practicing physician and was for many years a syndicated newspaper columnist who urged patients and readers to try this approach to weight loss.

As with many of the home remedies Dr. Gott champions—Vicks VapoRub for toenail infections, bars of soap under the sheets for restless leg syndrome—his diet is simple and inexpensive. You need not count or weigh anything, but you must read labels. If flour or sugar is an ingredient, it is off-limits. Its simplicity is appealing: "It is a wonderful diet that was easy for me to follow," says Jayne, a friend of mine who used it to lose 20 pounds.

In this case, avoiding flour means not just white flour but any kind of flour, including rice, wheat, or corn—this is different from many diets that swap in whole wheat flour. Sugars on the banned list include cane sugar, glucose, sucrose, beet sugar, honey, maple syrup, high fructose corn syrup, and molasses. In their place, Dr. Gott suggests whole grains such as brown rice and starchy vegetables like corn and potatoes; and for sweets, fruits, and sugar substitutes. In addition, Dr. Gott's diet includes lean meats, legumes, low-fat dairy products, and fresh vegetables, with an emphasis on nutrient-dense foods that satisfy hunger.

To estimate your calorie level for weight loss, Dr. Gott suggests multiplying your current weight in pounds by thirteen if you are inactive, or fifteen if you are physically active. To lose one to two pounds a week, Dr. Gott suggests reducing that number by 500 calories a day and exercising for thirty minutes a day. Losing more than one or two pounds a week jeopardizes the body's need for nutrients and energy, he believes.

His book includes a chart for more closely determining your caloric intake based on your level of activity. It also has recipes, as does his companion book, *Dr. Gott's No Flour, No Sugar Cookbook*.[7]

This plan might work for me because . . .

- ☑ Avoiding flour and sugar sounds simple to me.
- ☑ I would consider a ban on all flours, not just white flour.
- ☑ I think that counting calories would be helpful for me.
- ☑ I can figure out an exercise plan on my own.

Chapter Ten

I'm Out
of Options

Going with Bariatric Surgery

Not long ago, weight loss by means of surgery was considered cheating. Obesity was viewed as the result of a simple lack of willpower, something that could be overcome if you only tried hard enough.

Today, while acknowledging that overconsumption is a contributing factor to obesity, doctors also recognize that genetics play a factor in a person's body shape and weight and that hormones such as appetite-regulating ghrelin and leptin actively work against one's best efforts to lose weight and maintain a healthy weight.

Often, the condition of obesity creates a classic catch-22. Obese people modify their diet, but their bodies fight the perceived starvation and cry out for nourishment. They need to exercise, but they cannot because their weight and overstressed joints prevent them from accomplishing meaningful movement.

The cold, hard fact is that for morbidly obese people, weight loss through behavior modification alone, although possible, is a tough road with limited possibilities.

"A perfect storm of factors works against weight loss," said Dr. Scott A. Shikora, chief of general surgery and bariatric surgery at Tufts Medical Center in Boston, in an interview with me. "Fewer than 10 percent of morbidly obese people will see meaningful and sustainable weight loss without surgery."

As early as the 1990s, the National Institutes of Health declared surgery the only effective sustained weight loss treatment for morbid obesity.[1] By then, weight loss surgery already had a long history; the first gastric bypass actually was performed more than forty years ago by a doctor at the University of Iowa.

Once the backwater of surgical specialties, weight loss surgery—also called bariatric surgery—is a growing medical specialty today. Dr. Shikora, senior past president of the American Society for Metabolic and Bariatric Surgery (ASMBS), says the organization has seen a 600 percent growth in membership over the last decade.

For the person who is 100 pounds or more overweight and has a Body Bass Index (BMI) of 40 or more, or whose BMI is at least 35 and who has life-threatening health conditions, weight loss surgery is becoming an increasingly accessible solution. In 2009, the latest year for which statistics are available, the ASMBS estimates 220,000 people underwent bariatric surgery. Still, that number represents just 1 percent of the estimated 15 million people in the United States who are morbidly obese.[2]

The explosion in interest is the result not only of an increasing rate of obesity but also of the influence of high-profile individuals who have talked publicly about their experience: Al Roker, Carnie Wilson, and Muhammad Ali's daughter, Khaliah Ali, are a few of the better known celebrities who have undergone weight loss surgery.

Where we used to hear vague stories of "stomach stapling," patients today have a choice of surgeries, including gastric bypass, gastric banding, and duodenal switch. Each of these procedures alters the size of the stomach and, therefore, the amount of food one can eat. Some procedures also bypass parts of the digestive tract, decreasing the time food spends in the system, so the body absorbs fewer calories.

Gastric bypass is the most popular choice these days, Dr. Shikora says, but a relatively new procedure called sleeve gastrectomy, which removes about 85 percent of the stomach but doesn't bypass any of the digestive tract, is gaining interest. Gastric banding, though an adjustable and even reversible procedure, is decreasing in popularity, he says.

Whatever surgery is chosen, it is just the beginning of the patient's weight loss journey. As with any weight loss program, a person must change eating habits and activity levels for life. The good news is that studies show weight loss surgery patients have been able to maintain a 50 to 60 percent loss of excess weight ten to fourteen years after surgery.[3] The two women whose stories follow have had long-term success following weight loss surgery, too.

Allison Bottke

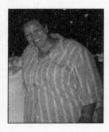 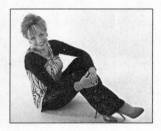

Dallas-Fort Worth, Texas
Age: 55
Occupation: Author and speaker
Accomplishment: Lost 120 pounds
How She Did It: Gastric bypass surgery

How's this for an unreal scenario? Your boss calls you into her office and warns you that unless you *gain* 20 pounds, you'll be out of a job.

It's hard to imagine, but that's exactly what happened to Allison Bottke. In the 1980s, Allison was the Wilhelmina Agency's first full-figured model. She worked for some big names in fashion, including Gloria Vanderbilt, and modeled for many well-known brands, such as Levi-Strauss, Pendleton, and Sasson Jeans.

Living in California, Allison was in her early thirties and wore a size 20. At 5 feet, 7 inches, she weighed about 220 pounds. At the time, department stores carried nothing for large women—Lane Bryant and muumuus were the only thing going—but Allison trolled consignment shops, deftly using color and accessories to create a unique style. As a cosmetologist who had once worked for Estée Lauder, Allison knew how to style hair and apply makeup, skills that served her well personally and professionally.

"I had a sense that what I was doing to help people mattered," Allison says. "I didn't look frumpy, and it made me crazy that fashions for large women were so poor."

Allison was also a fundraiser for nonprofit organizations and spent her days with "people whose job in life was to look beautiful and spend money." She loved her job and led a whirlwind life of charity events, modeling gigs, and parties. She was raising a son and, on the side, earning a college degree in theatre arts. Hers was a life to envy.

But what looked from the outside like an exciting and fulfilling life felt very different on the inside for Allison. A survivor of childhood molestation in a foster home that nearly ended her life, Allison was raised by her single mother and ran away at age 15 to marry a boy she met at a Dairy Queen. "I wore a size 6 blue lace mini dress," Allison remembers.

But Allison's Prince Charming turned out to be an abuser. Allison became pregnant at 16 and ran for her life, moving thirteen times in a single year to ensure her safety. Looking for love and comfort, Allison tried drugs, alcohol, relationships—anything she thought would satisfy.

"I believe that we have a void in our hearts, and if it is not filled with God, we try to fill it with something," Allison says. "I was such a mess emotionally."

In her pregnancy, Allison had gained 100 pounds. On welfare and receiving care at a clinic, Allison didn't see the same doctor regularly, so her weight gain didn't elicit much response. After her son's birth, Allison tried many ways to lose weight, including calorie counting, starvation, liquid diets, and in-patient clinics. An obliging doctor prescribed amphetamines—so-called "Black Beauties"—for weight loss and Valium to help her sleep.

The following years brought relationship failures, an abortion, alcohol and drug use, and a turbulent time with her son, who rebelled as a teen, became addicted to drugs, and was often arrested. In one of her darkest hours, Allison attempted suicide by swallowing her pills. Finally, she began to see a therapist. Ironically, it was the help she got in counseling that led to the crisis in her modeling career.

"I was seeing my photos, what I really looked like. I was around very positive people in my work, and therapy was helping me sort through my issues," Allison says. "I was becoming a whole person. I started eating better, stopped the drugs, and began losing weight."

The day Allison was called into the Wilhelmina offices, she had dropped to a size 16/18. "If you don't gain 20 pounds," her agent warned, "you're going to be out of work."

Undaunted, Allison abandoned her modeling career. Still, she struggled with her weight over the next five years, gaining and losing through many life changes—a conversion experience at age 35, a move to Arizona, writing gigs for magazines like *Cosmopolitan, Ladies' Home Journal*, and *Woman's World*, and eventually remarriage, a move to Minnesota, and the creation of *God Allows U-Turns*, a thriving book series and speaking ministry. At one point, she checked into a Minirth-Meier New Life Clinic, seeking relief from her struggles.

At her highest weight, Allison reached 280 pounds. She managed to lose 30 pounds one year through strict calorie counting but was distraught when she gained back 35 pounds in just two months. She suffered from sleep apnea and underwent surgeries to her neck, knees, and feet. One day at her doctor's office, Allison caught sight of her chart.

"Next to my name, the doctor had written 'morbidly obese 40-year-old woman,'" Allison recalls. "I had never seen that term applied to me, and I thought, *That's what's going to be on my death certificate.*"

Soon after, Allison saw a commercial for gastric bypass surgery. Although it was a relatively rare procedure then, Allison felt sure it was the answer to her struggles, especially when she found that one of its top surgeons lived in Minnesota. Again, she sought the help of a therapist, who confirmed for Allison that weight loss surgery was a valid treatment plan.

Allison opted for the Roux-en-Y procedure, because of its high success rate. She prepared for the surgery for about nine months, attending support group sessions, researching, cutting back on fatty, high-calorie foods, and losing 30 pounds as ordered. In October 2000, she underwent the surgery that bypassed a part of her intestinal tract and reduced the opening of her stomach to the size of a pencil eraser and the size of her stomach to that of an egg.

Although Allison was careful, she suffered complications and was hospitalized once for dehydration and once to remove scar tissue blocking the opening to her stomach. At times, she could barely swallow water, she couldn't quench her thirst, and she had to constantly monitor her food choices and intake.

"I would stand in front of my refrigerator and just cry," Allison says. "I kept praying, *'Let that day come when I don't have to think about food all the time.'*"

Yet within six months, Allison lost 90 pounds and after a year had dropped 120 pounds. Her career continues to thrive, with the addition of the series *Setting Boundaries* and *God Answers Prayers*, among other books and ongoing speaking engagements.

Today, she maintains her weight at about 160 pounds. She does suffer a common side effect of the surgery known as "dumping syndrome," a sort of shock to the system in which sugar and fats enter the bloodstream too quickly, and she has had two reconstructive surgeries. She monitors her protein intake, takes nutritional supplements, and keeps one step ahead of anemia. But her prayer has been answered.

"About two and a half years after the surgery, I was working one day, when I thought, *Oh gosh, I haven't eaten,* and I realized it had been quite a while since I had been so focused on food," Allison says. "I would do it again in a heartbeat. It is a quality of life issue, and I feel great."

Thanks To

Therapy and counseling: Find a trustworthy professional and get the help that you need.

My Tips

I didn't tell anyone other than my immediate family and my best friend about my surgery. You don't need people giving you their opinion and saying, "So-and-so died from that." I am a big believer in counseling. Don't be afraid to deal with the stuff in your life, or the weight is just going to come right back on. Do what it takes!

Gastric Bypass Surgery

In gastric bypass—also known as Roux-en-Y bypass—a surgeon creates a small pouch at the top of the stomach and a bypass around the rest of the stomach and the small intestine. Gastric bypass is considered when people are extremely obese—a BMI of 40 or higher—or obese to a lesser extent (BMI between 35 and 39.9) and have a serious related condition such as diabetes or high blood pressure.

Gastric bypass surgery works in two ways. First, it reduces the stomach to about the size of a small egg with the capacity of about half a cup of food. This gives the patient a quick feeling of fullness when eating, and therefore allows him or her to stop sooner and eat less. Secondly, the surgery bypasses a portion of the body's intestines, so it reduces the body's ability to digest food and absorb calories.

The patient cannot eat for a specified time after the surgery—sometimes several days—after which food is gradually reintroduced, starting with liquids and moving on to pureed and soft foods. In the six months following surgery, eating habits must be carefully controlled, as eating too much or too fast can cause pain, nausea, and vomiting.

After the surgery, people can expect to lose 50 to 60 percent of their weight within two years. But to accomplish long-term weight control, they must follow strict dietary and exercise guidelines. The guidelines are familiar to anyone wanting to lose weight—that is, limit high-sugar and high-fat foods and exercise regularly.

Bariatric surgery patients must also chew food well, eat small and frequent meals, and avoid too much snacking or grazing, which can result in excessive calorie intake. They must also pay attention to when and how much liquid they drink to avoid dehydration or unpleasant digestive side effects such as dumping—a premature passing of food into the small intestine that can be accompanied by nausea, vomiting, dizziness, and sweating. Some food prohibitions will be a matter of trial and error. Nutritional supplements are needed to overcome possible vitamin and mineral deficiencies.

Debra Anderson

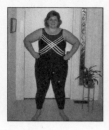 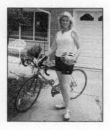

Dayton, Ohio
Age: 47
Occupation: Bariatrics program service director
Accomplishment: Lost 140 pounds
How She Did It: Duodenal switch surgery

Trained as an occupational therapist, Debra Anderson saw the debilitating effects of obesity up close.

"Every day I saw people who had diabetes, who had lost limbs, had heart attacks, neuropathies, strokes," says Debra. "I saw that many of these folks were significantly overweight, and I thought, *If this is happening to them, this is in my future.*"

Debra didn't want that kind of future; her past carried enough pain and failure. A "chunky" child, Debra had enrolled in her first weight loss program by fifth grade. At 5 feet, 2 inches, she weighed more than 130 pounds.

"I was definitely a part of the 'clean plate club' and food was a reward. You had to finish all your dinner to have dessert. That was ingrained in me," she says. "And it was Ponderosa if you did well on your report card and McDonald's for special treats."

Although she says it was agony to go to meetings alone, and to eat separate meals at home, Debra lost 35 pounds within six months on Weight Watchers when she was in the fifth grade. She was active in her school and college years, dancing, biking, swimming, and running for exercise.

157

But after college, Debra moved to Chicago to take her first job. There she started eating a lot of fast food and convenience food. She knew it wasn't good for her, and she tried just about every diet out there to get her weight under control. "Almost everything but fen-phen and acupuncture," she admits.

Every year brought another ten pounds, though, until Debra, now 5 feet, 8 inches tall, weighed about 210 pounds. At one annual physical, while waiting in the examining room, she heard her doctor outside the door.

"I heard him say, 'My gosh, she weighs more than I do,'" Debra recalls.

Crushed, Debra worked with a dietitian to adopt the American Dietetic Association's eating plan. Even so, the pounds rolled on.

By the time she was 42, Debra weighed 308 pounds. She would routinely wake up at night gasping for air, and she made a few visits to the emergency room suffering from chest pains. She was desperate, but she couldn't find the way out of her dilemma.

"I tried everything to lose that weight," Debra says. "But every time I lost 10 or 20 pounds, it would return to hound me, with extra 'dividends' in the bargain. I'm pretty smart, but I couldn't outsmart it."

Moving back to Dayton and working in a hospital environment, Debra began to hear about weight loss surgery. A thorough and careful person, she researched the various surgeries and settled on biliopancreatic diversion with duodenal switch because it had the highest success rate, in terms of pounds lost. She also thought it would fit into her lifestyle the best.

"I was single, and I ate out a lot with friends," she says. "I didn't always have control over the recipes, and I didn't want to be limited to dollops of food, as you are with some surgeries." On May 4, 2004, she underwent the procedure.

All went well, and Debra recuperated at her mother's home. Within a few days, she was eating small amounts of soft foods—cottage cheese, scrambled eggs, string cheese, yogurt, and puddings made with protein powder. Gradually, she reintroduced meats and vegetables to her diet. Surprisingly, she found herself satisfied with her limited diet.

"I thought, *Gee, did he do surgery on my stomach or my brain?*" she says. "After the surgery, I didn't want to eat the same things I had before. I wanted fresh fruits and vegetables, not deep-fried foods or anything like that."

Even now, when Debra wants a treat, it's a small one. She admits to a weakness for chocolate-covered peanut butter "buckeyes," a regional favorite.

"A couple of weeks after the surgery, I went to a Cracker Barrel, and for dessert, I ordered a buckeye. I cut it in fourths and I ate a quarter of it," she says, marveling even now. "Before, I could have had half a dozen or twelve of them, easy."

Within a year and a half, Debra had lost 140 pounds, 90 percent of her excess weight. She credits her success to the surgical changes to her digestive system. "I really needed malabsorption to lose weight and keep it off," she says.

Today, Debra maintains a healthy weight of about 175 pounds. Once a size 28, she now wears a size 14. In the years since her surgery, the hospital hired the doctor who performed her surgery, created a weight loss surgery program, and promoted Debra to director of the program's Bariatric Service Line. Her personal life is thriving, too; she was married in 2009.

Living an active life today, Debra sails with her brother, something she could barely do before. Two weeks before her surgery, she bought a bike and set a goal. "I wanted to ride that bike within a year," she says. She began by walking, building up her strength until she was doing twenty minutes on the treadmill. Ultimately, she got on that bike.

Debra didn't stop there. Sixteen months after her surgery, she competed in the Chicago Triathlon, swimming nine-tenths of a mile on Lake Michigan, biking 24 miles, and then running 6.1 miles. That was one of three international distance triathlons she has completed to date. It was at the finish line of her first triathlon that the beauty of her new life hit Debra full force.

"I was coming around the final corner, when everything that had happened hit me and I started bawling," she says. "I just hope people think, *If she can do it, so can I.*"

Thanks To

My mom, Nancy M. Anderson, for your love, support, and encouragement every step of the way.

My surgeon, Dr. John P. Maguire, for your wisdom, compassion, skill, and gifted ability to improve the lives of others.

The Weight Loss Surgery Team at Miami Valley Hospital, for your commitment to high-quality patient care and the long-term success of every patient.

My Tips

Whatever weight loss option you're considering, choose what's going to fit your lifestyle. Commit to it 110 percent. It needs to be a lifestyle that you can honestly commit to for the rest of your life.

Biliopancreatic Diversion/Duodenal Switch

The biliopancreatic diversion with duodenal switch (BPD/DS) or gastric reduction duodenal switch (GRDS) procedure, often simply called the duodenal switch, surgically reduces the size of the stomach so that it holds about one-third to one-fifth of its original capacity. It also reroutes the small intestines so that a separate path for bile and food join together near the large intestine. During the surgery, the gallbladder and appendix may also be removed.

The surgery is restrictive, which means the patient's capacity for food intake is cut back. But it also reduces the amount of time the body has to capture calories and absorb fat from food in the small intestine. Because of changes to the digestive tract, the body no longer absorbs all the nutrition from ingested food. Patients must take vitamin supplements for the rest of their lives. Protein intake must also be carefully monitored.

Patients who undergo a duodenal switch typically lose 75 to 80 percent of their excess body weight, a success rate that many people considering weight loss surgery find attractive. Postoperative eating patterns may not be as strict as for other weight loss surgeries. Patients may begin by eating soft foods, rather than a liquid-only diet. Many times, the surgery is done laparoscopically, which also cuts down on recovery time.

One long-term side effect of the surgery can be that eating too much can cause diarrhea. But many patients often prefer this surgery because dumping syndrome is not a common side effect. And, although the size of the stomach is reduced, patients generally report being able to eat more normally than patients who have undergone bypass or banding surgery.

Chapter Eleven

You're Never Too Young

Catching Childhood Obesity Early

In one of my interviews with a man who had been overweight as a child, he made an interesting point. He recounted that when he grew up in the 1970s and 1980s, he was the target of cruel comments and hurtful exclusion by other children because he was "the fat kid." But today, he speculated, kids might not have it so bad.

"Today, you're not the only fat kid in the class," he said. "You're just one of many fat kids."

If this is true, maybe it's not so bad to be an overweight child these days.

But if it's true, there are a lot more fat kids than there used to be.

In fact, that's just what health researchers have found. In a survey undertaken for 2007–2008, the latest year for which statistics are available, the National Center for Health Statistics calculates that about 17 percent of children from age 2 to 19 are overweight or obese.[1] That number has more than doubled in the last few decades.

Having a child myself, I don't want to believe that the blame lies solely with parents. And, in fact, I don't think it does. All you have to do is read up on the food industry—*Don't Eat This Book* by Morgan Spurlock or *Fast Food Nation* by Eric Schlosser, for a start—to come face to face with the powerful corporate forces that are battling us for our children's health.

But we are not blameless. One Cornell University researcher has quantified just how much responsibility we as parents do bear. In his book *Mindless Eating: Why We Eat More Than We Think*, Brian Wansink examines the influence within the family of the person he calls "the nutritional gatekeeper." For most families, that means the parent who does the menu planning, grocery shopping, and cooking. Through extensive studies, Wansink found that this person is responsible for about 72 percent of a family's food choices.[2]

I was somewhat heartened by that number, because it means that in our house we can control all but 28 percent of the food our child eats. But if I'm going to be honest, I'll have to admit that the decisions we make aren't always good. Grilled sausage-and-cheese sandwiches. Donuts. Cheese puffs. Pepperoni pizza. Of our own free will, we abdicate some of the 72 percent responsibility on a daily basis.

At some point, the bad choices and external forces catch up to our children. And when they do, the issue of weight control can become a flash point for just one more parent-and-child conflict, piled atop the towering heap of arguments about clothing, music, video games, friends, tattoos, body piercing, cigarettes, drugs, and alcohol. It's hard to know how to help or where to find the strength to begin.

As with adults, more often than not the child must come to the decision to help himself or herself, regardless of the good intentions—or the nagging—of parents. And that's just what these teens did.

Cassie Bordner

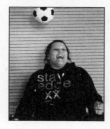 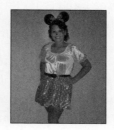

Waco, Texas
Age: 18
Occupation: Student
Accomplishment: Lost 70 pounds
How She Did It: Wellspring Camp

As a child, Cassie Bordner was teased mercilessly about her weight. Today, she'd love nothing better than for her tormentors to see what she's accomplished.

Born into a military family, Cassie was about 10 years old when her family settled in North Carolina after an overseas Navy posting. She had a tough time of it there. Though she says she was just "chunky" then, kids at school never let up on her about it.

"I was shy, always coming into new situations, and the kids were mean," she says. "I didn't have many friends."

Even at home, Cassie came in for teasing from her older brother, who was athletic, bean-pole thin, and able to eat anything he wanted without consequences. Cassie thought maybe if she ate the way her brother did, she would be thin, too. Not understanding anything about nutrition or metabolism, she tried it. But, of course, it didn't work.

In part, it didn't work because the family's food choices weren't the best. Her parents both worked and neither enjoyed cooking. Fast food or takeout was on the menu almost nightly—Taco Bell was a favorite. Lunches might be peanut butter and jelly, and snacking was a way of life. "Cheez-Its were my downfall," she admits.

At home, Cassie would snack while watching television and playing video games, either alone or with her brother. And, even though her weight increasingly bothered her, Cassie didn't really know what to do about it. For a while, she was vegetarian, not for weight loss but as a matter of conscience. Even then, she made the wrong choices. "I loved Mexican food—beans, cheese, chips," she says. "I ate onion rings, french fries, grilled cheese sandwiches."

Yet Cassie understands that choosing the wrong foods wasn't her only problem—her emotions were causing problems as well.

"The constant teasing started a downward spiral for me. I cried almost every day," Cassie says. "Food was how I comforted myself."

As a teenager, she and her mother tried a few fad diets—cabbage soup, diet shakes—but nothing seemed to work. "I'd lose 10 pounds and then gain 20 back. These diets never taught me how to eat," she says. "And how long can you eat cabbage soup, anyway?"

Even well-regarded programs based in weekly meetings didn't work for them. In their busy family, finding time to get to meetings was difficult. Eventually, a family move to Texas brought some relief. There, Cassie suffered less teasing. "People here in Texas seem more accepting," she says.

Yet Cassie still hated how she looked.

"I felt so big all the time. I could shop at the stores my friends did, but just barely," she says. "I bought the biggest size they carried. I wore hoodies all the time—I didn't want anyone seeing more than they had to."

On top of that, Cassie had chronic health problems. She had high blood pressure and her knees bothered her. They popped in and out of joint easily, causing her a lot of pain. She was plagued by depression and anxiety and had even gone to the emergency room after one anxiety attack.

"I felt so trapped in my body," she says. "It was like my soul was trapped."

One day, 16-year-old Cassie stepped on a scale and was shocked to realize that she weighed more than 200 pounds—more, in fact, than her father did. She never let her dad know how much she weighed, but it was her father who stepped in to help. He began researching weight loss camps and found Wellspring's camp in San Marcos, Texas.

"My first thought was, *Fat camp! I don't want to go to fat camp*," she remembers. "But my summers were really boring anyway, so I decided to give it a chance."

At Wellspring, Cassie weighed in at 211 pounds. Just 5 feet, 3 inches tall, she wore an XL top and size 13 pants. These facts might have discouraged another teen, but they only gave Cassie the determination she needed to finally succeed. "I just decided I'd had enough," she says. "I was ready to give it my all."

Cassie had been active as a young child, and she was happy to engage in the athletic activities the camp offered—swimming, dancing, dodgeball, basketball, obstacle and ropes courses, and rock climbing. She enjoyed the camp's healthy meals and snacks, tracked her food choices, took the camp's cooking classes, and enjoyed the camp's "dine-out challenges," the field trips in which campers learned to make healthier choices at restaurants.

Perhaps the biggest breakthrough, though, was her counselor's encouragement to stop looking to food for comfort. Cassie began to express herself artistically instead. She kept a journal, wrote stories, and participated in arts and crafts classes. In group sessions, campers were encouraged to compliment each other, and gradually her self-esteem recovered from all the hits it had taken.

Over eight weeks, the healthy meals, physical activity, and behavioral counseling enabled Cassie to drop 31 pounds. She wasn't "supermodel thin," she says, but she was on such a high from camp that she dropped another ten pounds after she returned home. She fixed her own meals—and even managed to work around her dislike of salads, a staple in most weight loss menus.

"I made fat-free pancakes, sandwiches with egg substitutes, veggie burgers. And I love veggies like asparagus, broccoli, and corn," she says. "I just don't like lettuce."

Wellspring worked so well for Cassie that she went back for a second year, this time for ten weeks as a mentor. "A lot of kids told me I was the most motivational person they knew," she says. She ramped up her exercise program, running in the morning and whenever she could throughout the day. She became even more enthusiastic about running once a counselor showed her how to run without rolling her feet inward, a habit she had acquired to accommodate her extra weight. That summer, she lost another 29 pounds.

At home, just like at camp, Cassie fills her days with activity. She goes to the gym four days a week, where she likes Zumba classes. She used to be afraid of group activities, but now she is active in her school's Spanish Club and in the National Honor Society, with which she does community service projects. In college, she expects to enroll in ballet classes.

While Cassie has had her ups and downs—in the stress of studying for AP exams, she gained back ten pounds—she remains as committed as ever to her weight loss. Although some people have suggested that her goal weight of 110 pounds might be unrealistic, that is what she is aiming for. Today, 30 pounds shy of that goal and wearing a small top and size 8 pants, she isn't backing down. "I am so close now, and I've come so far," she says.

Cassie is once again an outgoing person, willing to talk in class and not as shy about making friends, both boys and girls. Not only that, but in her senior year of high school, she joined the cross country team. "Me! On a sports team!" she says, with wonder.

"For the first time in my life, I'm being looked at as the athletic kid," Cassie adds. "I've always wanted to be that kid! I can truly say that going to Wellspring is the best decision I have ever made. I am a new person—70 pounds lighter, healthier, happier, and excited about my future."

Thanks To

Myself and my inner motivation: No one wanted this as much as me!

Liz, my behavioral coach at Wellspring.

Tips

Keep a journal of everything you eat, and research the nutritional value of what you eat. You'd be surprised at what's in some foods! I look for fat-free options wherever possible—low-fat doesn't count. Even low-calorie foods can be high in fat. The fat-free Frappuccino at Starbucks tastes exactly the same as the full-fat one. When I eat out, I usually go to Subway, where I choose a low-fat option, like the veggie sub.

Wellspring Camps and Academy

"The Wellspring Plan isn't a specific diet; it is a pathway to a better life. You'll find plenty of bumps along this road; but through the Wellspring Plan, you'll learn how to overcome the inevitable obstacles and master one of life's most difficult challenges."

—The Wellspring Weight Loss Plan: The Simple, Scientific and Sustainable Approach of the World's Most Successful Weight Loss Programs for Overweight Young People—and How You Can Achieve Lifelong Success With It by Daniel S. Kirschenbaum, MD (Dallas, TX: BenBella Books, 2011)

Most people know Wellspring Camps as the setting for The Style Network's reality television show *Too Fat for 15.* Wellspring began in 2004 and today has eleven locations. Camp programs are divided into three demographics: camps for children, teens, and young adults ages 11 to 24; family camp for families having children ages 5 to 15; and a women's program for adult women age 25 and up. One location, Wellspring New York, is exclusively for girls.

The camps offer sessions of varying lengths of time, from three weeks to twelve weeks, depending on location and camper choice. Family camps offer weekly sessions, while women's camps start at two weeks in length. Wellspring Academy offers programs of ten to thirteen weeks year-round that combine academics with weight loss and fitness for students ages 11 to 24. Those campuses are in North Carolina and California.

Wellspring's program is fashioned around strategies that, if followed, promise sustainable weight loss over the long term. Dr. Daniel S. Kirschenbaum, Wellspring's clinical director and director of Chicago's Center for Behavioral Medicine & Sport Psychology, maintains that on the Wellspring Plan campers consistently lose on average four pounds per week and 30 pounds total over eight weeks of camp. In six- to twelve-month follow-up studies, the average camper maintains the weight loss or loses an additional five to eight pounds. Wellspring estimates that 70 percent of campers maintain their weight or lose more weight upon returning home.

While the camp regulates most of its campers' food choices and activities during its programs, it provides some opportunities for campers to make their own choices. Wellspring aims to give campers tools to regulate their food intake and activity levels on their own once they return home. In group counseling and through mentoring, they also focus on emotional and social growth.

After camp has ended, Wellspring offers several choices to help campers and their families make lifestyle changes at home. A two-day Family Workshop covers healthy food choices and how to shop and cook in ways that support a healthy lifestyle. Families learn to keep track of food intake, receive pedometers and calorie counters, and go home with an individualized plan for the family. Behavioral counseling is also offered at the workshops. A yearlong Continuing Care option is also available. This online program enables campers to self-monitor and record their daily choices and offers private online conversations with their behavioral coach.

This plan might work for me because . . .

- ☑ I would like to be totally immersed in a weight loss program.
- ☑ To succeed, I think I need a support team of friends and mentors.
- ☑ I would like to have healthy eating and activity habits modeled for me.
- ☑ I can devote a summer to achieving my weight loss goals.

Daniel Greenlees

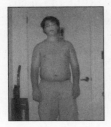 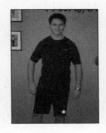 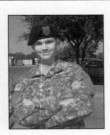

Myrtle Beach, South Carolina
Age: 22
Occupation: Military
Accomplishment: Lost 70 pounds
How He Did It: Personal trainer at a gym

From the age of 12, Daniel Greenlees's family lived on a 65-foot sailboat. His bedroom measured 7 feet by 4 feet. You'd think that this space crunch alone would be reason enough for a person to slim down. For Daniel, though, it was where the boat docked one day that mattered more.

In November 2006, the boat was damaged in a storm, and the family was forced to dock in Norfolk, Virginia. They rented an apartment in nearby Virginia Beach while they waited out the repairs. One day in the apartment, Daniel took off his shirt, and his stepfather looked at him in alarm—ugly stretch marks sprawled across the boy's chest. "We've got to do something about that," he told Daniel. At 5 feet, 7 inches, Daniel weighed 236 pounds.

Daniel had always struggled with his weight. As a homeschooled teen, he would sit at the computer fourteen or fifteen hours a day, studying, eating, surfing, and playing games. Not attending a traditional school and moving every few years, he had no friends and little contact with others. He didn't mind that so much, though. When he was younger and attended public schools, he often found his interactions with other children painful.

"I had no trouble at a small school I attended, where there were maybe only 180 kids and no one picked on me," Daniel says. "But at one large school, I had only one or two friends. Kids were not nice to me at all. They acted like a mob."

A few times, Daniel and his mom tried to do something about the extra pounds. But good intentions can backfire.

"I remember once my mom decided we were going to eat healthier food," he says. "But instead of just buying some good things, that night for dinner she made her own pasta from scratch . . . from eggplant! It was awful."

In Norfolk, the family's apartment was just steps away from Jim White Fitness Studios. The day after his stepfather commented about his weight, Daniel and his mother went over to check it out. He liked what he saw, and he knew it was time to act. "I knew this was the best opportunity I'd ever have to lose weight, and so I took it," Daniel says.

Jim paired Daniel with personal trainer Eric McGlaughlin. The first thing they did together was clean out the boat's pantry and refrigerator. "We threw out pancakes, waffles, Toaster Strudels, Hot Pockets, Pop-Tarts, a lot of different things," Daniel says. He and his mom went shopping for fruits, vegetables, lean meats, and other healthy foods and began cooking low-fat, low-calorie meals.

Although his starting weight initially hampered his ability to exercise for long periods of time, Daniel quickly fell into an ambitious routine. At the gym, he worked two days a week with Eric and three days by himself, each time for 45 minutes to an hour and a half, splitting his time between cardio workouts and weight training. As a homeschooled teen, Daniel's days were flexible enough to accommodate as much time at the gym as he could manage. Although he was self-motivated, he credits Eric with much of his success.

"I worked out as hard as I could, and Eric wouldn't let me slack off," Daniel says. "He could tell when I was getting bored, and he'd change things around to keep me motivated."

Daniel loves being outdoors now, and he participates in sports. He's still amazed at how much he's changed, when not so long ago his future looked hopeless.

"I used to see people jogging or playing games outdoors, and I'd think, *Why do people want to do that?*" he remembers. "I was always tired before, and I'd think to myself, *Why bother?*"

Despite the current popularity of recipes that sneak healthy ingredients into otherwise unhealthy foods—cauliflower puree in macaroni and cheese, spinach puree in a batch of brownies—Daniel believes that's the wrong approach. "We can tell the difference, anyway," he says. "It's better just to give kids veggies from the start so they'll like them."

As with any of us, Daniel has some regrets about his past and wishes some things had been different.

"They don't teach you anything in health classes. I wish someone had told me that 3,500 calories equals a pound," he says. "If I had the knowledge, maybe I would have done something sooner."

And he wishes his family had shopped differently. "If we didn't buy the bad stuff, we wouldn't have eaten it," he reasons.

After their stop in Virginia, Daniel's family docked in Myrtle Beach. For a time, he would give Eric a call or shoot him an e-mail when he needed a little advice. Today, Daniel has joined the Army, where fitness is a must, and he is stationed overseas.

"It's nice fitting into decent clothes now. I'm able to get places—I can run up stairs!—instead of moving at a waddling pace," he says. "I can't sit still all the time, like I used to. There are people out there I want to meet."

Thanks To

Eric McLaughlin, ACE, CPT, personal trainer at Jim White Fitness Studios, Virginia Beach, Virginia, who says, "We really care about our clients. I couldn't go to bed at night if I felt that I hadn't helped someone that day."

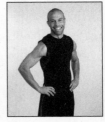

My Tips

Order the grilled chicken or turkey. Hold the mayo. Throw away the bun. Have an apple instead of the chips. Drink diet soda or water. Avoid burger places.

Me: The Nutritional Gatekeeper, Asleep

We were coming to the end of our conversation, when Daniel blurted out that he wished his mom had given him healthier food to eat as a child. That statement cut like a knife to my heart.

In his book *Honest to God?*, Bill Hybels tracks a hypothetical teen to assess her daily intake of sugar.[3] Her day goes like this: sweetened cereal, cider, and buttered toast with jam for breakfast; cream of chicken soup, lemonade, and Jell-O for lunch; a frozen beef entrée with french fries and a dish of ice cream for dinner. For snacks, the girl has chocolate milk, two cupcakes, and a soda.

Her total? About 81$\frac{1}{2}$ teaspoons of sugar! I was floored to read that.

I want to believe my child eats better than that. But I'm not sure he does. I haven't thought much about it, because at age 13, Evan is a slender child who weighs barely 90 pounds. So I conducted a similar experiment to see how we stack up. I piled the kitchen table high with boxes, bags, bottles, and packages. Here is Evan's typical daily menu:

- **Breakfast:** buttered toast or kids' cereal, 1 strip of bacon, half a cup of 1% milk
- **Lunch:** 6 ounces low-fat yogurt or half a cup of sweetened applesauce, snack crackers, 1 pack fruit snacks or a 100-calorie snack pack, bottle of water
- **Snack:** handful of red grapes or half a banana or apple, toaster tart, half a cup of milk
- **Dinner:** 8 homemade chicken nuggets with 1 tablespoon catsup, half a cup of mashed potatoes with butter, a quarter cup of peas

- **Dessert or snack:** 4 Oreos and half a cup of milk or 1 cup of ice cream
- **During baseball season:** one 20-ounce sports drink

To estimate his sugar intake, I looked at the food labels, where ingredients are listed in grams—4 grams of sugar equals one teaspoon. Counting only the added sugars—that is, not foods' natural sugars—here's Evan's total in teaspoons:

Breakfast: 2 ½ to 5½
Lunch: 8 to 8½
Snack: 6½
Dinner: 1
Desserts or snack: 7 to 13
Sports drink: 8½

TOTAL: 25–43 teaspoons

Whew! That's better than 81½ teaspoons! I'm pretty proud of the fact that there are no soft drinks on the list, but it's eye-opening to see how much sugar is in a sports drink. (And don't even think about so-called healthy "vitamin water." Another 8 teaspoons down the hatch.)

Remember, though, Dr. Wansink estimates that parents, as nutritional gatekeepers, control only 72 percent of a child's diet. Add in birthday cupcakes, pizza parties, lunch trades, team celebrations, and other splurges, and Evan's consumption could increase by almost 30 percent. At its worst, that's a total of about 56 teaspoons a day! For comparison's sake, consider that the U.S. Department of Agriculture advises us to eat no more than 10 teaspoons of added sugar a day.

I took out a measuring cup. Those 56 teaspoons pile up to one and a half cups of sugar. As if that weren't shocking enough, I then converted the sugar into calories, at a rate of 16 calories per teaspoon. Evan's total now? About 900 calories!

Estimate that an active child under age 14 might consume 1,000 calories a day, plus up to 100 calories per year of age. That means Evan's diet could contain up to 2,200 calories a day. If so, he could be getting about 40 percent of his calories from sugar.

Keep in mind that this tidy bit of math doesn't address the fat and sodium in his diet, which I can see is considerable. And it doesn't take into account the other danger of a high-sugar diet—that it usually translates into a low-fiber diet.

It's clear that we have a little pantry cleaning of our own to do.

Chapter Twelve

It's for My Health

Losing Weight as a Secondary Goal

In order to move in the right direction, I had to trick myself into it. Although deep down I really did want to lose weight, I had to convince myself that I simply wanted to improve my health. I had failed enough times at weight loss that I didn't want to admit I was trying again.

There was a good bit of truth to that. My back problems were severe enough to require physical therapy, and my blood pressure was high enough that medication was always just one reading away.

So, lap after lap in the pool, I shut out thoughts of smaller dress sizes. I told people I was doing this for my health. And eventually, as I began to get up in the morning and realize that pain wasn't the first thing to enter my consciousness, I actually did stop thinking about weight loss. I did jump the chasm to the other side—good health became my motivating goal. And the pounds gradually dropped away.

Given our national obsession with weight, I was surprised to find that the message of health may once have gotten more press than that of weight loss. At a garage sale, my husband picked up a copy of *You Are What You Eat*, Victor H. Lindlahr's 1940 ode to healthy living.[1] While weight loss is mentioned on the cover, it gets barely five sentences in the book. Ninety-nine percent of the book is devoted to the idea—so shocking then!—that the body needs fruits and vegetables more than it does stick-to-your-ribs starches and meats.

The fact is, of course, that losing weight vastly improves your health and quality of life. So many health problems are created or exacerbated by excess weight: diabetes, cancer, heart disease, stroke, gout, sleep apnea, gallbladder disease, acid reflux, degenerative disc disease, blood clots, osteoarthritis, high blood pressure, and high cholesterol, to name a few of the most damaging maladies.

Even the mundane routines of life become an immense challenge. "I could barely walk up a flight of steps without stopping to catch my breath," more than one person told me. Nighttime was a never-ending struggle for breath and sleep. Several people admitted getting a peek at their medical chart and being stopped cold by the term *morbid obesity*, even though they knew all too well their bodies' aches and pains.

With these conditions and limitations in mind, some people define success not only as weight loss but as gaining control over their health. Some people have no debilitating conditions themselves, but their family has a history of them. "It haunted me that all the men in my family died young from heart attacks," one man told me.

But, of course, by adopting new eating habits and exercise routines, people often discover that weight loss is a desirable side effect. I talked with two people whose quest for health has caused the pounds to drop away.

John Bellemer _____

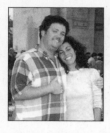 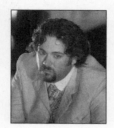

Brooklyn, New York
Age: 42
Occupation: Opera singer
Accomplishments: Boosted his energy, lost 70 pounds
How He Did It: Body-*for*-LIFE[2] and Eat to Live

John Bellemer may sing opera, but it's Hollywood that calls his tune.

A lyric tenor, John relies for his living on roles that cast him in the role of romantic lead—Romeo in *Roméo et Juliette*, Don José in *Carmen*, the Duke in *Rigoletto*. And these days, with the influence of the big screen, even opera-going audiences want their heroes to be buff.

"Because of Hollywood, everyone's looking for matinee idols for my roles," John says. "The guy has to be believable as a romantic lead."

At 6 feet, 1 inch, John believed he carried his 260 pounds well. He knew he was overweight, but he felt that his girth gave him a stage presence that tenors often lack. "If you're small, you can disappear on stage," he says.

Yet, increasingly, John also suspected he was losing jobs he coveted to singers he felt were no more talented than he. "I wasn't getting the amount or type of work I needed to make a living," he says.

His suspicions were confirmed one day when he auditioned for the role of Alfredo Germont for the Portland Opera's production of *La Traviata*. He was thrilled to be one of two finalists under consideration. But his manager had crushing news for John.

"The director thinks you look more like a truck driver than a lover," John recalls his manager saying.

While that comment stung, John later did win the role of Alfredo for the Opera Theatre of St. Louis. But before rehearsals began, John crossed paths with the conductor for the performance—a longtime friend of John's—who put in a call to the director of the company.

"He said to the director, 'It looks like John has gained weight. I'm not sure this is the direction we want to go,'" John recalls.

The honesty of his friend and mentor moved John to action. It was time to find out whether his career was foundering because of his weight.

John picked up Bill Phillips's book Body-*for*-LIFE, and in January 2001, he began a 12-week challenge that included a meal plan of lean protein and complex carbohydrates, along with aerobic exercise and weight training. In that time period, John lost 27 pounds. By October, he had lost 56 pounds.

Not only did he look better, but John saw a huge difference in his singing. "When I lost weight and built abdominal muscle, I found my singing was stronger," John says. "Singing is all about breathing, and I was able to get better air, and there was more strength in my sound."

Not only that, but John felt his newfound health improved his stage performance as well. Opera is a very demanding profession, one that requires ten-hour rehearsal days and physical endurance on stage.

"In *The Magic Flute*, Tamino is chased around the stage by a serpent, and then five minutes later he has to stop and sing 'Dies Bildnis ist bezaubernd schön,' one of the most beautiful tenor arias Mozart wrote," John says. "A number of my roles are very physical, and they were difficult to perform when I couldn't get a breath."

After his weight loss, John got feedback that was more to his liking. Following his performance in *Rigoletto* with Idée Fixe in Belgium, the director cut a video that ultimately made its way around France. "People were asking, *'Who is this tenor?'* I know I wouldn't have gotten that reaction if I hadn't lost that weight," John says.

For seven years, John's career flourished, yet he was not content to stop there. Although he was free from illness, John was mindful of his family history of heart disease, stroke, and diabetes. He wanted to forge a plan for eating in a way that promoted health and became convinced that he needed to eat less protein.

John heard about Dr. Joel Fuhrman's Eat to Live plan, which calls for eating almost exclusively fruits and vegetables. In March 2008, he and his wife, Sarah, adopted it. Having maintained a 30-pound weight loss for about 20 years, Sarah was just as eager to try the plan as John was.

For breakfast, John and Sarah would have a fruit salad or oatmeal, using natural coconut as a sweetener. For lunch, they'd have an "enormous" salad with chickpeas, and for dinner, they made recipes from the book, such as bean burgers or chili, and served them with a green or fruit salad. When they went out to eat with friends, they'd have a meal that often included a small amount of meat.

"It's an intense plan, but I really felt more energetic, and in the first week, I lost seven and a half pounds," John says.

John says the pared-down meal plan worked out well for a long time, but eventually he and Sarah felt they needed to adapt the plan to be sustainable for life. Their diet still is weighted toward fruits and vegetables, but they've added in more sources of animal protein, such as chicken, fish, and steak. Their philosophy is to consider no foods off-limits and to enjoy everything in moderation.

Because they live in Brooklyn, John and his wife walk a lot, both to get around and to walk their dogs. When at home in Brooklyn, he bikes about 100 miles a week, mostly on bike paths along the water or around Prospect Park.

With his career thriving, John is on the road about ten months of the year. He often stays at hotels lacking gym equipment, so he has begun his own program of yoga, which he can do in his room. Often, when working in an unfamiliar city, John will walk until he deliberately becomes lost and then find his way home, generally covering about five miles that way.

These tactics, coupled with the grueling nature of rehearsal schedules, often boost John's weight control efforts. "I generally lose weight more quickly on the road than at home," he says.

Although John isn't watching the scale anymore, he believes he weighs in the low 200s and is poised to dip below that benchmark. He has worn size 36 pants for a while, but now "they're falling off of me," he says. Not knowing the exact numbers, he is nevertheless delighted with the change he sees and how good he feels.

"Before, when I went into an audition, I would be thinking, *They think I'm fat*, and already I was in an uphill battle," he says. "The other day at an audition, I walked past a mirror and caught sight of myself. I thought, *I can't believe that's you!* That whole element of negative thinking is erased. I feel so free now."

Thanks To

My friend, conductor Stephen Lord.

My family, who passed the *Eat to Live* book around.

My wife, Sarah Blaze, also a professional singer: I don't want people saying, "What is she doing with him?" I want people to say, "These two look great together."

My Tips

I think every single weight loss program should have a "free" day. It is my saving grace. I know I'm not restricted forever, that there is light at the end of the tunnel. Both Bill Phillips and Joel Fuhrman have free times when you can eat what you want. My free day is Sunday. Sometimes I wake up on Monday feeling hung over from food. But I think it's important to throw your body a curve, feed it something different, put your metabolism into overdrive.

Eat to Live

"Regardless of your metabolism or genetics, you can achieve a normal weight once you start a high-nutrient diet style."

—*Eat to Live: The Revolutionary Formula for Fast and Sustained Weight Loss* by Joel Fuhrman, MD (New York: Little, Brown & Co., 2005)

Dr. Joel Fuhrman believes that a diet of foods that are high in nutrients and low in calories is the key to weight loss and health. In the process, he believes you can also maximize longevity; reverse heart disease, hypertension, and diabetes; and avoid medical intervention.

The Eat to Live diet represents a dramatic change from the typical American's diet. Dr. Fuhrman advocates an entirely, or an almost entirely, vegetarian diet. His 90-10 guideline calls for eating 90 percent of your diet as fruits and vegetables and the remaining 10 percent in proteins and fats from legumes, nuts, or a small amount of animal protein. If you follow his plan exactly, your diet should contain no more than 300 milligrams of cholesterol and six grams of salt per week.

The six-week meal plan is intended to produce speedy and dramatic results. Dr. Fuhrman believes that moderate changes are not sufficient to produce results. Although the plan is intended to improve overall health, it is advertised as a plan for people who want to lose 50 pounds quickly. Yet he also states that the diet is designed as a lifelong "diet-style."

This plan might work for me because . . .

- ☑ I want to improve my health as well as lose weight.
- ☑ I need a total break from my current eating habits.
- ☑ I can see myself thriving on an almost entirely vegetarian menu.
- ☑ I am looking for dramatic and speedy results.

Gwen Mergian

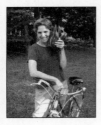

Troy, New York
Age: 50s
Occupation: Nurse and writer
Accomplishment: Lowered her cholesterol, lost 20 pounds
How She Did It: Ornish Program

Numbers are powerful. Just ask Gwen Mergian how powerful.

The first number to slap Gwen in the face was the number 50.

"When I reached my fifties, I felt like I was living on borrowed time," says Gwen. "My father died at age 49 from a massive coronary, and my grandmother had a sudden fatal heart attack in her fifties."

The second number that stopped her cold was 303.

"I was aware of my family history, and so I felt that I chose a fairly healthy diet, even though I didn't really exercise. I had no chronic disease, although I was maybe 10 to 20 pounds overweight," says Gwen. "But the results of a routine blood check came back showing that my total cholesterol was 303. Something about that number bothered me."

That number, in fact, put Gwen in the American Heart Association's highest risk category. The AHA says that having total cholesterol of 240 milligrams per deciliter of blood or higher presents a person with twice the risk for coronary heart disease as someone whose cholesterol level is 200 mg/dL or below.

Faced with the facts, Gwen's doctor recommended starting Gwen on a cholesterol-lowering statin drug.

Trained as a nurse, Gwen didn't like the thought of drugs as the answer to her dilemma. At the same time, Gwen socialized with friends who were in the medical field, among them research scientists with whom she regularly discussed the findings of health studies. Turning her focus inward, she decided to bring the scientific method home.

"I read up on all the little things that are supposed to lower cholesterol, and I thought to myself, *I could conduct an experiment of my own. I could be the subject, the researcher, and the reporter,*" she says.

Gwen proposed to her doctor that she try to lower her cholesterol through some of these means. If at the end of six months, her numbers weren't satisfactory, she would go on the drug. Seeing her as a walking time bomb, her doctor wasn't thrilled, but she agreed to let her try. As least Gwen would be healthier when she went on the drug, the doctor reasoned.

Gathering dust in Gwen's basement was an old copy of *Dr. Dean Ornish's Program for Reversing Heart Disease*. The program is a low-fat diet rich in vegetables, fruits, whole grains, and legumes, combined with regular exercise and stress reduction techniques. She decided to adopt the Ornish plan as her guide.

Gwen's goal was ambitious—and it involved another number. Not focusing on her total cholesterol of 303, she targeted her LDL cholesterol, the so-called "bad cholesterol," which can be a more accurate gauge of risk. Her LDL was 193—again in the AHA's highest risk category—and she set a target level of 130, which is still borderline high.

"I was committed to the experiment, but I didn't really think I could do it," she admits. "I am a very stubborn person, though, and when I put my mind to something, I'm like a tenacious little dog."

Although Gwen felt that overall her diet wasn't bad, she admits she had a weakness for pizza, "the hardest thing for me to give up." She also liked meat and cheese, eggs, and omelets and had ice cream maybe three times a week on average. But the real hurdle was a big one: she didn't really like vegetables.

Nevertheless, in March 2007 Gwen switched to a plant-based diet. She stopped eating meat, except one to two servings of salmon a week, which she wanted for the healthful omega-3 fatty acids. She prepared huge salads and incorporated new grains into her diet, such as kasha, quinoa, and couscous. She loves to bake, and she has adjusted recipes to cut down on the fat and sugar of her muffins and other baked goods.

The six months went by fairly quickly, Gwen feels.

"I wanted to see what I could do," she says. "I didn't want to cheat. If you do, you have to think about it: *Well, I cheated yesterday, so today maybe I'll.* . . . I cheated only twice in six months, once when a very kind woman made a pie and I had to accept a piece."

How did Gwen do? In September, at the end of the six months, her total cholesterol had dropped to 177, well below the 200 mg/dL benchmark. Her LDL cholesterol came in at 96, almost 100 mg/dL below her starting number and 34 mg/dL below her target of 130.

In addition, Gwen found she had lost about 20 pounds. At her highest weight, Gwen had been 140 pounds, and at 5 feet, 5 inches tall, a size 14. Always having considered herself "chubby," Gwen is satisfied with her weight now, even though she has regained five pounds, and she doesn't feel she needs to lose any more.

Still, Gwen continues on the Ornish plan. In addition, she takes a multivitamin and supplements such as red yeast rice and flaxseed, which are said to lower cholesterol naturally. She drinks white and green tea, pomegranate juice, and a drink she mixes from apple cider vinegar, grape juice, and apple juice. Three or four times a week she has a scientific dose of red wine with dinner, about 25 milliliters.

Gwen admits that exercise has not been a priority in her life, although she fondly remembers roller skating and tap dancing as a girl. She will sometimes walk the two and a half miles home from work. At the gym, she works out two or three times a week, usually speed walking on the treadmill.

One day, Gwen saw a bicycle in a shop window, a chestnut-brown, 1970s, five-speed bike that reminded her of her mother's, and she had to have it. She began biking around her neighborhood, and eventually she worked her way up to an eleven-mile ride suggested to her by a friend.

"It was on my tongue to say no, but before I did, I thought, *You can try, Gwen,*" she says. "I had to stop four times and walk my bike up the hills, but I did it."

Gwen has also tried several means of lowering stress, such as tai chi, mindfulness meditation, and yoga, with mixed success. Again, focusing on making change fun, she has tried activities like writing with her left hand or sketching upside down and left-handed, to stimulate the right side of her brain. For several years, she blogged about her progress in the Albany (New York) *Times Union*.

What started as an experiment has turned into a lifestyle for Gwen, and she's grateful for the opportunity she's had to expand her horizons.

"This experiment took me in directions I wouldn't have expected. It brings me such joy and pleasure," she says. "As you age, it's easy to get into a rut and experience things as diminishing. I find myself embracing new things, and as I look ahead, I want to be healthy and I feel like there are good things to come. That's the blessing and the bounties of this way of life."

Thanks To

My husband, Harout: When I made the switch, he came along 100 percent. He didn't make a peep. He was so supportive, and he's the real secret to my success.

My Tips

The whole construct of an experiment made this fun for me. It always helps me if I feel like I'm playing. It is more expensive to eat this way—I buy good organic produce—and it takes a lot of time to shop for and prepare meals. You have to be organized. I chop massive amounts of vegetables, so I use a Toss & Chop, a gadget that allows you to chop greens and veggies right in the bowl. I cook in quantity over the weekend so I have meals ready for the week. Here's a muffin recipe that I adjusted to lower the fat and sugar. It's my favorite.

Recipe for: **Healthy Heart Muffins**

1 ½ cups whole wheat flour

1 teaspoon baking powder

1 teaspoon baking soda

¾ teaspoon cinnamon

1 teaspoon vital wheat gluten

dash of salt

1 cup fruit (e.g., blueberries or chopped cranberries)

¼ cup oats

¼ cup oat bran

¼ cup wheat germ

2 teaspoons sugar (more, if you like)

½ cup chopped nuts (I prefer walnuts)

1 cup almond milk

1 ripe banana, mashed

2 egg whites

1 tablespoon canola oil

1 teaspoon vanilla

In a large mixing bowl, sift together flour, baking powder, baking soda, cinnamon, and vital wheat gluten. Stir in sugar, oats, oat bran, and wheat germ. Add nuts and fruit, mixing gently with a wooden spoon.

In another mixing bowl, mash banana. Mix in two egg whites, canola oil, and almond milk. Gently mix wet ingredients into dry ingredients. Do not overmix.

Spoon batter into a greased muffin tin, making 6–12 muffins. Smooth out tops a little to shape into soft peaks. Bake at 350 degrees for 25 minutes for smaller muffins, 30 minutes for larger muffins.

The Ornish Program

"You really can eat more and weigh less—if you know what to eat. And . . . it's easier to make big changes in diet than modest ones, if you know what changes to make."

—*Eat More, Weigh Less: Dr. Dean Ornish's Life Choice Program for Losing Weight Safely While Eating Abundantly* by Dean Ornish, MD (New York: HarperCollins, 2000)

Published in 1990, Dr. Dean Ornish's original plan, *Dr. Dean Ornish's Program for Reversing Heart Disease,* was intended to help patients treat heart disease without surgery or drugs. His plan was one of the first to advocate cutting back substantially on fat intake and increasing the intake of complex carbohydrate foods.

As a weight loss plan, *Eat More, Weigh Less* is based on Dr. Ornish's original plan. The diet aims for consumption of few fats and little protein but plentiful carbohydrates. While the diet does not involve counting calories, if closely followed, it will be a low-fat, low-calorie diet.

Dr. Ornish recommends eating only 10 percent of calories as fat, 15 to 20 percent as protein, and 70 to 75 percent as complex carbohydrates. Whole grains, fruits, vegetables, and legumes can be eaten in unlimited quantities until you are full. Meat is either severely limited or excluded altogether. Dairy products are excluded, except egg whites, nonfat milk, and nonfat yogurt, as are all vegetable oils, nuts, seeds, and avocados. Caffeine is a no-no, while sugar, salt, and alcohol are OK in moderation. Cholesterol intake should be less than 5 milligrams per day. Nutritional supplements may be needed.

Although this way of eating can represent a dramatic change, Dr. Ornish maintains that big changes are often easier than small ones to make because people feel better so quickly that they are motivated by the joy of living. Many hospitals offer Ornish programs, which can help people find success on the plan.

By eating as much as you want as often as you are hungry, Ornish says, your metabolism stays level, or even increases, allowing for steady weight loss. The high fiber content also slows down the absorption of food into the digestive system, so you feel full longer than you would by eating calorie-restricted portions. The complex carbohydrates also stabilize the glucose levels in your blood, he says.

The Ornish program involves lifestyle changes that include moderate aerobic exercise, meaning 30 minutes every day or 60 minutes three times a week. He also favors stress management techniques such as meditation, massage, psychotherapy, yoga, stretching, or imagery. When the soul is fed, people have less need to overeat, he maintains.

Today, the Ornish diet is known as the Ornish Spectrum and is backed by Dr. Ornish's book, *The Spectrum: A Scientifically Proven Program to Feel Better, Live Longer, Lose Weight, and Gain Health*.[3] It stresses four areas of life in which you can make changes: what you eat, how you respond to stress, how much activity you engage in, and how much love and support you have.

This plan might work for me because . . .

- ☑ I want to improve my health as well as lose weight.
- ☑ I like the idea of having no restrictions on certain healthy foods.
- ☑ I think I can adapt to a radically different way of eating.
- ☑ I am willing to exercise regularly.

Chapter Thirteen

If Only I Liked Grapefruit

Do's and Don'ts from Those Who Did It

Over the course of a year, as I listened to one person's story after another, I became increasingly excited about the life-changing potential of weight loss. In fact, most people used that word—*life-changing*—to describe their experience. And, really, isn't that what we all yearn for?

So, now that you've heard from your fellow weight loss seekers, how do you get what they have? How can you grab onto that word *life-changing* and apply it to your own story?

Because the people in this book took very different routes to success—and because I am simply one of them and not a doctor or a dietitian—I can't tell you ten magic foods to eat or ten to avoid like the plague. I can't suggest the ultimate ten-minute workout or never-fail ten-step program. Something worked for every person in this book, but no one program worked for everyone.

Still, I can come up with a "Perfect Ten" conclusion for you. After months of interviewing people, I discovered similar touch points in the experiences of those who had succeeded at weight loss. While every person's story was different, ten distinct themes surfaced frequently. I'll share those themes with you here and trust that you will benefit from the wisdom of these remarkable people, just as I have.

1. When your moment of reckoning comes, don't shrink from it.

Why did you do it? I couldn't wait to ask people this question, the question that fascinated me more than any other. Most people, although not all, could point to a single moment in time that forced them to face their dilemma. This moment is so universal, it has a name—a triggering event. For some, it was a health scare, as when Allison Bottke imagined the term "morbid obesity" on her death certificate.

For other people, an honest comment from another person pierced their very soul—for example, when Nancy Sebastian Meyer's publicist told her that if she wanted more speaking engagements, she would have to lose weight.

Gwen Mergian's moment included the number 303—her total cholesterol level. "If it had been 295, I might not have had the same experience," she says. Adopting the Ornish Program, Gwen brought that number down to 177 and lost 20 pounds.

Some people expressed a strong sense of determination, even when no external forces pressed in. Teen Daniel Greenlees said he just knew instinctively that it was time to act, that he would never again have a chance like the one that presented itself when he found himself living steps away from a gym.

I felt horrible asking people about these experiences, these moments that humiliated them, or terrified them, or left them in despair. I know how these moments feel; I've had my own. That photo on the sidewalk haunts me to this day.

Each time I asked this question, I apologized, but everyone was gracious about sharing their experiences. These defining moments, although painful, gave people the courage to make the move they'd long wanted to make and provided them with the motivation they needed to succeed. "It is a moment of revelation, a good moment," says Ken Romeo, whose own moment of honesty in front of the mirror led to success.

2. Remove the word diet from your vocabulary.

"In this country, when we think of diet, we think it's something we do for sixteen days, and then we can go back to the way we were living," Dr. James O. Hill, co-founder of the National Weight Control Registry, said to me. "We know it's not right, but it's almost hard-wired in us."

Don't we all know *that*! I recently gave a friend a card that read: "I'm on a 30-day diet . . . already I've lost 15 days." We laughed because we've both been down that road. So have many others. "My mistake was to diet for a particular event—a prom or an upcoming wedding," says Debra Anderson, who lost 140 pounds after weight loss surgery.

The fact is that permanent weight loss—the kind of weight loss the people you've met in this book have experienced—rarely results from a short-term fix. It's important to wrap your mind around this fact.

The word *diet* has become a misleading four-letter word. It's not supposed to mean something you do to lose weight. It's just a word for the way we eat day in and day out.

Although the people I interviewed adopted new habits as dictated by the weight loss plans they chose, they did not abandon them once they reached their goal weight. They continued to use what they'd learned to adapt their eating and exercise habits for a lifetime.

"Every single moment matters," says Heidi Bylsma, who lost 100 pounds on Thin Within. "If I say this moment isn't important, that is what years of poor choices are made of."

3. Make weight control, not weight loss, your goal.

In our conversation, Dr. Hill went on to state a hard truth about weight loss.

"People go on the popular weight loss plans, and they do lose weight," said Dr. Hill. "The problem is that many of the plans don't help you keep off the weight, and that's the really hard part."

Uh oh. Just when we all thought losing weight was the problem, up pops this new challenge. Once you've taken the emphasis off short-term fixes, it's time to take the long view. Maintenance of a healthy weight should become your top priority for life.

"If what you're doing to lose weight isn't something you can continue long-term, then you're not likely to keep the weight off," Dr. Hill says. John Bellemer realized this when he adapted the largely vegetarian Eat to Live program to include more protein, a revision he felt could help him stay true to his eating habits over the long term.

Research into why it is so easy to regain lost weight increasingly shows that the brain, your hormones, and your metabolism work hard to force you into reclaiming your former size.[1] It isn't just a matter of flagging willpower.

Not only that, but a recent study suggests that if you want to keep the pounds off, you may have to work harder than you did to lose the weight. The less you weigh, the fewer calories you burn as part of your day-to-day activities, says Raina Mekary, a Harvard professor of nutrition and author of the study. To maintain your loss, she suggests, you may have to become even more physically active than when you were losing weight.[2]

Yet, while statistics about how hard it is to keep weight off are grim, those who succeed prove to us that it can be done.

"There are exceptions to everything we say about success rates," Dr. Hill says. "Success stories are motivating. People need to know they can do it." I say amen to that, Dr. Hill.

4. Resolve to look to the future and stop wasting time.

Many people exhaust themselves losing and regaining weight on one plan after another. Almost everyone I talked with had tried at numerous times and through numerous ways to lose weight. You may have, too.

But whatever you've tried in the past, and for whatever reason it has failed, put it out of your mind.

"Don't let the past dictate your future," said Eric McLaughlin, Daniel Greenlees's personal trainer at Jim White Fitness, in a conversation with me. "And don't be tempted by the gimmicks you see on television."

Ah, the gimmicks. These products—pills, herbal supplements, patches, exercise equipment—promise easy success. We have our doubts, but in our desperation, our hearts overrule our minds, and we can't whip out our wallets fast enough. We want to believe we can lose 50 pounds in a week without expending any effort—without even getting out of our chairs!—and certainly without giving up our french fries.

In 2003, the Federal Trade Commission suggested eight general guidelines for evaluating claims made for weight loss products and services.[3] The FTC said that no scientific evidence exists to support the claims of products that say they block the body's absorption of fat or calories and those that claim weight loss can be achieved by products you wear or rub into the skin. In addition, products said to eliminate weight from specific parts of the body are without merit, the FTC said.

Although the guidelines for weight loss can seem simple enough, that's not to say that success will come without effort. "If anybody tells you it's going to be easy, run the other way!" warns Dr. Hill.

5. Gear up to take on society, not just yourself.

All the people I interviewed stressed that to succeed they had to take responsibility for their own health. Yet it's too simplistic to lay the blame for overweight solely on the individual. Our entire society is set up to encourage a life of sloth and overindulgence.

"In this country, our communities are constructed such that we have to drive everywhere. If we decide we want to walk, there are no sidewalks. Even if we want to make healthy food choices, everywhere we go, there are unhealthy choices," says Dr. Hill. "To lose weight, we're asking people to resist these forces. You literally have to fight against the environment."

Registered dietitian Nancy Clark, a Boston-area sports nutrition specialist, agrees. Americans, she says, have some pretty destructive thought patterns to overcome, patterns that the American food industry is quite willing to cater to.

"The messages we get in America are that food is fattening, and we often don't have time to eat anyway, so we think we might as well skip a meal or two to try to lose weight," Ms. Clark said to me. "By listening to those messages, we get too hungry, and by that time we don't care what we eat, and there are numerous options—Starbucks, Cinnabon, you name it—when we get to that crumbling point."

Not only do you have to tune out those negative messages, adds Dr. Howard Eisenson of the Duke Diet & Fitness Center, but you have to stop looking to society to provide positive messages that will help you sustain your weight loss.

"While there are great long-term rewards for achieving and maintaining a healthier weight, some of the most motivating rewards for losing weight are short-term. People don't comment forever on how great you look, and you can't keep buying new clothes," he said to me. "The pull to return to the natural state of overeating and expending no more exertion than you need to is strong. You need to change your life in some very fundamental ways, not only your habits but your attitudes."

6. Listen to your body and the voices in your head.

Listening to voices in your head is generally frowned upon in polite society. But actually your inner voices have some very valid things to say.

For example, Nancy Clark advises people to consider one simple question before they pick up something to eat. "Ask yourself, *Does my body need this fuel to sustain itself?*" she suggests.

In fact, Ms. Clark's top tip for weight control is to eat healthy foods at regular intervals throughout the day, as your body signals that you are hungry, and then stop eating in the early evening and "diet" overnight. "It's a good sign if you wake up in the morning hungry," she says.

I keep that thought in mind all the time now. It's helped me lose my fear of the sensation of hunger. Before, if I felt hungry, to me it was an emergency. *Eat now—whatever you can find!* Now, I no longer feel I might die if I feel hunger. I know I have time to fix myself something healthy to eat.

But, as we've discovered in this book, what works for one person doesn't necessarily work for another. Hunger might be a motivating sensation for some, a debilitating condition for others.

"For me, hunger creates a personality problem," says Jimmy Moore, who lost 180 pounds on the Atkins plan. "Hunger makes me irritable. That's why I never succeeded on low-fat diets."

In the experiments he recounts in his book *Mindless Eating,* author Brian Wansink shows that how much we eat is often dictated by external signals—we eat because someone else is eating, or because it's noon, or because there's still popcorn left in the bowl, or because our TV show hasn't ended yet—when really we should be heeding the body's own internal signals of hunger and fullness.

In fact, most people I talked with reported being far more in tune with their bodies than they had ever been. Many of them told me, for example, that they had learned to stop eating before they felt the sensation of fullness, to allow the brain time to signal the stomach that they'd had enough. For some, it's a tough lesson to learn.

"Although most people say it takes 20 minutes for the brain to signal the stomach that it's full, I don't feel the sensation of fullness until almost an hour after I eat," says Lori Kimble, who lost 30 pounds through calorie counting. "I had to learn to stop eating way before I thought I needed to, or I'd overeat."

7. Banish your dread of exercise.

Some people are lucky. They like—even love—to exercise, sometimes to the point of obsession. In my interviews, I found this particularly so of runners.

"I am motivated by a challenge," says David Ireland, the pastor who lost 65 pounds and went on to run the New York City Marathon. "And there's something about running. It's a sort of 'runner's high' that you get from the release of endorphins."

In fact, of the 7,000 people who have logged their weight loss onto the National Weight Control Registry, the overwhelming majority report adopting a lifelong habit of exercise. Only 9 percent of people said they had lost weight and maintained their loss without exercise, says co-founder Dr. Hill. "You might be able to do it, but the odds are against you," he cautions.

It's a hard truth for many of us to accept. I grew up in Rochester, New York, a place famously noted for having just two seasons—winter and the Fourth of July. I just didn't go out much, because something nasty was always falling from the sky.

Not only that, but many people, particularly women of my age, were not raised to value athleticism. Title IX, the 1972 law enacted to correct the gender inequities of sports and other educational programs, hadn't had time to gather steam while I was in school. Sports were just not on my radar, especially given the humiliating field hockey scrums of my youth. (Those mustard-yellow gym uniforms haunt me to this day!)

In fact, only recently have researchers begun to understand the role childhood sports play in the development of what is called an "athletic identity." They've found that without participating in sports early in your life, you don't develop an image of yourself as an active person. I read about this phenomenon in the *Wall Street Journal* a few years ago, and suddenly my lifelong aversion to exercise made sense.[4]

In the end, though, I learned that it really doesn't matter what your excuse is, it's just an excuse. I had to stop using it and get moving. When I swim laps, I force myself to swim one more lap after I've decided I'm done, just to make peace with the idea of doing something I don't want to do. People like Lynne Modranski motivate me—despite her lack of interest in exercising, she is active every day, a fact that helps her maintain her 30-pound loss.

8. But don't count on exercise alone to lose weight.

It sounds contradictory, I know. But don't throw up your barbells yet.

"Exercise alone will not cause you to lose weight," confirms dietitian Nancy Clark. "You have to create a calorie deficit."

Simply put, you create a calorie deficit when you expend more calories than you take in. While many of Ms. Clark's high-profile clients, including members of the Boston Red Sox and Celtics and high-level college and Olympic athletes, expend a lot more calories than the average mortal, most who seek her help are humble beings who simply want to lose weight.

How does she advise people to create that calorie deficit? Not primarily by exercise.

"You have to get away from the kind of thinking that says, *I'm going to walk three miles so I can eat a 350-calorie brownie*," she says.

Of course, exercise can play a role in creating the deficit, but in Ms. Clark's experience, it's a tricky balance. For men, she says, exercise tends to dampen hunger. But for women, exercise tends to make food more appealing, which makes them eat more. "Too much exercise can be counterproductive," she says.

I heard several times from women that in their quest to lose weight, they fell prey to "exercise bulimia"—that is, an obsessive reliance on exercise to burn off calories, often to the exclusion of family and other interests. Heidi Bylsma admitted to missing out on huge chunks of her children's lives because of her former obsession with running.

The problem with relying solely on exercise to lose weight is that when injury strikes or interest wanes, the weight tends to come right back on.

What's an appropriate level of exercise? One that can be maintained for life, says Nancy Clark. That means choosing activities that you like and can commit to regularly. That's why so many people are drawn to walking and running. "It's easy, it doesn't cost anything, you can do it anywhere, you can be outside when it's nice, and it feels good," she says.

9. Realize that eventually new habits take hold.

After talking with Dr. Hill, I thought about how perfectly aligned his thoughts were with the study I mentioned in the first chapter showing that sticking with a weight loss plan—*any* plan—is a better predictor of weight loss than the particular method used to achieve it.

The people who shared their stories with me are living proof of that. Long after they'd read the book, adopted the plan, and lost the weight, they stuck with their new patterns. How long it took for these new habits to become second nature varied.

"It was shocking to me, how easy it was. I felt great right away, in the first week," says Stacy Merriman, who lost 220 pounds with Recovery from Food Addiction. "I was totally clean, and I lost all my cravings."

For most people, the process of transitioning to new habits is a little rockier. After much urging, the husband of a friend of mine finally agreed to eat vegetables, if he could start by having them on a pizza. So far, so good. But when the pizza arrived, he generously slathered the top with butter—"Because we are talking *vegetables* here!"

Roger Freberg, the former football player who lost 100 pounds on Jenny Craig, remembers fondly days of yore, when he could sit down at a restaurant and polish off a 72-ounce steak dinner—that's 4 ½ pounds of meat—with all the trimmings. "Well, I can't do that anymore," he notes, a little wistfully.

The problem with most diets, says Pam Smith, a dietitian and nutritionist who has worked with such high-profile clients as Shaquille O'Neal and the Orlando Magic, is that people try to break old habits without building new ones. "Most people don't plan to fail," she said to me. "They fail to plan." More than anything else, she says, having a plan is the key to establishing your new habits.

"Most people have vague goals like *I'm going to lose weight,* or *I'm going to eat better,* but they don't focus on the routines," she says. "You need to think instead, *I'm going to eat breakfast every day,* or *I'm going to eat brightly colored fruits and vegetables at every meal.*"

As habits do become established, many people find that eventually, even when the will wavers, the brain balks at overindulgence.

"On the Zone diet, you're allowed to pig out once a month," says Nancy Inglehart, who lost 165 pounds. "But pretty soon, you realize that if you do, the next day you'll feel like a Mack truck ran over you. So you learn to treat yourself in small ways and savor the choice you made."

10. Help someone else along.

Part of the allure of a twelve-step program is to get to the point of helping someone in the same way you've been helped. "Having had a spiritual awakening as the result of these steps, we tried to carry this message to others, and to practice these principles in all our affairs," the twelfth step reads. And many successful weight loss seekers live that truth.

"When I went to my first Overeaters Anonymous meeting, people greeted me, and everyone said, 'Please come back,'" remembers Marie M., who lost 60 pounds. "And I thought, *Oh, I'll be back.* I just knew." Today, Marie is both sponsored and a sponsor to others.

For those who are charged with the care of children, it will pay dividends in the future to guard their health now. In Colorado, for example, the nonprofit LiveWell Colorado is creating a road map for healthy living that cuts across the different stages of life, starting with child care and school settings and going on through work and community settings.

One Colorado school district, for example, made only water available in the classroom for children to drink. Another district created a "Harvest of the Month" plan in which fresh produce is available in the cafeteria according to what's in season, along with packets of information and take-home recipe cards.

It may be most difficult, though, to live the message at home. We parents and grandparents like to reward our children with food, love them with food, pacify them with food, busy them with food, give in to them with food. "We're just not going to do that anymore in our family," says Robert Hartwell, who lost 100 pounds using Nutrisystem.

It is easier said than done, though, as I found out from examining my son's diet. Trying to make better choices now, I give him fruit for a snack before offering him any of the carbs he so loves. We've switched to unsweetened applesauce, low-fat yogurt, and low-calorie sports drinks. I allow him only one daily sweet snack or dessert. He's not thrilled about it, so I have to steel myself for the blowback. "Just my luck to have a mom who's writing a diet book!" he complains. (You were right about the spaghetti squash, though, Evan. I shouldn't have tried to pass it off as pasta!)

When people begin to dramatically change their lives, it is often those around them who cannot adjust. "Although our weight is not their fault, there will always be those dear women who bring Heavenly Rice and Ambrosia to church dinners and urge you to eat," says Allison Bottke, who lost 120 pounds after gastric bypass surgery. Many people told me they were grateful to spouses, family members, and friends who encouraged them, rather than discouraged them, along the way.

～ ❧ ～

Some time ago, I came across a term that startled me. In an online summary of a new weight loss book, a reviewer said that the book was a worthy addition to anyone's "weight loss library."

Weight loss *library*? I was taken aback. Do people really have shelves groaning with weight loss books? Judging from the hype and success of every new diet book, I guess they must.

The truth is we're desperate to discover what works. One recent study found that about 65 percent of American adults are either dieting or exercising or both.[5] And it's true, what would the blogosphere do for content without weight loss seekers? It's a pretty good guess that many people do pack their share of weight loss tomes.

Still, I wondered, *Do people really need a weight loss library?* Isn't the point just to get out and do it?

Yes, of course that's the point. But if I've learned anything through writing this book, it's that what works for one person doesn't necessarily work for another. The more sources of information you have, and the more ideas you hear, the more likely it is that you'll stumble on the strategies that will work for you.

"How delightful is a timely word," says the ancient proverb.[6] In other words, you never know when something will "click," as Marie M. said about seeing a mention online of Overeaters Anonymous and Sandy Ward about seeing a First Place ad in church.

In my weight loss journey, I've encountered ideas that jumped out at me in the same way, almost as if they were meant just for me. Let me share a few of the thoughts and ideas that I personally have depended on to lose weight and maintain my loss.

- **Nothing tastes as good as thin feels.** This saying has been getting a lot of flack lately for supposedly promoting anorexia. But I heard this sentiment over and over from people who succeeded in losing weight. Taken in a healthy way, it is absolutely true.
- **It's calories in, calories out.** Not everyone—especially low-carb aficionados—would agree with this, but it worked for me. When I broke a foot a while ago, Heidi Bylsma encouraged me to keep this in mind, and I did. In the three months that I couldn't exercise, not only did I not gain weight, but I lost two pounds to boot.
- **Am I really hungry?** Once I began asking myself this question, I cut way back on aimless eating. In *Mindless Eating*, Brian Wansink says that in regard to food, Americans have essentially three states of being: 1) I'm starving, 2) I'm stuffed, or 3) I could eat more.[7] Too true! I'm trying to exist in a fourth state—the elusive state of contentment.
- **Salad fills you up as much as a piece of cake will.** This is another craving buster. Although cake might satisfy something in my psyche that salad doesn't (that's putting it mildly!), I don't need to reach for it when I am hungry.

Veggies and fruits do take care of hunger, and they keep it at bay longer.

- **I don't need willpower—I need strategies**. I always thought that losing weight was about toughing it out. Now I realize, as dietitian Pam Smith says, it's about planning ahead. Stock the refrigerator with the good stuff and take it with you when healthy options aren't available. I exercise early in the day, before the pull of inertia exerts itself. I brush my teeth in the early evening, so I'm less likely to snack after dinner.

- **There's more to life than steamed veggies**. Many people told me they no longer cook, except to grill meats and steam vegetables. I like to cook, and I need variety. So, I'll pan-sear or roast vegetables in a bit of olive oil. Steaming vegetables may be healthier, but I love the sweet, smoky taste of charred carrots, onions, green beans, asparagus, and snow peas. With a squeeze of lemon juice and a sprinkling of sea salt, I can eat a boatload of these veggies! I beef up my recipes with the high-fiber and high-water-content fruits and vegetables that can keep me full without a lot of calories. Soup—it's a miracle food!

- **Walking counts**. It's so silly! I'd drive to the gym to swim my laps, and then spend 10 minutes looking for the parking spot closest to the door. The irony of it struck me one day. Now I always park in a spot at the end of the furthest row. It's never taken.

- **Fifteen minutes is fifteen minutes**. As the mother of a young child, I didn't have an hour a day to devote to exercise. But I did have fifteen minutes, and my brief, fitful bouts of swimming added up over time. Even now, I rarely have extended periods free to exercise. I'll have to leave the marathons to Christina Chapan and David Ireland. A walk to the post office and back works for me.

⤙ ❧ ⤚

I wish I lived in Colorado. For one thing, there's Garden of the Gods. But more to the point, Colorado has the lowest incidence of overweight of any state in the nation. Less than 20 percent of Colorado's population is obese; in fact, no other state can make that claim.[8]

In part, Colorado's claim to fame can be attributed to its setting of rugged outdoor beauty and its lure for the physically active.

"Colorado is definitely a society of 'What did you *do* this weekend?' not 'What did you *see?*' or 'What did you *eat?*'" says Rachel Oys, who helped to create Colorado LiveWell.

So, it's notable that the state has implemented a sweeping health initiative that aims to change school, work, home, and community environments. Despite its relative health, Colorado has seen obesity rates double since the early 1990s.

The National Weight Loss Registry's Dr. Hill, who happens to live in Colorado and serves on the board of Colorado LiveWell, thinks that programs like this one bode well for the future.

"I'm an optimist," Dr. Hill says. "I think that when Americans really take on something, they solve it. Who would have said in the 1950s that we could cut the rate of smoking in this country? I think there is cause for hopeful optimism here."

Also looking to the future, Dr. Howard Eisenson of the Duke Diet & Fitness Center finds hope in ongoing obesity research.

"I am most interested in research that recognizes that we need to better personalize the approaches we take," says Dr. Eisenson. "Moderation may not be the right message for everyone; low-fat or low-carb is probably not the right message for everyone. It is with a sense of humility in the face of this huge challenge that we admit we don't have all the answers yet."

While we may not have all the answers, we do have one good answer to the challenge of weight loss. For everyone in this book, something *did* work. Take heart in this—believe that something *can* work for you! And when you discover what works, the surest way to success is to stick with it. My new low-carb friend, Jimmy Moore, perhaps expressed this thought best.

"Dance with the one that brung ya," advises Jimmy.

The people in this book have been on the dance floor for a while now. I hope that soon you will join us.

Acknowledgments

I have one person to thank for my personal transformation—my good friend, Sue Seferian. Sue gave me a certificate for a free week at her gym, Princeton Fitness & Wellness in Princeton, New Jersey. Seven years later, I'm still going.

Sue, I think of you every time I slip into the pool. I think of you as I put on clothes I never thought I could wear. When my dad exclaims, "Look at you! You're half the woman you once were!" I think of you.

Thank you for passing along that certificate, Sue. Who could have guessed how valuable that slip of paper would become to me? Let's make a date to meet on the treadmills soon.

It is a pleasure to work with the folks at Leafwood Publishers. Stop the treadmill—I want to get off here! Thank you, Leonard Allen, Gary Myers, Robyn Burwell, Seth Shaver, Duane Anderson, Phil Dosa, Ryan Self, and everyone who is working so hard to put my books out there.

Thank you, too, to my agent Bill Jensen, who realized the value of a book acknowledging that weight loss isn't a one-size-fits-all proposition. Yet if I lived close enough to Bill to benefit from his culinary skills, I'd soon be back in my one-size-fits-all clothing!

As always, my husband John and my son Evan provide unwavering love, support, and encouragement, which makes my writing life possible. To them, I just want to say—back away from the chips and eat your veggies!

Appendix

To enhance readability, the copyrights and registered trademarks of the weight loss plans mentioned in this book have not been included in the text. Following is a list of terms protected by copyright law.

Atkins® is a registered trademark of Atkins Nutritionals, Inc.

Body-*for*-LIFE™ is a registered trademark of HarperCollins.

CalorieKing™ is a registered trademark of CalorieKing Wellness Solutions, Inc.

The Carbohydrate Addict's Diet™ is a registered service mark owned by Dr. Richard F. and Dr. Rachael F. Heller.

Curves® is a registered trademark of Curves International, Inc.

DietPower® is a registered trademark of DietPower, Inc.

Dr. Gott's No Flour, No Sugar™ diet is a registered trademark of Hatchette Book Group USA.

eDiets® is a registered trademark of eDiets.com, Inc.

Jenny Craig® is a registered trademark of Jenny Craig, Inc.

Lean Cuisine® is a registered trademark of Nestle USA, Inc.

LIVESTRONG™ MyPlate is a registered trademark of The Lance Armstrong Foundation.

Naturally Thin® is a registered trademark of Jean Antonello, RN, BSN.

Nutrisystem® is a registered trademark of Nutrisystem, Inc.

Overeaters Anonymous® is a registered trademark of Overeaters Anonymous, Inc.

The South Beach Diet™ is a registered trademark of South Beach Diet Trademark Limited Partnership.

SlimFast® is a registered trademark of Unilever.

SparkPeople® is a registered trademark of SparkPeople, Inc.

Weight Watchers® and PointsPlus® are registered trademarks of Weight Watchers International, Inc.

The Zone® is a registered trademark of Zone Labs Inc.

Zumba® is a registered trademark of Zumba Fitness, LLC.

Notes

Chapter One

1. CDC National Center for Health Statistics, National Health and Nutrition Examination Survey (NHANES), "Prevalence of High Body Mass Index in U.S. Adults, 1999-2008," *Journal of the American Medical Association*, 303, no. 3 (2010), 235–241.

2. Jane Fritsch, "95% Regain Lost Weight. Or Do They?" *New York Times*, May 25, 1999. Today, New York Hospital is known as New York-Presbyterian Hospital.

3. Traci Mann, et. al. "Medicare's Search for Effective Obesity Treatments: Diets are Not the Answer," *American Psychologist*, 62, no. 3 (April 2007), 220–233. This comprehensive study analyzed data from thirty-one long-term diet studies.

4. G. K. Chesterton, *What's Wrong with the World* (New York: Dodd, Mead and Company, 1910), 37.

5. Michael L. Dansiger, et al., "Comparison of the Atkins, Ornish, Weight Watchers, and Zone Diets for Weight Loss and Heart Disease Risk Reduction," *Journal of the American Medical Association* 293 (January 5, 2005), 43–53. A later study published in the *New England Journal of Medicine*, "Comparison of Weight-Loss Diets with Different Compositions of Fat, Protein, and Carbohydrates," by Frank M. Sacks, MD, et al., 360 (February 26, 2009), 859–873, having 645 participants, came to a similar conclusion.

Chapter Two

1. Pew Research Center, "Americans See Weight Problems Everywhere But In the Mirror," press release, April 26, 2006. Pew Research Center telephone survey of 2,250 American adults conducted February 8–March 7, 2006.

2. Jeremiah 17:9.

3. Information following a person's story about the weight loss plan he or she used came from publicly available sources such as websites, books, brochures, and press releases. In some cases, the plans have been modified since the weight loss seeker had success with them. In these cases, updates to the plan have been addressed.

Chapter Three

1. Michael Jacobson, director of the Center for Science in the Public Interest, a low-fat diet advocacy group (1979).

2. "What If It's All Been a Big Fat Lie?" *New York Times Magazine*, July 7, 2002; "Hold the Lard," *Reason*, December 5, 2002; "Big Fat Fake," *Reason*, March 2003; Gary Taubes, *Good Calories, Bad Calories: Challenging the Conventional Wisdom on Diet, Weight Control and Disease* (New York: Alfred A. Knopf, 2007).

3. Eric C. Westman, MD, Stephen D. Phinney, MD, and Jeff S. Volek, PhD, *The New Atkins for a New You: The Ultimate Diet for Shedding Weight and Feeling Great* (New York: Touchstone, 2010).

4. Arthur Agatston, MD, *The South Beach Diet Supercharged: Faster Weight Loss and Better Health for Life* (New York: St. Martin's, 2009).

5. In 2011, the federal government replaced the former food pyramid with a new concept titled MyPlate. It is a graphic of a dinner plate divided into recommended portions of fruits, vegetables, grains and proteins, accompanied by a drinking glass representing dairy. The recommendations are based on the USDA's 2010 Dietary Guidelines for Americans, which can be found at www.dietaryguidelines.gov. MyPlate can be found at www.myplate.gov.

6. *Mastering the Zone* (New York: William Morrow, 1996), *Zone Perfect Meals in Minutes* (New York: William Morrow, 1997), *What to Eat in the Zone* (New

York: Harper, 2003) and *Zone Meals in Seconds* (New York: Harper Paperbacks, 2004). All of these books are authored by Barry Sears.

Chapter Four

1. To estimate how many calories you burn engaging in various sports and activities, see the section "How Many Calories Did That Burn?" in Chapter Nine of this book.

2. An explanation of the Atkins diet can be found in Jimmy Moore's story in Chapter Three.

3. Robert Pritikin, *The Pritikin Principle: The Calorie Density Solution* (New York: Time Life Medical, 2000).

4. Robert A. Vogel, MD, and Paul Tager Lehr, *The Pritikin Edge: 10 Essential Ingredients for a Long and Delicious Life* (New York: Simon & Schuster, 2008).

Chapter Five

1. To adhere to Overeaters Anonymous's tradition of anonymity, the name of this member has been changed to Marie M. and her photos obscured.

2. To adhere to Recovery from Food Addiction's tradition of anonymity, the name of this member has been changed to Stacy Merriman and her photos obscured. The name of her sponsor has also been changed.

3. Kay Sheppard, *Food Addiction: The Body Knows* (Deerfield Beach, FL: Health Communications, 1993). More information about the plan can be found at Sheppard's website, www.kaysheppard.com.

4. A complete list of approved and banned foods can be found on Sheppard's website.

5. *From the First Bite: A Complete Guide to Recovery from Food Addiction* (Deerfield Beach, FL: HCI, 2000).

Chapter Six

1. Charlie Shedd, *Pray Your Weight Away* (Philadelphia: Lippincott, 1957), 40.

2. Kenneth F. Ferraro, "Firm Believers? Religion, Body Weight and Well-Being," *Review of Religious Research* 39, no. 3 (March 1998), 224–244. Krista M. C. Cline and Kenneth F. Ferraro, "Does Religion Increase the Prevalence and Incidence of Obesity in Adulthood?" *Journal for the Scientific Study of Religion* 45, no. 2 (June 2006), 269–281.

3. Northwestern University's research was presented at the American Heart Association's Nutrition, Physical Activity and Metabolism/Cardiovascular Disease Epidemiology and Prevention Scientific Sessions in Atlanta, Georgia (March 2011). The study tracked 2,433 men and women for 18 years and found normal weight young adults ages 20 to 32 years old with a high frequency of religious participation were 50 percent more likely to be obese by middle age after adjusting for differences in age, race, sex, education, income, and baseline body mass index. High frequency of religious participation was defined as attending a religious function at least once a week.

4. See Dr. Ireland's story in Chapter Nine.

5. *Thin Within: A Grace-Oriented Approach to Lasting Weight Loss* (Nashville, TN: W Publishing Group, 2002).

6. Arthur W. Halliday, MD, and Judy Wardell Halliday, RN, *Get Thin, Stay Thin: A Biblical Approach to Food, Eating and Weight Management* (Grand Rapids, MI: Revell, 2004). Judy Halliday, RN, and Joani Jack, MD, *Raising Fit Kids in a Fat World* (Ventura, CA: Regal Books, 2004). Allie Marie Smith and Judy Wardell Halliday, *HEAL: Healthy Eating and Abundant Living: Your Diet-Free, Faith-Filled Guide to a Fabulous Life* (Loveland, CO: Group Publishing, 2008).

7. Carole Lweis and Marcus Brotherton, *First Place 4 Health: Discover a New Way to Healthy Living* (Ventura, CA: Gospel Light, 2008).

8. Carole Showalter with Maggie Davis, MS, RN, LDN, FADA, CDE, *Your Whole Life: The 3D Plan for Eating Right, Living Well, Loving God* by (Brewster, MA: Paraclete Press, 2010).

Chapter Seven

1. James A. Levine, et al., "Interindividual Variation in Posture Allocation: Possible Role in Human Obesity," *Science* 307 (Jan. 28, 2005), 584–586.

2. Pamela Peeke, MD, MPH, FACP, *Body-for-LIFE for Women* (Emmaus, PA: Rodale Books, 2005).

3. Bill Phillips, *Eating for Life* (Golden, CO: High Point Media, 2003).

4. Bill Phillips, *Transformation: The Mindset You Need. The Body You Want. The Life You Deserve* (Carlsbad, CA: Hay House, 2011).

5. An explanation of the First Place 4 Health program can be found in Sandy Ward's story in Chapter Six.

Chapter Eight

1. "Eating More; Enjoying Less," Pew Research Center, report, April 19, 2006.

2. "2011 Restaurant Industry Forecast," National Restaurant Association, February 1, 2011.

3. "The U.S. Diet Food Home Delivery Market," Marketdata Enterprises, Inc., May 2011.

Chapter Nine

1. You can find the study at www.nwcr.ws.

2. McDonald's lists the nutritional content of its menu items at www.mcdonalds.com/us/en/food/food_quality/nutrition_choices.html.

3. The Physical Activity Guidelines can be found at http://www.health.gov/paguidelines.

4. Adapted from the 2005 Dietary Guidelines Advisory Committee Report. The Dietary Guidelines for Americans can be found at www.cnpp.usda.gov. The ongoing publication contains the federal government's most up-to-date information on how good dietary habits can promote health and reduce risk for major chronic diseases. Updated every five years, the guidelines form the basis for federal food and nutrition education programs.

5. For the sake of the group's anonymity, Sandee prefers not to name the twelve-step program she attended. It is a group for people who consider themselves either compulsive eaters or food addicts. In place of information

about the group's eating plan, I have included information about a well-known flour- and sugar-free plan by Dr. Peter H. Gott.

6. 1 Chronicles 4:10 NKJV

7. Peter H. Gott, *Dr. Gott's No Flour, No Sugar Cookbook* (New York: Wellness Central, 2000).

Chapter Ten

1. "Gastrointestinal Surgery for Severe Obesity," NIH Consensus Development Conference Consensus Statement 9, no. 1 (March 25–27, 1991).

2. "Metabolic & Bariatric Surgery Fact Sheet," American Society for Metabolic & Bariatric Surgery, June 2010.

3. Walter J. Pories, et al., "Who Would Have Thought It? An Operation Proves to Be the Most Effective Therapy for Adult-Onset Diabetes Mellitus," *Annals of Surgery* 222, no. 3 (1995), 339–352.

Chapter Eleven

1. Cynthia L. Ogden, et al. "Prevalence of high body mass index in US children and adolescents, 2007-2008." *Journal of the American Medical Association* 303, no. 3 (2010), 242–249.

2. Brian Wansink, *Mindless Eating: Why We Eat More Than We Think* (New York: Bantam, 2006).

3. Bill Hybels, *Honest to God? Becoming an Authentic Christian* (Grand Rapids, MI: Zondervan, 1992).

Chapter Twelve

1. Victor H. Lindlahr, *You Are What You Eat* (New York: National Nutrition Society, 1940).

2. An explanation of the Body-*for*-LIFE program can be found in Christina Chapan's story in Chapter Seven.

3. Dean Ornish, MD, *The Spectrum: A Scientifically Proven Program to Feel Better, Live Longer, Lose Weight, and Gain Health* (New York: Ballantine Books, 2007).

Chapter Thirteen

1. Shari Roan, "Why It's Hard to Maintain Weight Loss," *Los Angeles Times*, June 2, 2008.

2. Rania A. Mekary, et al., "Physical Activity in Relation to Long-Term Weight Maintenance after Intentional Weight Loss in Premenopausal Women," *Obesity Journal* 18 (June 4, 2009), 167–174.

3. "Deception in Weight-Loss Advertising Workshop: Seizing Opportunities and Building Partnerships to Stop Weight Loss Fraud," FTC Staff Report, December 2003, www.ftc.gov/os/2003/12/031209weightlossrpt.pdf.

4. Tara Parker-Pope, "Why Gym Class Matters: Kids' Attitudes Toward Sports Affect Their Adult Health," *Wall Street Journal*, Personal Journal, September 2, 2003.

5. "In the Battle of the Bulge, More Soldiers Than Successes," Pew Research Center, press release, April 26, 2006. Pew Research Center telephone survey of 2,250 American adults conducted February 8–March 7, 2006.

6. Proverbs 15:23 NASB.

7. Brian Wansink, *Mindless Eating*, 48.

8. "F Is for Fat: How Obesity Threatens America's Future," Trust for America's Health and the Robert Wood Johnson Foundation, annual report, July 2011. The study is based on data compiled in 2010. Colorado's obesity rate just barely came in under 20 percent, at 19.8 percent. Mississippi reported the highest rate of obesity, at 34.4 percent of the population, and a dozen states top the 30 percent obesity rate. Perhaps the most sobering statistic of the report is that prior to 1995, not a single state had an obesity rate above 20 percent.

Index

E

Eat to Live, 179, 181, 182, 183, 194
Eisenson, Howard, MD, 37, 73, 196, 205

F

First Place 4 Health, 103–104, 116, 117, 119, 219
FormulaZone, 53, 54, 55, 56
Freberg, Karen, 128–133
Freberg, Laura, 128–133
Freburg, Roger, 128–133, 200
Fuhrman, Joel, MD, 181, 182, 183

G

Gastric Bypass, 150, 151, 152, 154, 156, 202
Gott, Peter H., MD, 145, 146
Graham, Kristin, 120–133
Greenlees, Daniel, 171–174, 192, 195

H

Hartwell, Robert, 123–126, 201
Hill, James O., MD, 135, 193, 194, 195, 198, 200, 205

I

Inglehart, Nancy, 52–55, 201
Ireland, David, PhD, 93, 137–140, 198, 204

J

Jenkins, Jerry B., 57, 59
Jenny Craig, 128, 129, 130, 131, 132, 133–134, 200, 209
Jim White Fitness Studios, 172, 173

K

Kimble, Lori, 60–64, 197
Koop, C. Everett, MD, 11

About the Author

Nancy B. Kennedy worked in newspapers for many years, including a stint as an editor for Dow Jones's pioneering electronic news service. As a freelance financial writer, she worked for many newspapers and magazines, including the *New York Times* and the online *Wall Street Journal,* and for the financial services firm Merrill Lynch. As an editor, she worked for such well-respected publishing houses as Princeton University Press and Ecco Press.

Most recently, Ms. Kennedy authored *Miracles and Moments of Grace: Inspiring Stories from Military Chaplains* (Leafwood, 2011). She also has written two children's books, both teacher resources that combine science activities with stories of faith—*Make It, Shake It, Mix It Up* (Concordia, 2008) and *Even the Sound Waves Obey Him* (Concordia, 2005). She writes articles and personal essays for books, magazines, and newspapers. Many can be found at her website, www.nancybkennedy.com.

Ms. Kennedy is a member of the Authors Guild. She and her husband, John, live in Hopewell, New Jersey, with their son, Evan.

EARLY PRAISE FOR
GROUNDED SPIRITUALITY

"Jeff Brown is an iconoclastic visionary about intimate matters. There aren't many of those around, since most modern geniuses seem devoted to seemingly more glamorous and critical matters like artificial intelligence, 3-D printers, and smart chips implanted in our brains. But the truth is—at least in my view—revolutionizing the way we do our inner work and craft our intimate relationships is the most important action we can take to transform the world. And Jeff provides potent ideas to help us do just that. His rigorous imagination is in service to creating a more emotionally intelligent culture. When I read his words, I get riled up in all the best ways. He disrupts my habitual thought grooves, which inevitably leads to unexpected healings and inspirations. These days the word 'soul' gets carelessly bandied around by many lazy and sloppy thinkers, but Jeff is not one of them. He is reverent and impeccable, an astute connoisseur of the soul and its needs."

—ROB BREZSNY, author of the weekly column "Free Will Astrology" and the book *Pronoia Is the Antidote for Paranoia*

"Jeff Brown never disappoints, and his latest book, *Grounded Spirituality*, is no exception. Jeff is a uniquely human sage-preacher-man for the most cutting-edge, revolutionary, evolutionary take on human spirituality. There is nothing more needed in this broken world than the re-emergence of a human culture that deeply honors that which is real—the worthy dirt of this earth, the smile from a stranger, the tears we all shed at the moment of a loved one's death, our flesh and bones... these are the sacred meditation objects of Jeff Brown's *Grounded Spirituality*. In this book, Jeff offers his vulnerable and ever-so-human heart, through his own personal story of spiritual struggle and revelation. He also takes on the role of a wisened sage, reminiscent of an ancient Vedic teacher-student conversation style. Most impressively, this book places its finger on the exact pulse of cutting-edge spiritual development—a place that honors tradition, while at the same time, dramatically breaking from its harmful patriarchal shackles. While reading this book, I could feel the Goddess smiling."

—KATIE SILCOX, New York Times Best-Selling author of *Healthy, Happy, Sexy—Ayurveda Wisdom for Modern Women*

"Anyone who has felt the least confusion on their spiritual path should immediately get a copy of *Grounded Spirituality* and start reading. With laser precision, Jeff Brown dissects what passes for wisdom in much of today's spiritual teachings, slices away the illusions, and lays bare the simple truth: to grow into your spirituality is to grow into your humanity, in all its connected, tender, messy, luminous embodiment. And simple as that truth is, Brown doesn't pretend that the path to a fully embodied humanity is a piece of cake. He renders the pitfalls and rewards of that journey poignantly clear in a fictionalized dialogue that carries the reader towards a personal renewal of their own sacred purpose. The clear-eyed passion that fueled this book helps bring us closer to the future we all need."

—PHILIP SHEPHERD, author of *Radical Wholeness* and *New Self, New World*

"This is a crucial book that needs to be thoroughly read, explored and discussed. Jeff Brown eagerly invites us to look into the utmost importance of a grounded spirituality. At a time when much of spirituality has diverted us away from our true individual self, our authenticity, and our sense of social and ecological solidarity, this book orients us back to a spirituality rooted in our humanity and in our participation in the struggle of the world for greater freedom and justice. This book is a much needed masterpiece!"

—CHRIS SAADE, author of *Second Wave Spirituality*, and co-author of *Evolutionary Love Relationships*

"With absolutely naked transparency, Jeff Brown, in *Grounded Spirituality* shares his complicated spiritual journey—the good, the bad, the ugly, and everything in between. He recounts the twists and turns of his path without any narcissistic indulgence, but with an outpouring of broken-open vulnerability and courage. Jeff shows us that we are already divine, and our work is not necessarily to become 'more spiritual,' but to immerse ourselves in the life-altering process of becoming wholly human, wholly here, wholly present to our embodied existence on this planet."

—CAROLYN BAKER, author of *Dark Gold: The Human Shadow and The Global Crisis,* and co-author with Andrew Harvey of *Return to Joy,* and *Savage Grace: Living Resiliently In The Dark Night of The Globe*

"Jeff Brown's wisdom in *Grounded Spirituality*—the idea that 'life is the only real spiritual teacher'—resonates deeply with my own lived experience and with what I have witnessed with my clients and students. He articulates so well how our truest path includes our stories, our emotions, and especially our bodies... that our bodies not only house our souls—they are inseparable from them while we walk this earth. The exercises woven with the story will support any seeker to become a 'finder.' I believe Alexander Lowen and John Pierrakos would proudly recommend *Grounded Spirituality* if they were still embodied. I know I will recommend it to my students."

—KATE HOLT, RN, Core Energetics Practitioner and Teacher, Executive Director, Institute of Core Energetics

"There are certain themes that wash through the works of Jeff Brown. They touch the reader with different colors and textures, but the intention remains the same. His message is grounded in human vulnerability with the desire, the longing, for a connection to the wonder of the Divine whilst remaining utterly true to our human nature. He is a breath of fresh air in these times of rapid and uncompromising change. This book is like a warm hand that reaches for yours with the promise of safe passage."

—ANAIYA SOPHIA, author of *Sacred Sexual Union*, and *Fierce, Fierce Feminine: One Woman's Journey to Find Her Authentic Voice*

"Jeff Brown, who has long been known for his bold, passionate, and grounded approach to life and spirituality, has written an epic saga about truth, freedom, spirit, and what it means to be divinely human. He blends wisdom, humor, and illuminating moments of autobiography into a lively conversation that takes people out of their heads and returns them to their bodies—where our messy human emotions live. This is a book that vibrates with life, sensuality, and a willingness to embrace our humanity without apology. Jeff's compassion for the human condition may well be the antidote for the kind of apathy that has torn people away from their tenderness and ability to care for themselves, one another, and our planet. But don't expect easy answers here—Jeff's generous account of his journey emboldens all of us to step whole-heartedly into the questions and accept the call to adventure that life is offering. This is a book I want every human being, young and old, to pick up and read!"

—KELLY MCNELIS, Founder of Women For One, and author of *Your Messy Brilliance*

Other Books by Jeff Brown

Soulshaping: A Journey of Self-Creation

Ascending with Both Feet on the Ground

Love It Forward

An Uncommon Bond

Spiritual Graffiti

GROUNDED
SPIRITUALITY

JEFF BROWN

FOREWORD BY
ANDREW HARVEY

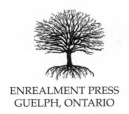

ENREALMENT PRESS
GUELPH, ONTARIO

Published by Enrealment Press
PO Box 64,
Acton, Ontario
Canada L7J-2M2

*Note to Reader: The optional exercises in this book are designed to promote self-aware-ness and self-improvement. Please note that they do not constitute psychotherapy or psychiatric health care in any way, and they are not a substitute for psychotherapeutic or medical advice in diagnosing or treating any stress or mental disorder or mental health condition you may have. Always consult with your psychotherapist, medical doctor or health care provider about any mental health care concerns you have or think you may have. Please also note that the Service Providers (Publisher and Author) expressly disclaim any and all warranties and conditions of any kind, whether express or implied, including, without limitation, the implied warranties or conditions of fitness for a par-ticular purpose. Your participation in the exercises may elicit strong emotions. By doing them, you expressly understand and agree that in no event shall the service providers be liable for any damages whatsoever, including without limitation, direct, indirect, incidental, special, consequential or exemplary damages, whether based on breach of contract, breach of warranty, tort (including negligence) or otherwise, arising out of or in connection with your use of the exercises.

Cover photo by Susan Frybort
Author photos by Tarini Bresgi and Paul Hemrend
Cover and book design by www.go-word.com
Publisher logo by Brad Rose (www.facebook.com/GetSeenGraphics)
Printed in the USA

From *The Way to Vibrant Health,* by Alexander Lowen, M.D. and Leslie Lowen, published by the Alexander Lowen Foundation, Vermont. Copyright © 1977 by Alexander Lowen. Reprinted by permission of Frederic Lowen. http://www.lowenfoundation.org/

Library and Archives Canada Cataloguing in Publication

Brown, Jeff, 1962-, author
        Grounded spirituality / Jeff Brown.

Issued in print and electronic formats.
ISBN 978-1-988648-03-3 (softcover).--ISBN 978-1-988648-04-0 (PDF)

        1. Spirituality. 2. Self-actualization (Psychology).
I. Title.

BL624.B744 2019   204   C2018-906446-3
                                          C2018-906447-1

For Susan Frybort Brown

The weaver of my heart.
The love of my (every) life.

Contents

Foreword

This is a book we have all been unconsciously waiting for. It is a book written by a man who has truly understood the dereliction of our time. The collapse of any real moral or spiritual reverence, and the bankruptcy of the religious and guru systems. It is a book written by a man who has not only understood this but stayed profoundly faithful to the vision that was being birthed in him, of a path to the Divine through the body. This may seem small, or in some ways, fascinating but not profound… but the reality of our situation is, as all the great evolutionary mystics have shown us, that we are going through a massive and necessary global "dark night" in order to fulfill the evolutionary will of the Divine: to co-create the birth of a new embodied divine humanity. It is this birth—this extraordinary miraculous amazing birth—that is our greatest hope. And if you want to understand how this birth works, read this book.

In this book, you will find someone who truly understands that the divinization of the body is the key to the birth of a human race that can respond from the fullness of itself to the problems now erupting everywhere. What Jeff Brown understands is that this birth of the Divine in the body is the hardest path of all. Because in order to take this path, we have to unlearn all of the religious and mystical messages we have been given about the illusory nature of the body, the sinfulness of the body, the ignorance and illusion steeped in the body. Unlearning these messages is an excruciating business because it forces us to look at the ways in which we have treated our bodies. To re-enter the body, as Jeff Brown brilliantly shows both in his own writing about his own journey, and in the amazingly passionate, rustic, and nakedly honest conversations that he has with the character in the book, Michael—requires extraordinary courage.

This is true for three reasons. The first reason I have already suggested: It is deeply challenging to unlearn all the messages that we have been given about our body. In my own case, this was a frightening reality and adventure because it compelled me to understand the ways in which mystical reality had been manipulated for power for millennia. This was a very sobering and devastating recognition. The second reason is that to re-enter the body, you have to confront all of the trauma, karmic terror, grief, and deep suffering that your body has stored over your lifetime. This is part of the reason why so many people are refugees from the body, and why so many people embrace transcendental philosophies that deny the body. The work of actually going down into the body to listen to the screams that have been suppressed by our wounds and that are hidden within the body is a devastating process... necessary but painful and very, very demanding. The third reason why going down into the body is so demanding is that the body itself resists transformation by the light. Sri Aurobindo has written brilliantly of the four sheaths by which the body protects itself. They are very real, and not easily dissuaded from their protective mission.

Through this book, you will find ways of being so inspired by what living in the body can open up for you, that you will become not only willing to do the work, but thrilled to do the work. Because Jeff Brown's genius is to open up to us such an exciting and invigorating vista of what we can experience if only we arrive here—in full integration of mind, heart, soul, and body, that anyone reading these words with an open heart will long to do whatever is necessary to come into authentic human fullness. This is because he speaks from true lived experience. He has seen and known the joy of what it is to live in a full beingness. And he communicates this, as well as the difficulties, the suffering, the bewilderment, with such reverence that we cannot help but do whatever we must to reclaim our wholeness.

The work of embodiment is not just one more game the human race has to play. Not merely one more version of enlightenment. It is the only way we can possibly go forward. Because until we are united with our bodies, we will never love the body of the earth enough. Until we are living in the pulse and vibrancy of our bodies, we will never love other bodies—the bodies of our friends, and the bodies of our lovers, and the bodies of our parents, and the bodies of our grandparents, and the bodies of our beloved animals. We will never love them enough, because we will never savor the beauty of their presence with enough adoration to do everything we can to save them and the world we live in.

For me, Jeff Brown is a modern-day alchemist. And by that, I mean he has embraced the ancient alchemical path. The ancient alchemical path has 3 stages. First, profound experience of transcendence that reveals divine identity. This makes obvious the truth of what's written in the Upanishads—*You*

Are That. The patriarchal traditions have mistakenly taken this stage for enlightenment. But the alchemists knew that this was only the first stage. The second stage is the stage that Jeff is such a master of: this is where the deep knowledge of the transcendent and the forces aroused by that knowledge, are consciously integrated step by step with mind, heart, soul and crucially, and most importantly, the depths of the body. As this second stage progresses, the third stage which is called "the simple thing," starts to emerge… and for this third stage there are very few descriptions, because very few people have truly matured in the mystery of profound union with all that this stage brings. Jeff Brown knows the glowing fringes of this stage and has experienced the truth of the revolutionary birth that happens through the choice to ground transcendence in the depths of reality. And that's why this book is so important. Because in its rugged, ragged, and absolutely contemporary way, it models the ancient path to transfiguration that was known by the ancient alchemists, and by a small number of grounded mystics that have blessed us with their wisdom. This path for transfiguration now needs to be known everywhere, because everyone needs to align themselves with the evolutionary will of the Divine—not to destroy us, but to transfigure us so that we can become conscious embodied co-creators of a wholly new way of being and doing everything.

What I find wonderful about Jeff Brown's book, is not only that it offers us a searing indictment of patriarchy on all levels, and not only that it is the most comprehensive dismantling of the superficiality, and bypassing, and voluptuous indulgence, and inanity of the new age… but the real reason I love this book is that it provides a very down-home truthful basis of empowerment for potentially millions of people. If honest seekers can now use their deep mystical experience as a source of power to help them reintegrate their whole selves with the one, then millions of honest seekers can come together in a loving army of beings prepared to risk everything to start healing our world. As a sacred activist and the founder of the movement of sacred activism, I celebrate and salute this book because it will give anyone who wants to truly meet the challenges of our time with honesty, ferocity, and grace—the information, the practices, the vision, and the grounded rugged persistence that they are going to need to step up to the greatest evolutionary challenge humanity has ever faced. Read Jeff Brown's book, do the practices, saturate yourself in the wisdom that radiates from its pages, and go forward as an increasingly embodied divine human being who is willing to become a sacred activist on behalf of the Divine and the divine-in-humanity, to save our species and our beloved planet.

What one does for diplomacy is not what one does for truth. And Jeff Brown has written a book of truth—one that honors our humanity and offers us a co-creational path home. Join him.

—ANDREW HARVEY
November 12, 2018
Chicago, Illinois

Preface: A Spiritual Imperative

We are a magnificent species. Endowed with remarkable gifts and abilities, each of us carries a profound and luminous purpose at the core of our being. Each of us is here with an unlimited bounty of treasures to bring to the world. This extraordinary human birth, this powerful physical form, this uniquely nuanced personality, all the threads and strands of our consciousness—are not cases of mistaken identity. We are not accidental tourists on this planet. We are here because we have a sacred offering to bring. We are here because we are intrinsically valuable and wholeheartedly worthy. We are here because we are needed here.

And, at the same time, we are at war with ourselves. It's a nasty, insidious war, one that has left few of us unscathed. Somewhere along the way, many of us became separated from our authentic humanness. We became fractured, adrift, severed from what is real. We moved further and further away from the inner wells that nourish us. Our self-alienation is now bleeding out everywhere we look, showing up in the forms of: misplaced aggression, meaningless materialism, psychotropic drug dependency, a perpetual dishonoring of the Divine Feminine, a lack of reverence for the earth that breathes us, and a blatant disregard for those humans we share a planet with. As brilliantly as we have excelled and evolved on a technological and virtual level, many of us are still at war with our humanness. We are still not at home in our own sacred skin.

In the throes of this estrangement, it becomes difficult to see through to its source. It is easy to imagine that our self-alienation is caused by something outside of us. But make no mistake—most of this madness is a direct reflection of our unhealed and misaligned inner worlds. We are manifesting our individual fragmentation everywhere, and it has now reached a stage of dangerous perversity, threatening our very existence as a species. There is no time left to distract from the core questions of our lives. The present state of the world requires that we dig deep, and get to the root of our fracture. World events have made it perfectly clear that we can no longer find our answers independent of the self, itself. There is real work that must be done now, within each of us, to right this earth ship and to bring us into alignment. All self-avoidant flights of fancy must be grounded until further notice.

At the heart of this war is our fundamental amnesia as to who we are and why we are here. That is, what is our purpose here on earth? What does it mean to live a life of meaning? What is it to be a self-actualized species? What ways of being will bring us together, and into co-creative alignment—with ourselves, with each other, and with the natural world? What does it mean to be fully conscious, for this entire human experience? What is it to be fully alive? What is REAL spirituality?

To answer these age-old questions—we have often relied on systems of belief. This has taken manifold forms across the globe: world religions, scriptures, self-proclaimed masters and gurus, Father God in the sky, and a whole gamut of teachings and methodologies. With unrelenting determination, we have sought many of our answers outside of ourselves. And throughout the course of 2000+ years, these systems haven't managed to heal our fundamental divide. They may have served limited purposes, but they have not remedied our fractured awareness. In fact, many have made our fragmentation more pronounced and taken us further away from a healthy wholeness. One thing has become certain: If we continue to look for our answers and direction outside of our embodied experience—we will not find our way home.

It is time that we looked in another direction—right at the heart of our humanness. Not out there—in the alleged wisdoms of others—but deep within our own uniquely constituted human blueprint. Not the self-reflective brand of looking within that is confined to our thinking and rational mind, but the one that integrates every aspect of what we are into the equation: our emotional bodies, our flesh temples, our intuitive knowings, and yes, even our often misunderstood ego-self. I am not talking about a narcissistic honoring of the self—I am talking about a healthy and reverential regard towards our manifold components—in the full spectrum of what we are. Deep within our brilliant natural-born selfhood lie the answers as to who we are, and why we are here. We don't just have those answers—we actually *are* those answers. They make their home at the heart of us, continually feeding us information about our path and purpose. We just have to learn to attune to the subtle intonations and intimations of our inner knowing. We have to learn how to recognize and honor our inherent wisdom. We carry the information we seek.

This perspective runs counter to the culturally embedded tendency to diminish and desacralize the self. If we weren't born 'sinful,' we were born histrionic (women) or violent (men). We were born allegedly wild, and the only way to contain our unstoppable life-force was to condition and repress the self, making us dependent on religious institutions and marketing constructs to frame our lens on reality. When we are in a weakened state of fragmentation, it is easy to be subjugated. If you are not standing in the strength of your own embodied intactness, you will invariably seek a sense of wholeness from outside systems. You will have no other choice but to look to them to direct your path and purpose. Someone else's version of God, someone else's idea of truth, someone else's idea of where to spend your money, someone else's version of purpose, and someone else's idea of your inherent worth.

It is time to put an end to this delusion. It is time to restore power back to the individualized self and to see it for what it is—as the only authentic course in miracles. Far too many of us are spending our precious lives apologizing for our wondrous humanness. It has been systemically and collectively shamed—and somewhere along the way, we bought into it. Yet, the truth is—we are no mistake. We are a benevolently intended miracle in process, each here with a uniquely constituted sacred purpose residing in the bones of our being. Our life's work is not to shame and shun our magnificent selfhood—it is to celebrate and embrace it. It is to plumb its depths for encoded information as to who we are and why we are here. It is to embody and integrate all of the gifts and callings that we came into life to manifest. This is how we regain our sovereignty and how we evolve as human-beings.

Before we can identify our reasons for being, we have to arrive *here*, in the most inclusive sense. If we are disempowered, distracted, dissociated, or in any way fragmented—our experience of the here, now, will be intrinsically limited. And through that limited lens, we can only access a tiny splinter of possibility for our lives. We can only see the whole picture—and actualize the full range of our destiny—to the extent that we are, ourselves, whole.

In order to truly arrive *here*, we must first acknowledge something that the powers-that-be often want us to forget. That we are all wounded. That we are all trauma survivors (to one degree or another). That we all long to be healed. The age-old established structures that were built on a maligned sense of self—are dependent on us forgetting this. When we focus on our own healing, it severs their reins of control. It empowers our voice. It strengthens our intuition. It reminds us that our hunger for personal meaning cannot be satisfied by religious edicts, media sound-bites, or substitute gratifications. Our buried wounds and feelings keep us fractured and easily manipulated. Healing them brings us back into a strong, stable and rooted selfhood. Once there, we can no longer be controlled, and we begin to see more clearly the ways that all of us—even those in positions of authority and power—have been imprisoned by a divisive consciousness. It may have served some of us on certain levels, but it has served none of us from the perspective of a wholly integrated human-being.

The truth is that we have been denying our woundedness for centuries, and it has only made things worse. We are pretending all is well, while stockpiling our grief and anger. Denial has trapped us deep within our woundedness. A few more generations of unacknowledged trauma, and we will all be lost at sea. The weight of our undigested baggage is making us mad. Because we all know where the unresolved material goes—back into destruction. It builds into a cache of weapons that turn inward against the self, or outward against others. It is imperative that we clear the trauma stockpile before it reaches a tipping point where we no longer care about our impact on the planet, or each other. We must address this at the root. Healing is the only thing that can save us. Time's up, in more ways than one.

Why This Book

For the past three decades, I have been deeply engaged—both within my own personal process and at the heart of my work in the world—with a quest for wholeness. This has taken me into a rigorous examination of the spiritual paths and models that play a role in addressing our fragmentation. I have found that many of these core beliefs actually perpetuate and intensify our state of internal division. The focus of this book is to critically examine some of these philosophies. And to bring forth perspectives and models that honor a healthy selfhood, aligning our spiritual philosophies and practices with the most holistic and inclusive ways of being possible.

In service of that intention, I engage in a ruthlessly honest—and sometimes uncomfortable—examination of some of the fundamental tenets of spirituality that have guided us for centuries. How these models have, in many ways, held us back from achieving an authentic wholeness. How they have dangerously negated and diminished our humanness. How these traditions haven't been grounded in the body, and in the honoring of our personhood. How many of them have just been fleeting bliss-trips or dissociative forays into unity-consciousness. These perspectives will be specifically examined, deconstructed, and then reconstructed—with an invitation to move into an authentic and 'enrealed' version of spirituality.

As more humans turn towards spirituality for answers, it is essential that we investigate all paradigms and perspectives to assess if they serve us going forward. To explore if they truly answer the depth, breadth, and scope of what we are. To inquire into whether they meet our current needs as a species. Do these models grow us forward, into a more evolved humanity, or hold us back? At this point of desperation, one where we are at a collective and planetary crossroads—it is particularly essential that we look closely at those models that distinguish our spirituality from our humanness. Since time immemorial, spirituality has been characterized—and not *only* by mystics, saints, and cave-dwellers—as a way of being that is above and beyond our 'faulty' humanness, and certainly separate from many of the chaotic and unpleasant aspects of our life experience. It is clear that these paradigms are no longer serving us, and will not be our answer or our remedy. It has been my revelation—through extensive self-exploration and truth-telling—that if we can come to embrace our spiritual life as indistinguishable from every aspect of our human life—and that includes the healing of our traumatic material—we will begin to organically develop practices that will both serve us, and save us, going forward. As with any of the social structures that influence us, the more narrow the model, the more imprisoned our consciousness and limited our possibilities. The more expansive the model, the more liberated our consciousness and limitless our possibilities.

At the end of the day, when all the other debates have been resolved, we will be left with the one that threads through them all: Human Consciousness. What does it mean to be wholly human and to live a truly spiritual life? In what ways are we the same, and in what ways are we uniquely constituted and intended? What is an inclusive, wholly integrated consciousness? If we continue to limit our visions of possibility to compartmentalized spiritualities, we will most assuredly obstruct our collective expansion. We will imprison ourselves in our own alienation. And many more of us will be led astray, walking a path that is not truly our own.

To avoid this, we must embrace a conscious scrutinization of that which is said to be 'spiritual.' Nothing accepted at face value, no stone left unturned.

We must examine and critically review the true implications of the teachings: Do they make us more, or less, human? Do they encourage and energize our quest for our own unique path, the purpose we were born to live, or do they enable us to hide-out in a disembodied haze? We do not approach this inquiry carelessly or with an arbitrarily rebellious agenda, but we approach it discerningly—honoring lineage only to the extent that it truly resonates with our present-day circumstances, our intuition and our common sense. People in the spiritual community often use "lineage" as a kind of bulwark against legitimate queries into the underpinnings of their core beliefs. A conscious scrutinization bows before no lineage, unless it honestly reflects and genuinely supports our individual and collective evolution. If we don't acknowledge dangerous spiritual teachings, the world of sacred possibility that we seek will never come to pass. The only sacred cow is truth.

At the heart of this debate must be a bold and brave willingness to examine the leaders, teachers, and influencers themselves. To look beyond their charismatic or hypnotic presentation, to the person beneath. To do a deep dive into the psychological factors that shape their perspective. To look closely and honestly at any possible interface between their unresolved issues and the models they advocate. To challenge the conditioned belief that 'spirituality' is above and beyond confrontation and reproach. To courageously call out the untruths wherever we see them. Just because they call themselves spiritual teachers or leaders doesn't mean that we shouldn't critically review their perspectives. It doesn't mean that we shouldn't get to know the human-being below their revered identities. If anything, it's all the more imperative that we do.

This level of cutting honesty and discernment will require us to pierce the veils of protection that shroud many spiritual teachers. Repression is an industry and the ungrounded spiritual community is one of its primary merchants. A form of spiritual fascism has developed, one that benefits only a small few. If you call out the lying guru, you are met with the 'no gossip' mantra and, for those who are intoxicated by them and subjugated to their teachings, the irrational fear that they will sic their shakti-powers on you. If you feel triggered by their teachings, or violated in any way, you are reminded that spirituality should not include anger or negativity. You are handed back the burden of blame—that it is just your own 'issues and resistances.' I had always imagined spirituality a quest for truth, but that is not the all-pervasive consensus. There is widespread investment within the spiritual community in having particular opinions protected.

Even common sense judgments, acts of conscious discernment, evidence of wrongdoing firmly grounded in reality, have been conveniently mischaracterized as anti-spiritual, a philosophy that plays right into the hands of ill-intentioned gurus. If we can be persuaded that it is unspiritual to judge the teacher, if we can be conditioned to believe that our judgments about their integrity are merely a reflection of our own issues, then anything goes. We can easily understand why gurus and spiritual leaders would want to put a protective veil around themselves. It preserves their market share egoically and financially. It grants them permission to sell their teachings as impenetrable gospel. Yet they aren't. Not even close. They are as worthy of debate as any other concept or notion. Better we speak our truths and let the karmic chips fall where they may. Every voice and perspective matters.

Examining the real-time implications of spiritual teachings also means looking closely at their distorted cultural roots. At some point on my own journey towards wholeness, I began to see the parallels between much of the 'spiritual' world—particularly those communities fixated on transcending their humanness, and the greedy capitalistic structures that permeate our Western society. It became clear to me that it is all part of the same power-seeking patriarchal system—one that focuses on individual mastery at the expense of connectiveness, one that focuses on being *above* rather than being *among,* one that denies the value and significance of the world of feeling, one that refuses to honor the earthy and relational wisdom of the Divine Feminine. We see this unhealthy self-centeredness in the single-minded focus of the unconscionable capitalist—who seeks to accumulate at the expense of all else. On the endless quest for more, his obsession with achievement and accumulation is grossly confused with self-actualization. And we see it just as vividly in the ungrounded spiritual movement, where a vast cadre of pseudo non-dualists seek to master a unified field of consciousness while bypassing the very substance of their humanness. Simply put, if one is driven to conquer the economic realms at any cost, or if one sees the whole world—including their humanity, and that of others—as illusion, they are unlikely to notice or care about their impact on the planet, nor are they likely to contribute to the healing of our world. So busy imagining themselves actualized or enlightened, they do nothing to advance humankind. So busy pondering their no-navels and trivializing our human story, they are oblivious to the impending threats that are looking us square in the eyes. And oblivious won't get us anywhere good. If we keep pretending that the self is an illusion, if we keep pretending that others don't matter, soon we will be right. There won't be any left. It is time for dominant patriarchal structures to surrender their power to a more heartfelt and wholesome way of being.

For inspiration on our journey of exposing antiquated patriarchal structures, we can look in the direction of the #MeToo movement. A bold escape from Patriarchial Penitentiary, this movement is a firm step in the direction of the kind of deep healing and inclusivity that our world needs. Both in their refusal to bury their truths, and in their brave willingness to boldly call out toxic masculinity, empowered women world-wide are marching us toward a more self-honoring consciousness. One where every individual is free to acknowledge their victimhood. One where every individual has the same rights and protections. One where every individual is invited to heal. One where the struggles and liberation of the self are championed. One where no one has to hide beneath their shame-shackles—but can be heard, seen, acknowledged, and ultimately… celebrated. For me, this is a truly spiritual movement because it brings us closer to a humane world.

Of course, as we expose those philosophies that don't serve—we must also seize the opportunity to delineate spiritual models that offer the greatest liberation for all. We must work together to develop consciousness paradigms that reflect a more horizontal and connective way of being, that celebrate an intuitive and empathic way of relating, that revere the role that emotional healing plays in transformation and in the fostering of awakening states. We need models that understand that healing our stories and growing in relationship are as, or even more, fundamental to our spiritual development, as solitary path pursuits. We don't need more disembodied men meditating in caves while the village suffers. We need embodied humans healing together, communing and exploring the relational field as the grist for our spiritual development. We need accomplishment to become a relational construct; that is, we co-create together, with mutual benefit as our shared goal. We need models that lead us back into our hearts, into a deep and reverential regard for the self. These models may invite us to detach momentarily, in an effort to see ourselves through a different lens, but they will not leave us stranded out there, floating into the eternal emptiness and calling that a life. We need models that invite us to integrate what we find 'out there' with who we are 'in here.' Without this new paradigm, we are at risk of inviting humanity further and further away from the field for our soul's expansion—human life, itself. If we don't humanize our spirituality, how will we humanize our world?

It is time for a version of spirituality that is rooted in whole-humanness, fiercely unafraid to embrace all that we are. At the core of these new models must be the assertion that real spirituality exists right at the heart of our daily lives. From this perspective, the most spiritual being will be the one who is the most engaged in and connected to all aspects of the human experience. For too many years, we have been leading humanity away from the place where the answers reside—the embodied, enheartened, enrealed, enlivened SELF. It's not outside the self, for God's sake—it IS the self. The magnificent purpose-full self. The self that is in the everything, the self that is our portal to divinity itself. The self that is no accident, the stories that are no accident, the difficulties and challenges that are no accident, our nitty-gritty physical composition (imperfections and all). Not self-realization that leads us to find our awakening outside of the self—but that finds it deep within it. Grounded Spirituality.

From this truly self-honoring vantage point, one cannot ignore our impact on each other and the planet—because one understands that all of it is sacred. That all of it MATTERS. That we are not connected in theory—but connected in fact. And then we are inspired to take action, in every sphere of society, to craft structures, systems, and laws that honor, encourage, and connect us. With those in place, no one gets left behind, and every human gets an opportunity to participate and improve their life conditions. Inclusivity—within and between us, and at the heart of a humanized notion of spirituality—is not just a 'politically correct' progressive notion. It's a way of being where every one of us matters. Every struggle. Every wound. Every dream. All sacred. And when we believe that the plight of the self matters, we cannot help but work together to grow our humanity forward.

About This Book

I have divided this book into three parts: *The Journey, Here, Why*. In an effort to frame and contextualize the perspectives on spirituality presented later in this book, I begin by sharing their origins in my own personal story—my decades-long quest to understand the true meaning of enlightenment. It's one thing to briefly detach from personal story in the hopes of gaining a different perspective—it's quite another to deny our storied roots altogether. What will we stand in, then? At a time when our stories have been shamed and shunned in the spiritual community, it is all the more imperative to revive them and make luminous their sacred, transformative properties.

The past is not an illusion, as many would suggest. It is the ground of our being, the karmic field for our soul's transformation, a living vibration that echoes on, the mystery that threads right through our history. Story is where we come from. Story is what roots us in the present. Story is how we arrive at the next place intact. A spirituality without story is like a body without breath. Dead to the world.

Parts 2 and 3 consist of a dialogue between myself and a caricatured seeker named Michael. Although Michael is a 'construct'—I am not. I speak my truth, as it stands at the moment of writing. And while Michael does not actually exist, he is an amalgamation of various ways of being I have directly encountered—including myself at different stages of my own journey. He conveys a hodgepodge of common spiritual philosophies, past and present. During the writing process, he came so alive for me that I could almost see his form sitting in front of me, or hear the unique tenor of his voice. I would finish writing one chapter, and feel an eagerness to get to the next one—so he and I could sit down and re-connect. And when the book was complete, I felt a real sadness—like I had lost a true and dear friend. Parting is never easy, even when we are parting from a seemingly fictitious relationship.

In the same way as I used personal sharing in part 1 as a tool for critical review and the expression of ideas, I utilize our dialogues in parts 2 and 3 with the same intention: to critically review particular spiritual philoso- phies, and to forge new ideas to support humanity going forward. I don't for one moment feel like I have come to a point of completion with many of the ideas presented, but I believe this book succeeds at planting a seed of grounded possibility for humankind. Throughout my journey, I always longed for a spiritual model that was more self-honoring and grounded in the reality of daily life. This book is my best effort to craft that model. It will take time—and a varied palette of contributors—before we can form a more relational and inclusive framework of possibility for humankind. If this book contributes in some small way to that co-creation, then my sacred purpose has been faithfully honored.

As you read this book, I invite you to paint your own picture of possibil- ity. What does a spiritual life mean to you? If you were seeking to find the sacred in everyday life, what form would it take? What, if anything, have you been excluding from your spiritual equation? Have you differentiated your spiritual life from your daily life? Connect in with every aspect of your experience—your senses, your feelings, your body, your mind, your toes, your practical challenges, your relationships, your callings, your sensual nature, your pleasures and your pains. Imagine being alive to it all at one time. What would it mean to unite your spirituality and your humanness? How would you look, move, talk, relate, prioritize, feel? What would it mean to live everything as Godly? What would it mean to be truly *here* for all of it?

I wrote much of *Grounded Spirituality* in a rough-and-tumble library near my home. I sat front and center in the section where many of the downtrodden and disenfranchised come to sit and nap. Some of them stared at me, some of them said hello, some of them looked like they wanted to give me a punch in the head. I would sit amongst them, and it would help me to stay grounded and connected to why I write. It also made it impossible to get too airy-fairy, somehow imagining that love and light will resolve all of our problems. I would look at them, and sincerely wonder how we can construct a world where every one of us is intimately aware of why we are here. Where we realize our magnificence, and where we are invited to actualize it. Where we are all sacred advocates for each other. And where we understand the grounded steps that we must take to accomplish this. I understand why so many of us check out of this world—it's so severely painful—but I also know that we are remarkable beings, treasure chests of sacred possibility, hopeful and brave. The day that I give up on us, is the day I stop writing. I'm not giving up anytime soon.

I am sitting at my desk right now, in a cabin near my home. I have written this preface, after drafting the book itself. A great and vibrant peace exudes from my bones. I feel alive to this book in my body, I feel it in there, visceral proof that creation exists and that I am but one of her many limbs. At the same time, I feel intimately connected to the space itself. I sit at an old wood table, in a small cedar cabin. My back is pushed up against a comfy office chair, my bare feet firmly planted on the solid floor. I look out at a dense and fertile forest of green. I experience myself both distinct from—and blended into—the natural environment. And I also feel the ways in which I am not fully present for this moment—the tightness in my hips that blocks my energetic flow, the anxieties that visited this morning and continue to capture my attention. I feel all of it happening at the same time—my connected *and* my disconnected places, my broken pieces *and* my seamless aspects. The full spectrum of life experience. And I am deeply pleased. Not because I have achieved some perfectly integrated state—but because I am more comfortable than ever with all that is real, and with my offerings in the heart of it. It is my greatest hope that you receive this creation with the same generosity of spirit that I wrote from. I love humanity, and I am grateful for the opportunity to co-create with you.

—November 15, 2018
Eden Mills, Ontario

PART ONE

THE JOURNEY

I have something to share with you. Something I have arrived at in the heart of an arduous life journey. This sharing carries no illusion of absolute knowing. It does not imagine itself enlightened or perfected. And it is not something channeled or transmitted from above. It is much too grittily human for that. It was birthed right down here on Mother Earth, in the hard-worked entrails of this aging body temple. I have only been here for a moment in historical terms, but it often feels like centuries, eons. Perhaps it is, in ways I don't quite yet understand. This is not a complaint—my soul wouldn't have had it any other way—but it's my way of telling you that I come by my ideas honestly, after much lived experience. I have spent an inordinate amount of time in the School of Heart Knocks, enduring and integrating lesson upon lesson of rigorous study. Welcome to my humanness. I make no distinction between it and my spiritual life. This is the place I will share from.

Seeking *Here*

I have lived much of my life as an inquiry into what it means to really be *here*. Not here in the physical sense alone, but *here* in the most expansive and deeply felt form available to my consciousness.

In every stage of my life, no matter how fragmented and misguided I appeared on the outside, I was somehow questing toward a way of being that was truly, madly, deeply present for every moment—the real *here*, now. For reasons that I do not fully grok, this little guy wanted to be *here* bad. It was only later in life that I realized that my quest to be *here* was also a quest for an inclusive spiritual path.

This inquiry took root in infancy. As early as age four, I clearly recall having an experience of presence that brought me great satisfaction. I would lie in the backyard of our suburban Toronto home, staring up at a vast sky, earnestly trying to imagine what lay beyond. I would stay like that for a while, my mind flashing with vague imaginings, until it began to feel like a frustratingly incomplete vision.

Then I would breathe deeply and wiggle around inside of my animal body, stretching it as wide open as possible while rooting firmly into Mother Earth. And, finally, I would *feel* into whatever was true for me in the moment. I would feel it and, if called for, release all that wanted to be expressed. I would laugh, I would cry, I would tantrum, writhe, squirm. I would invite my animal body to let go of what no longer served it.

Although it might have appeared as madness to anyone watching, I somehow knew better. Because whenever I would release what I was holding in my compact little body, I experienced a profound feeling of calm and the sense that I had tapped into a far more expansive universe. It was like a door had creaked a little more open to the all-that-is every time I opened the gate to my heart.

Early on, I had the knowing deep in my bones: *Presence is a whole-being experience.* I didn't have language for any of it then, but I felt as though I was holding all the threads of human experience simultaneously—my heart wide open, my mind centered and clear, my body grounded and spacious. And through that portal, I experienced a rich and far-reaching connection to a unified field of awareness. One that was mutually dependent and intertwined. At the same time, the antennae, the source-spring for my most comprehensive experience of reality, was not the mind. Somehow, even as a mentally astute little kid, I intuitively knew that reality lived in the earthing, opening, and energizing of the physical and emotional bodies. This seemed to set everything else in motion.

For some years thereafter, I defended this knowing, and this state of being, like my life depended on it. Where many children broke off from the feeling realms at an early age, I clung to my feelings with ferocity. When my difficult parents came at me with hateful words and unfounded accusations, I resisted them by steadfastly refusing to bury my emotions. I had every reason to dissociate from my feeling-body in my volatile family of origin—it would have made life much more manageable in the short-term—but I refused, choosing instead to cry, tantrum, and truth-tell in the face of their madness.

It made for a blistering childhood, but I believe it saved my life. Although

I was punished for acting out, I avoided the biggest punishment of all—a lifetime sentence inside a prison of repressed emotions. And, just as I had experienced lying ass-flat on the backyard lawn, every time I moved my feelings and fully expressed my emotional truths, I found myself coming back to a fluid and seamless experience of the moment. Heart open, deeply present.

And then the overwhelming world got to me—as it does to so many of us—and I found myself retreating to my defenses as an adolescent. It was just too painful to be here for all of it. The open little boy that refused to be shut down had to split off from his heart in order to survive. Soon enough, I was stockpiling emotions rather than releasing feelings. No more lying on the grass opening my heart to God. I needed to keep my armor tightly fastened. To make it easier for myself, I turned to my favorite hiding place: my mind. A head-tripper extraordinaire, I then spent years in a state of emotional numbness, surviving by my wits. I couldn't feel the moment any longer—I *thought* it.

Then I found refuge in visions of a self-actualized reality, one where the world I inhabited would be in a state of perfect order. Like one of my idols, humanistic psychologist Abraham Maslow, I found great comfort in heightened imaginings, particularly as my family environment became more and more combative and abusive.

When the world disappointed me, I envisioned the world as it ought to be. When physically assaulted by my violent father, I imagined myself an achiever of super-heroic proportions. When the sheriff came to seize our family car, I disconnected by imagining the pristine home of my dreams: a glass house where I lived alone, high in the mountains, far above the fray.

Anywhere but *here*.

Although dissociative, these escape fantasies allowed me to transcend unbearable suffering and provided a vision of possibility to strive toward. With my eyes on the mountaintop, I was able to look away from the messy battlefield that I stood upon.

When I turned 19, I broke away from my family and went to university, fiercely determined to craft a self-actualized reality on my own terms. For many years thereafter, I would write my goals for the week in chalk on my bedroom wall and, like a good little actualizer, methodically check them off every Sunday, berating myself for anything I had failed to achieve, congratulating myself for every clever step forward. Although my unprocessed emotions were leaking toxic fumes everywhere, I stayed true to my heightened vision of possibility. One day, me and the spirit of

Abe Maslow would hang there together, safely held in the womb of our self-actualized consciousness.

At the age of 24, I was admitted to law school. I completed one year, and then requested a healing sabbatical. My undigested emotional material was beginning to push its way into my daily life, and it became clear I needed to re-connect with my inner world. Soon thereafter, a little voice inside broke through my habitual consciousness and whispered words of wisdom into an early morning dreamscape. The words startled me awake, and I quickly grabbed a marker and wrote them on the wall, so as not to forget.

Excessive analysis perpetuates emotional paralysis

In other words, "Stop limiting your experience of the moment to your thinking mind!" Although I wasn't quite ready to integrate the message, it kept at me like a mantra of remembrance—an echo of a lost key—until I was once again ready to embrace my emotional body in all its totality.

Three years later, right after being called to the bar, I stepped back from my chosen career as a criminal lawyer. I loved the law, and had enjoyed a remarkably engaging apprenticeship year under Canada's most famous criminal lawyer, Eddie Greenspan. Still, there was this feeling, deep in my bones, that I had to shed my warrior armor and explore other pathways of possibility in this lifetime. It was the hardest decision I ever made. After a childhood living in lack, my ego was gratified by the prospect of a presti-gious professional career path, and my poverty consciousness was finally quelled. I also was driven by a strong desire to do good work in the world, with a long list of things to accomplish in the legal system. But here was this other quiet subtle voice, nagging at me, calling me in another direction. The little voice that knows.

69 Easy Seconds

Immediately after making the decision to step away, I naturally turned right back to the thing that had saved me as a child: emotional release. I devoted much of the next few years to a therapeutic process, thawing out and releasing many of the feelings that I had repressed during the previous two decades. I had what I now call a *nervous break-through*, as waves of deep feeling turned everything that I identified as reality upside down. The process was greatly relieving, but it is worth noting that it was nothing like the underlying sense of wholeness that I had known as a child. It was more like that cathartic feeling you get when you have a good, deep cry and still feel like there is so much more lying in wait. It was different now, and I wasn't sure why.

I then embarked on a two-pronged, 20 year-long quest for meaning. During these years, I made my living from a window business I had opened in law school. A gruff, ass-busting, and humbling contrast from my intellectualized endeavors. Between selling door-to-door and the income derived from a small sales and installation crew, I was able to generate the money and find the space that I needed to explore my life's purpose. It wasn't easy, but it worked.

The first path of inquiry was a familiar one: the quest for *here*. That is, what is true presence? What does it mean to be truly *in* the moment? And, most pressingly—what on earth is this thing called "enlightenment?"

The second path was less familiar: the quest for clarity as to *why* I am here. That is, what is the purpose of my existence? Is this life an arbitrary adventure—the perpetual journey of an accidental tourist—or am I here with purpose coursing through my veins? I'd had many glimpses of possible paths: Jeff as humanistic psychologist, Jeff as author, Jeff as lawyer, Jeff as garbageman... but were any of them real? How do we find our true path?

The default stop on my quest for answers was in my mind. Still a highly proficient head-tripper, I hunted for enlightenment deep inside my thoughts, somehow imagining that realization would arise in the form of a concept. I spent copious amounts of time reading classic spiritual literature. I went for long walks in the woods, contemplating the principles of classical Buddhism, Hinduism, Taoism, and Sufism. I dialogued with others and debated concepts with great panache. And yet, none of it added up to much. I felt more like an observer of life than an active participant. An idea of enlightenment was not the same as an experience of enlightenment. Not even close.

Then I swung in the other direction and explored Tantra, seeking nirvana in the ecstasies of the flesh. From crown chakra to root chakra, in 69 easy seconds. Well, not really Tantra—just the sexed-up version that horny young people prefer. A counterfeit version of the authentic practice that truly embraces the light *and* the shadow.

Like a good little bliss-tripper, I jumped from one pleasure to another, dating a number of women and riding a wave of euphoria as long as it would last. It didn't last very long. Before I knew it, I was caught in a polyamorous web of reactivity, one where the painful material that fueled my non-attachment philosophy had come back to haunt me. I wasn't interested in polyamory as a conscious exploration of connection and a genuine spiritual practice. I wanted it to sidestep my attachment issues. Although joyous on the outside, I was actually a boiling cauldron of unresolved feeling in the deep within. This little game wasn't getting me anywhere good.

A Master of None

I subsequently turned to meditation in the hopes of finding my answers. I regularly attended a neighborhood Buddhist temple, where I practiced diligently under the tutelage of a particularly rigid monk. He would give a talk at the beginning of each gathering—touching on various Buddhist principles—and then we would sit in silence, sometimes for hours at a time.

At first, I loved the opportunity to leave my "monkey mind" at the temple door while exploring a singular point of focus. It was calming and clarifying. And then something shifted. While meditating, I would be overcome by a fierce degree of resistance. No doubt, some part of my resistance had to do with the persistent teaching emphasis on the "realization of non-self" (one of the three marks of existence according to the Buddhists, along with "impermanence" and "suffering"). This was entirely incongruent with the therapeutic work I was doing to build a healthy sense of self.

But there was something else. As the classes progressed, I found myself arriving at the distinct sense that the calmness I was experiencing was not actually authentic. I felt calm and peaceful on one level, and entirely agitated on another, like some fundamental part of me was being left behind and crying out for inclusion. I just didn't know what that part was yet.

One evening, in the heart of yet another restless meditation, I flashbacked to an interaction I'd had some years before. I was in my late twenties, on vacation in Mexico, when I met an older man by the pool. He was a sharp, crisp guy, the kind of man that emanated societal success. He asked me what I wanted to be when I grew up. I gave him a very lengthy answer that included a broad range of possibilities. He made a strange, disappointed face and replied, "Oh, a Jack of all trades, master of none. We don't need any more of these. We need masterful men."

And then he walked away, no longer interested in speaking with me. This brief conversation struck me, fortifying my perfectionist tendencies and perpetuating the patriarchally conditioned belief that the best way to survive and thrive on this planet was to both follow and master a singular path to the top of the mountain. I was particularly attracted to this manner of being, because it allowed me to focus on one prize while negating all the difficult material that I didn't want to deal with.

Later that evening, I recognized why this interaction had come into memory. I was lying on my bed with my eyes closed, when I saw myself standing before a large white-capped mountain. It had one clear path ascending up to the highest and most distinct peak, and a number of secondary paths meandering in a myriad different directions: up, down, and spiraling across its breadth. I imagined myself walking the clearly marked path up the mountain, and it held no interest. I understood that it was the most expeditious way to arrive, but I was more interested in exploration than efficacy. I felt captivated by the question of how one unique path led to another, led to another. I imagined myself traversing its winding trails, wandering its valleys, discovering the manifold ways to reach its staggered peaks. And then I saw myself finally arriving at the summit after a long, arduous journey, looking out at the world with a more multidimensional perspective because of all the different paths I had taken, and all I had learned along the way.

I soon realized that I had been walking the wrong way on my spiritual quest for enlightenment. I was focused on excelling along a singular path, rather than treading diligently across many paths. And though each thread yielded fruits, none of them brought me into the inclusively connected experience of the moment that I remembered from early life. In fact, it seemed like the opposite. The tantric bliss-trip left me energetically charged and entirely ungrounded, the head-trip sharpened my focus but blocked my heart, and the meditation trip both calmed me and left me feeling uncomfortably self-severed.

In and of themselves, they weren't enough. It was like I was scaling one tree at a time, but they never revealed the entire forest. I recognized that this was not true for everyone—some do find their peace on a single trail. But living my life through one portal alone was not the way this soul wanted to roll. I wanted to find a way to walk them all. Explorer of many paths, master of none.

Alexander Lowen

Soon thereafter, I began a long-distance master's degree program in humanistic psychology at Saybrook University, in Northern California. Years of reading and loving Maslow's work had confirmed my desire to explore psychology as a possible career path.

And then—another game-changer. I met Alexander Lowen, the co-founder of Bioenergetic Analysis, and he reminded me that I had a body. Not just a body to utilize in order to achieve my single-threaded goals, but a body to surrender to and through on my quest for meaning. I had joined the Bioenergetics training program in Toronto some months earlier, and I began taking the train down to Connecticut to participate in therapy sessions with him.

At the heart of Bioenergetic therapy is the idea that mind and body are functional reflections of each other. Our behavioral issues and personality defenses are perfectly reflected in the body, manifested as chronic muscle tensions and obstructed expression. To support healing and integration, the client engages in a series of physical exercises that energize the body, enliven the breath, soften blocks and holdings, and unearth the emotional material that is trapped inside. When repressed memories arise, the client is encouraged to explore and express them in many ways, including tantruming, crying, spontaneous movements and sounds, hitting, punching, and kicking.

My own learning began right after I arrived at Lowen's home office in New Canaan, Connecticut for our first session. Before I encountered a human, I was presented with reminders of our animal nature: the horses circumambulating the property, the quacking geese on the front lawn, and then, upon entering the house, his Golden Retriever, headbutting my knees, and licking my hands. And, every few seconds, an impossible-to-ignore parrot shrieking from his perch in the living room. This house was alive!

Eventually Lowen appeared. His 87-year-old gait was strong and assured, like a man in his 30s. A force of nature, this man embodied his own theories. It was undeniable.

He took me into a little room with two plain chairs, a dusty old mattress, and a weather-worn wood contraption. The room itself was coursing with primal physical energy, wild and untamed.

We sat in the chairs. After listening to me talk about my feelings ad nauseam, he asked me the question he would ask every time we met: "Are you ready to get to work?" I nodded. "Good," he replied, "then stop talking and get yourself undressed."

I took off my shirt and pants and stood before him in my boxers. He began to scan my body—an approach fundamental to Bioenergetics—in an effort to make sense of the way that I lived. For a Bioenergeticist, the body tells the tale of our lived experience and the ways that we organize reality. A therapist can hear about someone's issues, but it doesn't mean a thing, analytically, or therapeutically, if they don't perceive how it is reflected somatically.

With an intimate understanding of the necessity for grounding our consciousness, Lowen instructed me to rub my feet into the carpet for an uncomfortably long period of time: "You walk in a way that tells me you don't want to be here." Wise man. Some part of me *didn't* want to be here. I didn't trust the human race. I had endured much trauma, and, as a result, I wanted to be only partially here.

Then he instructed me to spend another 15 minutes in a falling forward position with my feet sturdily rooted: "Remain like this, until you feel vibrations moving from your feet through the rest of your body. And then stay there even longer." As I did, I felt my consciousness more fully infiltrating the room. I had more access to what was around me, and more access to what was within me. And, with that, a broad range of uncomfortable feelings began to quake and rumble into my awareness, the gate steadily creaking open.

Lowen then brought me over to the contraption in the middle of the office. "Now that you are more *here*, you can access more of your feelings. Before, you couldn't access them because you were floating above your body." The contraption was something Bioenergetic therapists call a breathing stool—similar to a mini-pommel horse that you bend over, to enable the opening of armored places in the body. He instructed me to lie backwards over it and intensify my breath. Such simple instructions, yet so painfully difficult while bent backwards over his device. I tried to get off it but he would have none of that: "Stay right there and breathe, man… breathe yourself back to life."

Somehow, I trusted this man and continued. Then, he simulated the sounds of crying, coaxing me to cry, too. "Now—cry, man! Access your crying reflex."

I tried, but I couldn't access enough air upside down on the stool. I gasped. That didn't stop him. He continued to simulate the crying sound, softly whimpering and moaning. And then, the oddest thing happened: my whole lens on reality flipped upside down. *Literally.* The more deeply I breathed my tight chest open, the more intimate I became with a giant reservoir of unfelt pain buried within me. It was all right there, beneath the armor I had accumulated to contain it. Nothing I had come into contact with in my talk-based therapy, or on my spiritual quest, came close to accessing this depth of sorrow. Memories of buried trauma surged through my body, demanding to be remembered, felt, and released. I flashed to images of my father's violent attacks, my mother's verbal assaults, hundreds of moments of embittered conflict on the family battleground. And with them, a flood of heaving hopelessness, as I felt into what it was like to experience these assaults, before my young defenses were fully formed. And then, the tears. I sobbed and sobbed. And sobbed some more.

I remained upside down on his device for some time, startled by the depths of my self-deception. It was entirely clear. I had been moving through life alienated from much of my unresolved emotional experience. And that truth was not inside of my mind, it was locked inside my constricted musculature and shallowed breath. It was living inside of my bones. So many questions emerged: How had I lived this long without realizing what I had buried? How could my spiritual quest be an honest one if I was this detached from my inner world? How could I come into the now, if my heart was still back in the *then*?

Like a stern but loving Grandpa, Lowen kept at me. He motioned me to lie on the well-worn mattress at the edge of the room: "Stay with the release, kid. Don't resist now… just keep opening those tensions."

As I lay down, he instructed me to fully express the words and feelings I was holding. Not just express them with my mouth, but with my whole body: "Tantrum, kiddo. Tantrum it all out of you. Get your whole body involved." And so I did, hitting and kicking and crying and raging at the darkness for the longest time. Wow. It was feral and it was primal and it was long, long overdue.

As I took the long train ride back to Toronto, I recollected on the nervous breakthrough I had experienced some years ago. It had felt somehow incomplete, and now I understood why. I hadn't been in my body then. I may have thought I was, but what I *thought* was a far cry from reality. To clear 20 years of accumulated holdings, I would need to get deep inside my body, opening it wide enough to bring the subterranean levels of material to the surface. Back then, I had only released the feelings at the top layers, when what was needed was a much stronger excavation. Opening my body was that excavation, the only way to break through the armor to the material trapped inside.

Lowen and I met for three more sessions, each one excavating more unresolved material to be released. It was shocking that one body-mind could hold so much. The muck didn't seem to end—nor did the presence it unveiled.

Finally we arrived at our last session. It was clear I had extracted the fruits of true healing from our work together, and it was time for me to plod along on my own. But I was interested in something else, too. I was drawn to understand how my emotional life related to my spiritual life. I found it so fascinating that after each grounding and release session with him, I would feel much more spiritually present—as though the two realms were related, if not synonymous. I would look out over the horse farm, and then up to the sky, and everything felt connected and unified. It was undeniable: if I didn't include the healing of my shadow in my quest for spiritual meaning, there would be no peace at all.

During our last session, I posed the question to Lowen directly: "I would like to know how you define a 'spiritual life.' What does it mean to be spiritual?"

He replied, to this effect, "It's an open and energized body, kid. You wake up the body and you become naturally spirited. That's spirituality!"

And there it was. A truly spiritual life is not something that exists independent of our emotional life and physical form. Spirituality is an embodied experience. It's a felt experience. It lives right in the heart of the matter.

The Monkey Heart

The in-wakening continued when I attended an "Insight and Opening" workshop with Insight Meditation Teacher Jack Kornfield and Holotropic Breathwork Co-founder Stanislav Grof in Massachusetts at the Governor Dummer Academy. It was the perfect name for a place that would support my movement towards a less mind-full, and more heart-felt, way of being.

Insight Meditation, or *Vipassana*, is a Buddhist practice that focuses continuous awareness on bodily sensation and mental phenomena, with the intention of gaining insight into the true nature of reality. It is believed to be the meditative practice taught by the Buddha himself. By contrast, Holotropic Breathwork is a less observational and more dynamic approach to self-exploration and healing, combining accelerated breathing with accelerated music in a safe environment. Participants lie on a mat with their eyes closed, each person using their own breath and the music to enter various states of consciousness. Some individuals have non-ordinary or transpersonal experiences. Others have experiences of a psycho-therapeutic nature, often moving into vigorous forms of process and release. This eight-day workshop would encompass both approaches.

First, Vipassana. As we meditated, motionless like statues, I looked around the room and saw everyone from a Bioenergetics perspective. Where before I might have imagined my fellow meditators serene and peaceful, I now saw constricted bodies, compressed energy, unreleased grief and rage. I saw a bunch of caffeinated, agitated Westerners trying to shift from their uncomfortable bodies into their observational mind. Was staying still really the best way to find peace?

With Lowen, I had entered a unified field *after* enlivening my body and releasing emotional holdings. Could it occur any other way? Could we really be in the moment if we are all dammed (and damned) up? Can we clear all those blocks sitting upright and disciplined on a meditation cushion? Aren't we already rigid enough? Shouldn't we energize and empty first? What about emotional release as the path to presence? What about meditation-in-motion?

I turned off my inner cynic and tried to meditate. It's a curious thing— to *try* to meditate. In this moment, it felt futile. I was too agitated, and too much of me wanted to move. In fact, I just wanted to scream. I would soon have my chance.

Then we moved into the Holotropic approach. After one particularly resistant breathwork, I went further into the next one, riding the intensified breath deep into my body cavity. The breath served as a kind of shovel, bringing unexpressed feelings, words and shouts to the surface, particularly around my relationship with my mother. I surrendered to an hour-long, full-body tantrum, owning the truth that longed to be expressed through my bones.

After I was done, I went outside to be in nature. Before the breathwork, I experienced the natural world as distinct from me. Now, the veils of separation had fallen away, and I felt everything as one. Just as I had experienced with Lowen, my energized and embodied emotional release had removed my blockages to clarity. But this time it was different. Where a bounty of doors in consciousness had opened with Lowen, a more luminous bounty had opened here. Every full-bodied release seemed to unearth yet another subtle realm of existence, each more richly nuanced than the last. Each release peeled me like an onion, revealing more of my core and the heart of the universe. The further I traveled, the more deeply I was at peace within my feeling-body, and consequently, even more connected to the interwoven tapestry of reality.

It was now irrefutably obvious to me that spiritual experience is both a relative process—an ever-expanding foray into the great beyond—and one that could not exist independent of the dynamic flesh temple that housed it. The answer wasn't out there, or up there, or beyond here—it was right inside my bones. And the more thoroughly I enlivened my body temple, the more deeply I penetrated reality. The more open and energized my physical and emotional bodies, the more inclusive, and far-reaching, my consciousness became. In its invigoration, I was able to see just how significantly my unconscious decision to shallow my breath earlier in life impacted my access to the moment. This wasn't a self-criticism—shallowing the breath, like armoring parts of the body, was a necessary defense against feeling—but it was an essential observation going forward.

That night, I sat down to meditate. Where before I could barely sit still, now I was actually *in* my body. I closed my eyes and traversed the inner caverns of my consciousness, exploring my inner world without obstruction. Of course, it wasn't my mindful attention to the breath that had brought me into a meditative state. It was the no-mind-full intensification of the breath. It was the intimacy with, and the involuntary submission to, the body. The super-charged breath had acted as an excavation tool, busting through the blockages, re-opening energetic lines, and supporting a profound healing within my next layers of woundedness.

With my emotional debris cleared, I could finally meditate more completely. It was crystal clear: The way to calm the monkey mind is to open the human heart. I had spent so much time looking for peace outside of my own heart. In the end, it wasn't out there. It was in *here*. But only at the tail end of vigorous embodied release. It left me wondering if we are missing the mark by focusing on the mind as the primary obstacle in the spiritual world. Deeming the mind hyper-active or troublesome or illusory doesn't tell us why this is so. What if it's just a symptom? What if the real issue lives down below? What if it's the "monkey heart" that's the issue—the state of inner tumult and chaos that emanates from an emotionally constricted heart. If so, we don't need mind-full-ness techniques to calm it. We need heart-full-ness techniques. We need to open and heal our hearts.

I meditated into the early morning hours, descending into my inner world. It was then, from there, *only* from there, that the "Insight Meditation" component of the workshop was of service, as it allowed me to take my process to the next level. More specifically, I began to gain actual insight into the next steps on my life's path. Glimpses of paths floated past, like leaves on the river of time—Jeff as author, Jeff as tender-hearted lover, Jeff as surrendered being, Jeff as spiritual activist.

In other words, the more fully I touched the moment, the more clearly my reasons for being here—the *why* at the heart of my existence—began to reveal itself. Clearing the emotional and physical debris hadn't merely brought me more fully into the moment. It had also opened the space inside for my path to begin to show its face. With my consciousness all bound up with old pain, my way could not be made clear. Now its countenance was peeking into view.

The Queendom of Goddess

And then, a great love came into my life, turning my current trajectory upside down, yet again. She was a soulmate of epic proportions, adding an entirely new layer to my deepening understanding of spirituality. To this point, my forays into a vaster consciousness had been a primarily solitary process. I was a lone male wolf clarifying his inner world and expanding toward unity. And it was, through my conditioned masculine lens, a primarily vertical interface. That is, when I would open, I would not look off to the side, or down at the earth. I would look UP, as though the source of an enlightened consciousness was only in the sky above me.

In the presence of *Rebecca*, a much richer and more multi-layered universal interface was revealed. It wasn't a universe limited to a singular lens on reality—the heightened Kingdom of a patriarchal God—but one that also included the more horizontal ways of the Divine Feminine—the enheartened and relational Queendom of Goddess.

Within seconds of our first sighting, I was catapulted to yet another dimension, one where unseen universes rose into view, each one more vivid and far-reaching than the last. Simply being with her, and most certainly in the electric sexual field between us, I was ushered along a continuum of consciousness that was more vital and inclusive than anything I had experienced in isolation. It was as if we had entered a great temple together, with our connection as the master key. The more time we spent together, the holier the world became.

If ever I had imagined that I could reach the outer parameters of a unified field in my isolated process, I now knew otherwise. In loving her, I was introduced to exactly what I had been seeking to avoid when I first embarked on my hierarchical quest for an enlightened consciousness. I had wanted the Divine way up there, far above the maddening crowd, but she kept appearing down here, in my physical and emotional body... and now, on the vulnerable bridge between my heart and another's heart.

In this experience, I was also reminded of the relative nature of enlightenment. On the bridge between our hearts, what felt like unity consciousness at one stage of opening was revealed as a mere fragment of possibility in another. Clearly, there was no endpoint to this process. Not a chance. Just as soon as one gateway opened, another beckoned, embracing of, and yet one step beyond, the last.

I couldn't help but wonder: What if it is LOVE—not personal mastery, not mindfulness, not disciplined focus, not perfected asanas—that is the great door opener? What if the lone-wolf men have had it wrong all along and it actually is *relationship* that is the primary mode of transport on the royal road to divinity? And, going a step further: What if our experience of divinity is in fact more complete when we co-create Him together, when She arises alight and enheartened on the wings of our love? What if we are not just here together to keep each other company, but to show each other God? And even more startling, what if God actually is relationship, in all its myriad forms?

These were the questions that pervaded my next months… pulsing through my being, working me, tossing and turning me inside and out, opening inner regions I didn't even know I had. It was like being dropped on to unfamiliar and mysterious terrain with no previous footprints to follow. This was a pivotal marker on my spiritual journey—where the "me" that was prior, and the "me" that came after—were simply not the same.

Mending the Broken Heart

And then I learned a harsh lesson: It is very difficult to sustain great love at this stage of human development. This is particularly true if one or both of the individuals haven't done enough work on their personal issues. If there is too much emotional rubble, too many unsettled issues and unconscious patterns, too little willingness to work them through in connection, then the relationship will inevitably plummet back to earth with a thud. Perhaps this is one of the primary reasons why many spiritual seekers choose to limit their explorations to their own individual practice and process: It may not go as deep or as wide, but it is often easier to sustain.

Though this great love had ushered me into a more fertile universe of possibility, it was now time to learn through a different medium: loss and heartbreak. After Rebecca left me and my freshly expanded consciousness crumpled on the ground, I was pushed, as we often are by love's leavings, to the next stage of transformation. I was now faced with a choice between shutting down—the familiar path of the armored masculine—or keeping my heart open in the midst of the most excruciating pain and loss I had ever known.

To my surprise, I made the choice to go deeper into the feelings. Something in my inner reserves demanded that I stay in the heartfire and weave my broken, bloodied, shattered heart back together with whatever thread of hope I could find. It was no easy feat. If shattered was what I needed to grow, then I got just what the Soul Doctor ordered.

Much of this process happened at a renowned healing center in California. I had completed my master's coursework, and then arranged a lengthy retreat. After some resistance, I surrendered to a transformative healing process around my abandonment wound. I ran through the forest and howled, wailed and emoted until my voice went hoarse. I soaked in the healing waters and wept for hours on end. I writhed on the forest floor and punched the earth with ferocity. I dove into the fires of anguish time and again, staying with each release beyond exhaustion, and then dug in for more. And then I would wake up in the morning and break at the edges again, surrendering to a loss that was far beyond my comprehension.

On the other side of that deep dive was a significantly transformed emotional body. My suffering converted into expansion in love's messy karmic kiln. After all was said and done, I felt calmer and more present and integrated than ever before on my spiritual quest. It was like I had passed through the narrowest transformation tunnel possible—fraught and riddled with primal perils—before opening to a vast and entirely generous polychromatic field of possibility.

Where before I had imagined that opening my heart in love's presence had been the great transformational catalyst, I now recognized that that was only the first step. There was something more. The next step was opening my heart in love's absence, right in the heart of loss. This too was a deepening path.

This experience confirmed that there is a strong, alchemical relationship between emotional healing and spiritual transformation. Spiritual life was not something independent of emotional life—it clearly lives at the heart of it. I am not simply referencing the new vistas that arise after we release (finally, there is space inside!); I am talking about the more expanded consciousness that we *become*, after working issues through. Each issue, in its own way, was a seedling for transformation. Each was a portal to another unique thread of consciousness, a gateway to a pre-encoded landscape, rich with possibility. In this case, I was forced even further into the healing of an abandonment wound that had plagued me for decades, maybe even lifetimes. In the past, I had made many efforts to work it through, but I had always stopped short. I had always been good at naming the wound, but transforming it was another matter altogether. It was easier to flee it, than to actually confront it. Until the break-up. The severing of a soul-deep umbilical cord with Rebecca. The perfect stimuli for festering primal material to ooze to the surface. At that point, it became so painful that my only choice was to breakthrough to the other side.

Once there, it was confirmed that the story I had been told for years by the so-called spiritual community was wrong. It was not in the absence of the self that I grew my capacity to be in the moment. It was deep within it. The more deeply I embraced the self, the more deeply I embraced the moment. The further I went into the marrow of my healing, the more I matured as a spiritual being. What *is* spirituality, if not a deep dive into our raw humanity, feelings and all?

Glimpses Behind, Glimpses Ahead

After being inside of this transformed state for days, more fruits of my process were revealed. While sitting in stillness one afternoon before returning to Toronto, I saw vivid images of my life's journey in my mind's eye.

I didn't have words for it yet, but it was as though I had uncovered a web of soul-scriptures that lay within me. I didn't believe that every bit of childhood suffering was somehow useful or part of a divine plan, yet there indeed was a karmic directionality to much of it, which perfectly reflected my growing edge in this lifetime. Wherever these scriptures came from, they were intrinsic to my expansion and fundamental to my quest for meaning.

One of the most lucid understandings was the inextricable connection between specific personal relationships and my own transformation. Not just sexual relationships like Rebecca, but other significant connections as well. People who have had near-death experiences often say that their life flashes before them as they cross over to the other side. This was like seeing my life flash before my eyes, while still alive. Witnessing in awe the way each piece fits together in impeccable order, like a jigsaw puzzle completed by God's nimble hand. I saw a web of transformative opportunities within a whole rainbow spectrum of connections: close family bonds, deep friendships, and highly charged brief encounters. They were not all colossal universal mistakes, or random spinning particles happening to collide by coincidence, as I had once imagined. They were fields of intrinsic possibility. In the briefest of flashes, I saw the mother who pushed me to find the cutting-edge I would need to bring my purpose through in this distracting world. I saw the best friend who grounded and lightened my heavy heart as I wrestled with my many demons. I saw the homeless man who marveled in gratitude whenever I brought him lunch, repeatedly showing me the simple gifts in the little things. And so many more, fervently cascading past my inner scope, laden with wisdom and treasures.

As I looked back on nearly 40 or so hard-lived years, I saw how the lone-wolf warrior consciousness that saved me, also prevented me from seeing the most obvious thing: the relational nature of growth. One way or the other, we are always interfacing with something, or someone, outside of ourselves. Left to my own devices, I could travel beautifully far, but nowhere near as far, deep, and wide as I could if I truly surrendered to relationships as an opportunity for awakening and transformation. If I fled relationship, I remain trapped inside a tomb of trauma, triggers, and transference. I imagined myself free, but the unprocessed material could not help but block elements of my expansion. My inner child's evolving understanding of enlightenment had now added a new thread of knowing to the weave: our relationship to other humans is fundamental to our spiritual lives. And not lovers alone, but all meaningful connections.

As night fell, the next step on my journey rose clearly into view: the urgent call to write my first book. I had to share my story, my struggle to heal my heart and find my path. It came through with a rush of certainty, like a moral imperative, one that I could not possibly deny. Up to this point, I had always suspected that I would someday write, but I also knew that I wasn't ready. Yet something had shifted in the heart of this healing process. I was now able to see the precise form the calling wanted to take, and I felt better prepared—more mature, less obstructed—to bring it through. As I had learned after the Holotropic Breathwork workshop, the more we clear and open up space inside and truly arrive *here*, the more access we have to the *why* we are here. Perhaps because I had cleared even more emotional debris this time, an even more precise vision emerged. Something in the profound working-through of emotional material had opened space inside for a new chapter on my path to purpose to reveal itself. The next chapter was to write my way home.

Eckhart Tolle

I began to write a few weeks before the 9-11 calamity, in the back room of my Toronto home. After a brief period of self-doubt, an unstoppable writing voice began to roar through me—a force of expressive wonder that could not be quelled. I found myself incessantly scribbling passages on walls, calling new paragraphs into my voicemail, waking up in the middle of the night by an inner command to get back to the computer. The compulsion to write was ravenous, all-consuming, a tsunami of expression that would stop at nothing.

In order to create space to write, I would go through stints of intensely focused and rigorous work, going door-to-door aggressively selling windows in Toronto-area subdivisions, striving to achieve my sales quota, so I could earn enough to sustain me through a phase of intensive writing.

At this time, I was still lodged in the belief that my spiritual life—reflected in my call to write, and my practical life—reflected in the window business, could not co-exist. I was either the more surrendered creativist honing his craft at the computer, or I was the assertive warrior punching his way through the marketplace. I didn't imagine that I could be both.

Then, a soft-spoken man named Eckhart Tolle entered the spiritual scene. With his regular appearances on Oprah, he seemed to be changing the landscape and conversation of spirituality in the West. With an open mind, I decided to check him out. Perhaps he had something new and fresh to bring to the spiritual banquet table. It was curious to me: Why was mainstream society resonating so much with this man?

I read Tolle's introduction in his book, *The Power of Now* (PON), time and time again, finding momentary comfort in his story of shifting from suicidal depression to his "true nature" in the course of a single night. It was a hopeful notion. Part of me also wanted to leave my "false, suffering self" behind and spend two years on park benches in a state of tremendous joy. Much easier than the rigorous excavation work I had been doing for years. There was a way in which he represented the ultimate breakthrough to me—that blessed moment when all your anxieties and unresolved memories collapse into God. That moment when the fruit of your soul's labor falls from the bodhi tree of enlightenment into your ripe and ready consciousness.

I became particularly interested in his claim that all you have to do is "witness" your emotional pain (what he calls "the pain-body") to break your identification with it. This had not been my experience, but I was open to the inquiry. In his words, "So the pain-body doesn't want you to observe it directly and see it for what it is. The moment you observe it, feel its energy field within you, and take your attention into it, the identification is broken. A higher dimension of consciousness has come in. I call it *presence*. You are now the witness or the watcher of the pain-body. This means that it cannot use you anymore by pretending to be you, and it can no longer replenish itself through you. You have found your own innermost strength. You have accessed the power of Now."

For some time, I explored his reflections. I spent an abundance of time inside of my witness observer, just as he instructed, watching my mind at work. And not what I normally construed as my mind—a whirlwind of persistent thoughts—but what Tolle identified as "the mind":

> Mind, in the way I use the word, is not just thought. It includes your emotions as well as all unconscious mental-emotional reactive patterns. Emotion arises at the place where mind and body meet. It is the body's reaction to your mind— or you might say, a reflection of your mind in the body.

When my monkey mind swirl of thoughts and feelings would arise, I would pay close attention to them from my witnessing vantage point. I imagined myself a passive lifeguard, sitting up high in the tower, quietly watching the ocean rise and fall before my eyes. Just observing. Sometimes, I would be reminded, when I was able to crack through to an experience of a vaster awareness, that my mind was only a small part of the ultimate consciousness available to me. I leaned into the idea that the pain-body was not something you should identify with; rather, it was the misidentified debris that you sever from your consciousness so that you can live your real life. It was the mirage in your field of awareness until you finally wake up and remember. Just like Eckhart did that night. The pain-body was the trash you trip over on the way up Bliss Mountain. Just keep your attention on it and move it off to the side with awareness. It's blocking your view of the enlightenment at the peak.

At first, I felt a palpable sense of relief in the heart of his approach. Like I had come back from war and finally got to lay down in a safe and peaceful field to get some respite. When I would hear him talk, I fell into a restful and somnambulant state. When he wrote that "silence is an even more potent carrier of presence", I invited silence closer. When he stated that "past and future obviously have no reality of their own", I invited myself to surrender more genuinely into the moment. When he explained that our unconscious identification with the mind created "the ego, as a substitute for your true self rooted in Being", I earnestly attempted to disengage and disidentify with my ego. I would see my ego—a contained and concrete identity—and I would quietly witness it. I disengaged and became aware of a backdrop of stillness just beneath.

When people I knew encountered me, they wondered where "Jeff" had gone. My slight edge had vanished, my waves of reactivity had diminished, and even my way of speaking had lost its usual fluctuations. From my peaceful perch above it all in a kind of thoughtless, present-centered awareness, I no longer felt triggered by the inner content that had customarily plagued me. My chatter had been replaced with presence. With my attention effortlessly focused on my beingness, I felt comforted by an experience of equanimity that buffered me from the madness of the world, and perhaps as importantly, from whatever madness lay within me. Or so I imagined.

Eventually, I found myself resisting. It was clear as a Bonshō bell—something was amiss. As I leaned further into some of the practices he suggested, I began to feel like I was trapped in some kind of holding pen—not a place of deliverance but a hiding place from life's challenges. Without strong roots in my emotional body, I felt progressively more dissociative, and disconnected from the marrow of my humanness. Unhooking from the pain-body felt like it was actually deadening me, leading me up and away from the place where life was truly lived. I felt like all the healing and embodiment work I had done—Bioenergetics, Holotropic Breathwork, and the process of soul-deep love found, and lost—was now being nullified. The new fresh soil I was standing on was becoming homogenized and dulled. I realized this wasn't real progress. Like a child with his hands over his eyes repeating, "This is not happening," when there is something too painful to witness, I felt as though I was sidestepping reality altogether. It was one thing to witness for a time, but then what? No matter how genuinely I explored Eckhart's techniques and ideas, my emotional life would invariably leak up from my pain-body and drown my objective watcher in an ocean of feeling.

Was that so wrong?

Wasn't there a way to integrate a witnessing consciousness with the raw truth of my emotionally vital inner world? Wasn't there a way for pain, and vaster perspective, to fluidly co-exist?

And it wasn't only about the world of feeling. I also felt my writing voice—a vital voice connected to my deeper purpose, fueled and energized by an enlivened physical and emotional body—rising up, unwilling to die to the idea that all my personal identifications were mistaken. Some of them perhaps, but surely not all of them. The further I traveled on Tolle's observer-ship, the harder it was to ride the waves of creation and creativity. I needed my humanness along for the ride. Where to find my voice, if not in the bones of my being?

After some time, I decided to give the teachings another shot. I had a subtle inkling that there was still more to glean here. So I devoted a few weekends to Tolle. I spent my afternoons and evenings listening to him, and watching his talks on video. As I tuned in to him, I allowed my body to open and to absorb the teachings. What I could feel surprised me. I didn't feel stillness. I felt agitation. He talked about the perils of the mind, and all I could feel was a head-tripper trapped inside a watcher consciousness. When he talked about embodiment, all I could feel was his deadened body. He talked about being in the "now," and all I heard were screams from his unresolved past. No matter how hard he had tried to rid himself of his so-called pain-body, all I felt coming off of him was undigested grief. It is an odd version of presence when it feels as though there is no one truly home.

I thought of Alexander Lowen, and his deep conviction that until we actually energized our bodies and cleared our emotional detritus, we could not possibly be "spirited," as our consciousness was still trapped in the past. I thought of my sessions with him—among many other experiences—where I only arrived at a calm and expansive present-centered consciousness after intense, activated releases. Witnessing the pain-body was momentarily helpful at times but it was the working through it that actually calmed my mind and opened the door to the true here and now. The more work I did growing through my stuff, the more capable I became of holding the *now* gate open. I couldn't have one, without the other.

I continued to dip my toe in PON, still with the inexplicable sense that there was something for me to extract: "Free from the *illusion* that you are nothing more than your physical body and your mind. This 'illusion of the self,' as the Buddha calls it, is the core error. Free from *fear* in its count-less disguises as the inevitable consequence of that illusion—the fear that is your constant tormentor as long as you derive your sense of self only from this ephemeral and vulnerable form. And free from *sin*, which is the suffering you unconsciously inflict on yourself and others as long as this illusory sense of self governs what you think, say, and do."

The illusion of the self. This notion seemed to live at the heart of his perspective, as it did with many Buddhist and New Age teachers I had been exposed to. The idea that everything you feel, think, remember, and regret is unreal. It's all illusory, a misguided identification with a self that doesn't actually exist. And what is real, then? I continued reading: "As you go more deeply into this realm of no-mind, as it is sometimes called in the East, you realize the state of pure consciousness. In that state, you feel your own presence with such intensity and such joy that all thinking, all emotions, your physical body, as well as the whole external world become relatively insignificant in comparison to it. And yet this is not a selfish but a selfless state. It takes you beyond what you previously thought of as 'your self.' That presence is essentially you and at the same time inconceivably greater than you. What I am trying to convey here may sound paradoxical or even contradictory, but there is no other way that I can express it." He also stated, "... all the things that truly matter—beauty, love, creativity, joy, inner peace—arise from beyond the mind."

This instantly got my alarm bells ringing and reeked of an inconsistency I could not reconcile. On the one hand, he was stating that the mind—which he had previously defined to include thoughts, ego, and emotions (particularly emotions emanating from the so-called pain-body), are unreal reflections of the false self. Yet, on the other hand, what is real is the mind-less and joyous and pure state of present-centered consciousness that arises when we can somehow rise above our forms. In other words, the only thing that is real is the bliss, love, and inner peace that comes after we detach from the self. But isn't joy an emotion, too? Isn't creation as alive in the shadows, as it is in the light? Doesn't the human experience include the complete spectrum? Why are painful emotions deemed to be "the mind," and "unreal," but not the sweet blissful sensations one experiences when they are sitting on a park bench without a care in the world? And who is the one experiencing the bliss? The illusion of the self, or *the self, itself*? It seemed to me that it could only be the latter. Something actual had to feel it. If the self is registering the joy, it can only be the self that is registering the pain, as well. You can't have one, without the other. They are two sides of the same coin, rather than one being false and impure, and the other true and pure.

It couldn't be this simplistic, could it? False is what hurts, and true is what feels good? When examined closely, this felt more like a feel-good approach to spirituality than a path of real substance. In my experience, if bliss is your all-pervasive state, it's not authentic bliss you are experiencing. It's the relief of having found a mechanism to sidestep pain, confusing relief with transformation. I smelled something disturbingly familiar. Drug addicts are well-versed in this mechanism. And so are pain bypassers, like myself.

I could not help but wonder: Was this an enlightenment dance, or a trauma trance? Was Tolle actually an informed spiritual teacher, or just another pain averse head-tripper?

I didn't stop there. There was still more to undress. I went back in, listening to him for many more hours. Now I was a man on a mission. It was clear to me: It wasn't that I needed these teachings to augment my spiritual life. It was apparent that these teachings were serving as a laboratory for my exploration into spirituality. And the discrepancies were becoming glaringly obvious. In essence, Tolle purported that his teachings were leading us more into the *now* than our habitual consciousness. While in fact, his version of the now—floating in the meditative stillness severed from the emotional body—wasn't *now* at all. Certainly not the rich, colorful, multi-threaded experience of the here-now that I had intimately come to know. How does one step fully into the now while detaching from their humanness?

At the heart of the framework was an oddly robotic idea of presence, one where we spend our precious lives inside of a witness consciousness. Detachment surely has a place—as an opportunity to gain a vaster perspective on habitual ways of being, and as a temporary refuge from the world of feeling. But when relied upon consistently, it becomes another safe-playing head-trip: using one part of the mind to tame another part of the mind. At best, this was basic level Buddhism packaged for the West.

This doesn't mean it can't be useful, but the balancing act was to not take it too far and end up floating in the lifeless emptiness with no road map for our return. What do you do once you get too far out there? How does one come back into their selfhood and integrate this vaster consciousness with their humanness—their emotions, identifications, memories, issues, and patterns? Where's the bridge between the transcendent and the immanent? Unity consciousness meets self-awareness? Story bridged with timeless essence?

The Universe or God or evolutionary intelligence seemed to go to a lot of trouble to craft a distinct self. What on earth for? To float into the transcendent emptiness? Did we each come in unique human form with the sole purpose of discovering our peace outside of it? What then is real, if all of our personal identifications are false? The eternal stillness? Isn't that our inevitable destiny—when we die? What of the self? What of the ground? What of all those undigested emotions waiting at the gate of transformation? What of the alchemical relationship between dark and light, pain and pleasure? What about integrating our macro-lens with the hard-earned miracle of the self, itself? When does identifying with the impersonal support our healing, and when does it annihilate the jewel of the self altogether?

All of these questions swirled and flowed, like a sparkling river of insights. I went back into his book again, like a spiritual detective in search of clues that would break through the facade. The discernment didn't come solely from my mind—it was like an ancient intelligence encoded within my very own being. As I kept reading, I worked to unpeel each layer and uncover the presumption at the core. Wherever I looked, the teachings seemed to express the same thing: parceling off the comforting aspects of the human experience, from those that challenge us. The former, Tolle characterized as fundamental to a pure consciousness. The latter was vilified as symbols of our separation from a pure consciousness.

For example, he referenced, "the ego, as a substitute for your true self rooted in Being." Nowhere does he state that the ego can serve both a healthy and an unhealthy function. But was the ego really the problem, or was it just another scapegoat for our currently unresolved stage of human development? I couldn't write these words without an ego. In addition, Tolle had written of silence as "an even more potent carrier of presence," one that "immediately creates stillness inside you," when you listen to it. He concluded with the following statement: "And what is stillness other than presence, consciousness freed from thought forms."

In other words, only within the experience of silence and stillness, do we find peace. And yet, my most potent memories of presence were sometimes silent and still, and sometimes noisy and dynamic. I had often found an experience of presence in the heart of lovemaking, emotional release, breathwork, dance, *life*! Even in pain, there can be profound presence. For instance, when you find out someone you love has died, a wave of grief floods in, and carrying it along is *presence*. You are moved and stirred—in touch with the profound meaning of life in the very midst of your sorrow. Profoundly present.

Despite my points of disagreement, I understood why Tolle's message was being received so positively by the mainstream. It was perhaps the first time we as a society had been invited out of our limiting self-identifications to taste a vaster perspective of our inner and outer lives. Yet, other than the helpful tool of temporarily witnessing our patterns and issues, I had to wonder if this approach was actually taking us anywhere good? Was this the power of now, or the power of *then*? The New Earth or the New Mars? Were these teachings those of an enlightened master, or merely a master of self-avoidance?

I went back in and read the Introduction to PON with a more seasoned lens—eyes that had just been through a rich, explorative experiment. I now saw the intro much differently. Tolle's flash of sudden and instantaneous enlightenment that left him homeless on a park bench, surrendered in bliss, now registered very differently in me: "I understood that the intense pressure of suffering that night must have forced my consciousness to withdraw from its identification with the unhappy and deeply fearful self, which is ultimately a fiction of the mind. This withdrawal must have been so complete that this false, suffering self immediately collapsed, just as if a plug had been pulled out of an inflatable toy. What was left then was my true nature as the ever-present *I am*: consciousness in its pure state prior to identification with form."

If there was one thing I knew for certain from my own healing journey, it was that you don't dissolve your emotional material that quickly. You may find a temporary technique to buffer you from your pain, thus preserving your life, but it is not possible to work through that level of suffering in the blink of a (third) eye. There may be a momentary peek into a vaster perspective. But that is only the beginning of the work that lies ahead: in fully embodying, integrating, and re-assimilating those emotions and wounds. A suicidal man does not fully heal and transform his consciousness in the course of one night. The pain still exists in your emotional body, your memories, your somatic structure, your cells. Material doesn't just dissolve like 1-2-3 hocus pocus! It took a long time for the pain to form roots in your consciousness, and those roots won't be eradicated in one evening. Not a chance.

Tolle purported being "peace," but it was not the kind of integrated, enlivened peace that comes at the end of a long, transformative healing journey into the heart of the embodied self. This was either pure dissociation, as many therapists would identify, or an initial stage of awakening—the preliminary stage when we first realize that there is a vaster framework of perception that exists beyond the ever-familiar mind and its habitual way of thinking. But it was not enlightenment. This was not the more difficult, and ultimately satisfying path, of weaving the transcendent with the immanent, the sky with the earth, the truth of oneness with the truth of individual story. This was just one man's attempt to abate his suffering.

And yet, I understood the temptation. We live in a traumatized world. We are an overwhelmed and often over-stimulated humanity. For many of us, it's difficult to be here. In order to survive, detachment practices are truly essential. At least until the danger passes. But no longer than that, or we run the risk of making things far worse for ourselves.

There's a big difference between momentary peace and sustainable transformation. At some point we have to return home. Not our cosmic home, but our embodied home: our selfhood. The cosmic home comes later, when we die. Let's not go there before our time.

The Yogic Path

Around this time, several aspects in my life began to shift. First, it became near impossible for me to take long periods of time off from writing. The call to write had become so fundamental to who I was that it began to assert itself even when I was doing business. I would be inside a home making a sale and find myself writing notes on the back of contracts. I would be on the way to a sales appointment, and pull over to the side of the road to re-language a paragraph I had written months before. My juvenile tendency to bifurcate my consciousness between ways of being—in this case, aggressive salesperson versus surrendered creative—was being exposed as yet another unsustainable dichotomy. It was now imperative that both aspects exist simultaneously. A vital step towards integrating and unifying my consciousness. An essential step towards a spirituality that was indistinguishable from daily life.

While surrendering to the river of language, a peace would overcome me. It was the peace that prevails when you have found your way home. It wasn't a serene, ripple-less peace—it was alive to the touch, gritty and chaotically magnificent. In the heart of, and even long after each creative outpouring, I felt energetically transported—at once floating on a vast and unlimited sea, and simultaneously, heartfully affixed to my unique mission at the center of it. It was a remarkable experience of what I would later call "sacred purpose."

The call to write was both intrinsic to my sacred purpose in this lifetime—embodying and expressing the *why* I am here—and also another gateway to the Divine. It was evidence of the synergistic relationship between presence and purpose. Deepening into the moment reveals your purpose, while deepening into your purpose expands your presence. The *what it is* to be here, and the *why it is* that you are here, are essentially reflections of—and portals into—each other.

As the call to write firmly took root, I began to regularly attend yoga class. One of the unexpected and profound benefits of my practice, was that the more I energized my body, the more I energized the calling. Quite often, I would go to class and actually stop partway through to jot down ideas and sentences for the book. What was most interesting was the dynamic relationship between the potency of the *asanas* (yoga postures) and the breadth of the writing that arose. The more I opened and enlivened my body on the mat, the more clarified and multifaceted the language that emerged. The freer my body lines, the freer my book lines. It was as though the words and ideas were inscribed deep within my musculature, just waiting for their opportunity to be excavated and wordsmithed into tangible form. The mind may have been the instrument that interpreted them, but the body was the temple that expressed them.

Perhaps the most vivid testament to this happened one day while I was cycling to class. I had been ruminating on the book's title for weeks, to no avail. I then made the decision to stop thinking about it altogether. The next day, while pedaling with all my might in an effort to avoid missing class, the curious word, *soulshaping*, kept rising into awareness. There the title was, waiting inside my body to be written into being.

Soon, I encountered the limitations of traditional yoga. One day, while attending an Ashtanga class with a friend, we began laughing at a private joke at the back of the class. The yoga teacher glared at us from the front of the studio. That didn't stop us, so he proceeded to make his way to the back of the class, where he came up close and personal and said curtly, "There is no laughter in yoga." He was dead serious.

After class, I devoted some time to researching the roots of yoga. What I found fascinated me. Although the word "yoga" means "to unite," it is not premised on the broadly inclusive form of unity that I had been seeking on my spiritual quest. This was actually a version of unity that is bifurcated and fragmented—compartmentalizing our emotional lives from our spiritual lives.

In its origins, yoga was designed as a purifying practice, a disciplined series of exercises intended to control the mind and purify the toxic body beast. Only through the disciplined containment and mastery of the body—including the emotional body—could one touch pure consciousness. There was no place for laughter, or anger, or tears, or pain-bodies, on the mat.

I began to drop into classes at studios offering various brands of yoga. And what I found was consistent. Although some were more liberal with respect to humor, none emphasized the value of emotional engagement and expression as fundamental to the practice. This very controlled approach was perhaps perfect for the wildly unruly—desperately in need of emotional containment. But it was not particularly helpful for those, like me, who were already driven and disciplined, and more in need of a practice that would shake loose feeling and expression. And it could be a potentially dangerous spiritual practice for trauma survivors. The asanas would excavate their unresolved wounds—as Lowen's Bioenergetics techniques do—but they would be discouraged from feeling into and expressing these tidal waves on the mat. They would be all opened up with no safe place to release.

I started to take a little time after yoga class, to deepen and integrate any feelings that emerged. And then I explored my own custom-designed yoga practice behind closed doors. As I practiced in my private space, I began to invite my various feelings to the surface. If I felt anger rise into awareness during an asana, I expressed it. If tears emerged, I cried. And not just painful emotions. If I was tickled by humor, I laughed. If I felt inspired to dance, I danced. I would move into the asanas and then break into whatever form of movement and expression organically arose in me. It produced a remarkably different experience and outcome.

When I would contain my feelings, I would come to the end of the class feeling energized but incomplete. I could sense that part of my consciousness had opened, but I did not feel unified and broadly present. Yet when I allowed for the broadest range of emotional expression and release, I arrived at the end of the session in a palpable state of grace. Much like the same multi-threaded state I had known as a child on my backyard lawn, feeling the stars weave into my body. It felt like I was here for all of it. As with all "spiritual practices," it comes down to intentionality. That is, do you want to engage in a practice in an effort to rise above aspects of the human experience, or in an effort to engage with all of it?

Karmageddon

Time passed, and I began to grow more grounded and seasoned in my approach to human-beingness. I was no longer looking outside myself—or in need of anything—yet whatever came my way, served as the perfect fodder to develop and deepen my own solid foundation.

Soon, I found my next laboratory for spiritual exploration—in the form of a dreadlocked, bliss-tripper named Bhagavan Das (BD). He was a kirtan chanter and self-proclaimed guru made famous in the best-selling book, *Be Here Now*, written by former Harvard professor Richard Alpert (aka Ram Dass). An American exploring India in the late '60s, BD was the one who brought Richard to the feet of his guru, Neem Karoli Baba (Maharaji), where Richard had the consciousness-expanding experiences that he shared in his renowned book. By the time BD rolled into my house, he had been on the road for years, making his living leading kirtan chants and Nada Yoga workshops worldwide. Commonly practiced in India, Kirtan is the repetitive chanting or singing of God's name. Intrinsic to the Hindu *bhakti* path (the path of devotion), it invites us to nestle into a more unified consciousness. Nada yoga is the yoga of sound.

I had first encountered BD years earlier. Chanting with him at California's Harbin Hot Springs had the distinct effect of igniting my sexuality during an intimacy-avoidant stage with Rebecca. I had been entirely restrained… until the two-hour chant somehow got my juices flowing. So I began to see him when he came to chant in Toronto. Each time I experienced a strong vibration quaking through me, as the intense guttural sounds acted like a chisel that cracked my emotional armor from the inside out. I would often find myself discharging anger and tears, arriving at the end of the session completely renewed. It was the first traditional spiritual practice I experienced that entwined my physical and emotional selves seamlessly and effectively. I chanted, and it all came together inside me.

In addition, I found BD's adherence to Hindu philosophy congruent with my own inclinations. Whereas many of the practitioners I had become cynical about advocated the Buddhist principles of detaching from life on the quest for enlightenment—the forms of Hinduism and Sufism that he espoused were all about jumping into life and experiencing divinity everywhere, in the heart of everything. After Tolle and the like, I was ready to explore passion, energy, vitality!

BD was all that and more. He was a wild-man at heart, unruly, irreverent, uncontained, unrestrained. He spoke his mind. He acted impromptu. He swore. He loved mischief. This was all magically enticing to me after so many detours on the straight and narrow spiritual paths. Given that I had experienced my greatest openings when I was activating more, rather than fewer, threads of awareness, I felt confident that the wisdom yielded from his decades-long exploration of spirituality would bear many fruits.

Soon the idea of a documentary came into being: *Karmageddon*. I wasn't sure what the film would look like, but had a sense that it would unveil itself as we went along. BD, always up for mischief and a shot at the limelight, happily obliged to be my subject.

On the first filming stint, he stayed with me in my home. We filmed a long series of energized dialogues, biographical pieces, chants and rants. Eager to distill the most cohesive parts of his message, I told myself to just surrender to his wildness. It would all work out in the end. And it did—but not quite in the way I had imagined.

In the presence of the Wildman, I had a palpable experience of bound-arylessness, a uniquely chromatic immersion into a field of expansive consciousness. When BD said that the squirrel was also God, I really felt it. When he spoke of Maharaji and his powers, I felt myself transported some-where magical. When we walked the neighborhood, it no longer felt like the same place I had lived for ten years. It felt like a divinely orchestrated puzzle, one in which every single aspect served a unique and instrumental purpose. There was no one and nothing superior, every being, object and sensation was alchemically necessary and fundamental to the greater weave.

Before our second filming trip, I interviewed and dialogued with many members of the spiritual community. I was interested in their lens on BD, and particularly how they viewed the relationship between integrity and enlightenment. It was beginning to befuddle me that many spiritual seek-ers could claim to be enlightened while not acting in integrity in all areas of their life. Could someone truly be enlightened if they were unconcerned about their impact on others? Could you be a credible voice of spiritual authority if you were not aligned within *all* of your chakras and levels?

This was clearly my next phase of integration, and exploration.

Much to my surprise, many of those interviewed provided the same essential answer—particularly the men. I paraphrase the sentiment, "Enlightenment has nothing to do with morality—enlightenment comes to who it comes to."

In other words, you don't have to work on your emotional life, your blind spots, your inauthentic aspects, your fetishes, indulgences, obsessions, and infatuations—since enlightenment will simply land where it lands, kind of like a bird will just happen to shit on whichever head it shits on. No point in taking precautions or doing the rigorous work. It's all arbitrary. It comes to who it comes to, no matter where or what you are, and how you are acting. I was suspicious: Could this really be true?

Interestingly, many of the seekers I spoke with quoted the popularized contention that someone can have an advanced spiritual life while being psychologically underdeveloped. They seemed intent on distinguishing waking up from growing up. In other words, you can be the most immature human alive, and still be deemed spiritually advanced. Was this correct, or is it only based on how broadly or narrowly we define spirituality?

If we define spirituality as a transcendent or single-threaded conscious-ness, one can certainly become enlightened without healing emotionally and developing psychologically. That would be an easy definition to live up to. Yet, if we define it as an inclusive experience—self and spirit as mutually dependent threads of the same holy weave—then those who do not align their emotional and behavioral lives with their spirit are far from spiritual beings. And surely not enlightened.

Bhagavan Das returned later that year for the next stage of filming. During this time with him, I paid closer attention to the ways that my body responded in his presence. I had noticed a tendency to unground on the first visit; in fact, it took days after he left to really feel my feet and my connec-tion to my practical responsibilities. But it was a very seductive experience of ungroundedness, because I actually relished the heightened sensations I experienced. On this second visit, the allure had worn off, and I began to see that the version of unity consciousness I was experiencing around him was actually quite dichotomous. Although I did feel connected to a vaster terrain, I did not feel like I was actually *here* for it. I did not feel fully present in my body, and rooted in my localized reality. I was swimming in an ocean of oneness—without a body. I was like a tall building without a basement or ground floor. Reaching for the heavens while wavering in the wind.

While he was in my home, I frequently flashed back to an experience I had with him after one of his Toronto kirtans some years before. As usual, I'd had a profoundly embodied experience during the chant, feeling more, rather than less, grounded in my body by the time it was done. Afterwards, I went over to BD to thank him for the experience, but he was in no mood for niceties. He was too busy mindlessly and erratically looking for some-thing under the meditation cushions and yoga mats.

"Bhagavan, can I help you? What are you looking for?" I asked.

"I lost my damn shoes! Where the hell did I leave them?" he replied.

"You don't have any memory of where you left them?"

"Of course not, I just finished chanting. I never remember where I left my shoes after kirtan."

Although I didn't yet understand why this was important, I intuitively knew that it was.

After he left Toronto, I proceeded to write him a scathing email, expressing my disappointment in some of his actions while he'd been in my home on this trip. His behaviors were entirely consistent with his spiritual perspective, but incongruent with my comfort zone. The email moved some of my emotions—but there was more energy to be released from my body. It was time for the Bioenergetic hitting cube. I taped BD's face to the cube—and clubbed it with all my might.

I wasn't truly clubbing BD, the man. I was clubbing out ungrounded spirituality. Slamming guru-worship. But there was still more to be processed. Even after dispelling these emotions—something was unsettled. I plummeted into a phase of deep confusion—both trying to reconcile these contradictory spiritual experiences and perspectives, *and* trying to come to terms with why I felt so drawn to him.

A Meeting with the Godfather of Western Spirituality

My burning inquiry culminated in a flight to Maui, to film a dialogue with Ram Dass. When I arrived at his home, he was sitting in his wheelchair, debilitated after suffering a stroke several years before, eyes soft and open, modeling the inextricable relationship between the emotional body and spirit. I felt deeply touched by his presence.

We began to talk about his 30-year relationship with BD. I shared my confusion. Looking back now, it is clear that I was trapped between two perspectives. One was rooted in common sense. I saw through BD's actions, and did not trust his intentions. The other was more of a "karmic" lens, one that bought into BD's assertion that his actions were actually intended for the higher good. Over and over again, he would tell me that he was "upsetting the apple cart"—not because of his own issues, but because the suffering that we endured at his hands was precisely what we needed to wake up. He was merely a vessel of service. If we were upset, it was because there was something for *us* to look at.

Ram Dass set me straight. Through his dignified presence, and his wise words, he helped me to understand that BD's intention was not always honorable. He made it clear that anyone claiming to be a guru must live up to their highest teachings at all levels of awareness and action. Clearly, BD wasn't.

On the flight home, and in the weeks that followed, a degree of lucidity emerged. One of the clearest realizations related to the concept of "spiritual bypassing," a term first coined by author John Welwood in 1984 to describe the tendency "to use spiritual practice to rise above the difficulties of unresolved personal problems and emotions."

Based on my experiences with BD, it was safe to say that he was a classic spiritual bypasser. Rather than turning to spirituality in an effort to become more integrated with embodied life, he turned to it in an effort to transcend his localized experience—that is, to get the hell out of here. His actions spoke volumes. He had no interest in raising the standard of his emotional and behavioral life to meet his self-proclaimed state of enlightenment. He preferred to keep them conveniently separate. As a result, he was like a bird with one wing, flying in circles, eventually crashing back to earth. Because I felt more deeply rooted *here*, after chanting with him, I made the assumption that this was also the case for himself and everyone who chanted as a spiritual practice. My mistake. He couldn't find his shoes for a reason.

One of the most obvious indicators of the spiritual bypass was the prevalence of name-changing in various spiritual communities, as though assuming a new name will somehow change the story that lives in the bones of your being. Many of those I interviewed and connected with had been re-named by a guru, or simply by their own choosing. Bhagavan Das's real name was Kermit Michael Riggs, until Maharaji re-named him. And on it went, countless seekers with cool Sanskrit names. If only it were this simple—change your name and your insides change to.

But in reality, it doesn't do anything other than perpetuate the ungrounded belief that our "true self" is something distinct from our personal history. It's one thing to identify a name that symbolizes who we wish to become, but name-changing alone will not make it so. It may provide a momentary relief, or sense of a fresh start, but as we proceed with the course of our lives, our stuffed-down stuff will surely re-emerge. At some point, we have to come back into our selfhood and do the work to integrate and become that in real time.

Worldly Matters

One night, I had a dream. I saw an elderly guru sitting in meditative repose in a dirty old cave. There was a golden light emanating from him, a divinely inspired luminosity of spirit. Watching him watching his thoughts, I got the feeling he had been there for years. Soon a hunched, elderly Indian woman entered the cave with a small glass of milk in her hand. She walked over to him, opened his mouth, and lovingly supported his head while he drank the milk. A deep love radiated from her eyes. At first, the image moved me. A saintly man, sacrificing his personal life so he could reach enlightenment, supported by his loyal community. And then, the dream-scape turned dark, as the saint began to morph into a demonic and impure entity. His face contorted and distorted, taking on the form of a deceiver, someone who had pulled the wool over the eyes of the villager. She had been conditioned to believe that he was a great one, an enlightened being focused on heightened cosmic matters. While she and the other women in the village were mere mortals, focused on lowly human concerns— relationships, basic needs, worldly matters. As the dream progressed, the truth was revealed. His image faded entirely from view, now fully at one with the darkness he so determinedly fled. And his "lowly" servant, became more luminous, as the light of the heavens shone bright on her divine countenance, revealing both her self and her worldly engagements as the substance of God.

I woke up early and walked around Wychwood Park, a former artists' colony near my home. It was here that I had frequently filmed dialogues with BD. Stopping at one of the trees we filmed at, looking up at the sky, watching the clouds slowly drift, I thought about the word "heightened," a concept so prevalent in my personal conversations with BD, and with so many other men I had engaged in spiritual dialogues. What was it about this concept? Where on earth did they get the idea that the spiritual quest for enlightenment was a heightened one, literally or metaphorically? That our purest point of consciousness is up there, floating above the human experience? Why higher, instead of deeper, more grounded, or more authentic? Why top-down instead of bottom-up? Why in the vast sky rather than down here on Mother Earth, breath in the body, hands in the dirt, where life is actually *lived*?

As I looked up, I invited myself to feel into what it meant to look for it, up there. I stood more upright, replacing my habitual slouch with a heightened stance. I stayed poised for some time, allowing myself to settle into an odd sense of satisfaction that I no longer had to look for meaning down here, where it hurt so damn much, but, instead, up. In the cloudy sky and in the vast cosmic space. It was a great relief, albeit a momentary one. Soon I became bored; as beautiful as it was, there was only so much I could find up there. And then I became anxious, as I recognized that I could no longer connect with reality with my eyes pointed up above.

I got down on the ground and rubbed by feet and ass into the dirt. It felt good to be here. I was in human form, for a reason. And that reason was not to bypass my humanity vertically and stare into the void. It was not to imagine that the most evolved path was a heightened and metaphorically "higher than." Again, it was to live in the heart of the everything.

Daddy Dearest

Bhagavan Das returned for a final trip. Although I hoped for some form of relational resolution between us, there was something else I needed more. I needed to understand why I summoned this experience into my life. There is no question that I was learning essential lessons about spiritual life, but there was something else. I could sense it in my bones. It turned out it was something entirely unexpected.

As we walked and talked, it slowly dawned on me. Bhagavan was never my guru, never my teacher or guide. But he was something to me. He was my father. Not a spitting image, but similar in the ways that pull on our primal unconscious. Both tall, lithe, and muscular. They even smelled the same. And, I responded to him as I had responded to my father as a young boy—by denying his shadow and elevating him at every turn. A boy yearns for the fatherly presence so fervidly that he will ignore all failings, all shortcomings.

By the time Bhagavan left Toronto, I understood. He was a calling back to a yet-unhealed part of myself. In my years of therapy, I had focused primarily on my combative relationship with my mother. I had scarcely explored my father wound. But, as undigested pain always does, it refused to be buried.

In this way, my journey with Bhagavan was as much a journey of personal redemption as it was an opportunity to study spirituality. At its heart, it confirmed something that I had been coming to understand for years— that my own quest for emotional healing was indistinguishable from my quest for a more enlightened life. Left unattended, my unresolved father wound could not help but obstruct my spiritual access. Yet if I could seize the day and do the deeper work, I stood a chance of growing in karmic stature. Or perhaps stature is the wrong word. It was about growing more fully... human.

In the months that followed, I devoted time to working inside my father wound. My time with Bhagavan Das had peeled back the scab of a festering wound—and I knew it would be no quick fix. But the process had begun. In the heart of it, I arrived at a new depth of understanding about a life of purpose. Purpose is not just that great thing that calls us to certain offerings in the world. It is also the unresolved emotional issues that grow us. Simply put, wherever there is growth, there is purpose—and to the extent that we can heal and work through our emotional blocks, we mature in every regard.

The Pushcart Guru

I continued to sell windows and to work on *Soulshaping*. When the manuscript was finally complete—or so I imagined—I went online and searched for spiritual publishers. I filled in a query form on the first one that appeared. Within a few days, I received an email asking me to send the manuscript over. Weeks later, I received an offer to publish. It turned out that the publisher had rejected the book in its original form, but their savvy editor had worked on it for weeks, getting it to the stage where they would make an offer. But there was one catch—I had to accept a significant decrease in word count.

I took a step back to consider the contract. On one level, I was delighted—one publisher, one offer. On another, I was upset. I had spent over 6 years inside this book—how dare they cut it down without my permission?! I sat with the question for a number of weeks, before rejecting their offer. Although there may well have been many financial and egoic benefits, I had to remain aligned with the intention that sourced the book: The voice of the soul. And my soul's story didn't take kindly to being cut nearly in half.

I self-published *Soulshaping* later that autumn. Soon thereafter, I joined Facebook in an effort to promote my book. Although it felt overwhelming, it also felt entirely familiar. I had spent nearly 20 years talking to new people while selling product door-to-door. Now I got to do the same thing on the computer, one fresh face at a time.

Then, another unexpected twist. (Life is such a little monkey, you never know what's going to happen next.) When I would walk the streets of Toronto, I would often see a tall homeless man, skin the color of dark coffee, whom I dubbed the Pushcart Guru. At first I would just pass him by, not paying him much mind. Just another nameless, faceless panhandler, doing his thing. But one day, I actually stopped to see him. And listen. His name was Slim—and turned out there was far more to Slim than meets the eye.

Soon after, I bumped into him at a Starbucks. When I told him about my book, his eyes widened. We began to talk, and right before my eyes, something unfolded. Soon, we were discussing an unconventional way to distribute the book. It was a little glimmer of a bigger picture that gave me soul shivers. The bigger picture would be tucked away for the future—when the time was ripe. But for now, Slim would start to sell my book on the streets, as a way of earning income and bridging himself back to the world. A win-win for both of us, and for those who would be blessed to encounter his wisdom and infectious energy.

Soon enough, he instructed me to design a sweater for him with the slogan: "Buy a great self-help book here," and he went to work, selling hundreds of books in very little time. Media came to showcase him, and people began to order books from around the world. Their orders often came with one qualifier: "Ask Slim to sign the book." Not *me*... Slim! Humbled yet again.

Back to the Island Oasis

A few months later, the positive energy around the book attracted a publishing offer from North Atlantic Books in California. They accepted my primary stipulation—to leave the word count, as is. I signed the deal.

Just before the book was republished, I went back to visit with Ram Dass in Maui. Now that I had come to terms with my projected father figure, Bhagavan Das, I wanted to spend more time with the godfather—someone I had grown to love. He had been a great help to me during a personal crisis—offering advice that served me on a profound and meaningful level. I was very grateful to him for his compassion and his wisdom.

He had read Soulshaping, and we began to explore some its primary themes in his Maui home. One of the first things he expressed was the belief that my emphasis on psycho-emotional healing processes as intrinsic to the soul's journey was both "neurotic" and "incompatible" with a spiritual consciousness. He was particularly troubled by the Soulshaping Dictionary—a list of terms I had crafted and added to the back of the book—because it made little or no distinction between psychological and spiritual experiences.

Before going deeper into that question, we focused on the relationship between the ego and the soul—yet another point of deviation between us. Where Ram Dass had often referred to the ego as antithetical to the soul and had promoted the idea that our spiritual advancement depends on the dissipation of the ego, I was coming to believe that nothing fundamental to human development could be soul-averse. For example, we need a healthy ego to function. How could I express my voice in this book without one?

And, more precisely, I was coming to believe that the progressive evolution of the ego is functionally intertwined with the evolution of the soul. In other words, our ego state directly reflects our stage of soulular growth. For example, if one of my life lessons is the healing of my mother wound, does not my fragmented ego with respect to this issue reflect the fragmented shape of my Soul?

Ram Dass and I engaged in an animated discussion. I played ego's advocate, Ram Dass—soul's advocate. And he actually moved a few steps in my direction. He acknowledged some responsibility with respect to the perceived ego/soul split in the West. When he wrote *Be Here Now,* he was counter-balancing the unhealthily egoic nature of Western Culture: the materialism, the headiness, the marked disconnect from a soulful consciousness. We were identifying ourselves as our ego rather than understanding the ego as a vehicle for spiritual transformation. His calling demanded that he put the soul's journey front and center, in order to help bring us into alignment. We needed a strong shot of Soul to wake us up. But now, 35 years later, he was open to a wider and more nuanced perspective. He certainly didn't agree with my declaration that the soul and the ego are indistinguishable, ("They are two planes of consciousness," he said), but he did agree that they are not the antithesis of one another.

After a little more banter, Ram Dass grabbed his copy of the Soulshaping Dictionary, and told me to come back the next day to continue our dialogue. I agreed. As he wheeled himself out of the room, he again called out that I was neurotic to strongly emphasize the connection between psychological processes and spiritual development. He was agitated, and, at the same time, ready to bravely confront the question.

The next day, we put on our gloves and jumped back into the ring. To the best of my recollection, this was our conversation. I said, "Ram Dass, some of my greatest leaps forward spiritually arose through my emotional healings. When I healed parts of my mother wound during a Holotropic Breathwork, I took a quantum leap. When I threaded my heart back together after a shattering love experience, my presence deepened. It was all grist for the soul mill. Without it, no healing. No expansion. The heal was for real."

He disagreed: "Why do you have to focus in that direction? Life itself will bring you tragic events—a car accident, or a medical calamity—and they will be the grist for your transformation. They will awaken you."

I already knew that he referred to his recent stroke as "Fierce Grace"— his guru's way of bringing him more fully into the moment.

I responded, "Why must it go that far, just work through your emotional material and you will transform. Why wait for a stroke—just work on your family of origin issues. Repressed emotions are un-actualized spiritual lessons."

He agreed that we live our incarnation material through our bodies, but he resisted my call to therapeutic process as fundamental to the enlightenment journey: "The psychological and the spiritual are distinct planes of awareness."

He was acutely concerned that our tendency to wallow in the psychological would inhibit our spiritual progress. Fair enough.

"I agree. It's a fine line between self-pity and a healthy working through of the material," I said. "At the same time, we cannot shape our soul to the next stage, if we don't deal with our psychological material. Not identifying ourselves as our stuff, but identifying our stuff as a key to our transformation. What else grows us from the ground up?"

Eventually, Ram Dass came a little closer to my view. Not that psycho-emotional healing was the *only* path to awakening—but that it could be one of them. And I agreed with him—that there were a number of authentic paths to awakening. We had found a healthy middle ground to stand upon.

Returning to Toronto, I reflected on my visit with the godfather of Western spirituality. If anything, my respect for him had grown. I had challenged him on what I perceived to be a blind spot, which was never an easy dialogue. But his love of the truth had prevailed. He could have told me not to return after the first day, but he chose to meet me head-on and go deeper into the question. It was precisely this brave part of him that had done so much to help humanity: bringing Eastern wisdoms to the West, engaging in countless acts of charitable service. This was not a spiritual teacher who lived in an avoidant bubble. He was a remarkable person-of-action, for decades making tireless efforts to benefit humanity. And this hadn't ended when he became ill. He continued to spread the love and share his wisdom freely. He continued to move from his heart.

At the same time, I was perplexed. I already knew from our past interactions that Ram Dass was not a spiritual bypasser. He believed strongly in the relationship between personal integrity and spiritual awakening. He had made that clear when I interviewed him for *Karmageddon*. And, even in these conversations, he had done something far more grounded than other teachers I had connected with. He had allowed our awakening to come through the heart of the human story—in the form of illness and accident—rather than through its transcendence. This comforted me.

Yet here was this theme again: that our psychological and spiritual lives are on separate tracks. That one does not awaken or evolve spiritually through the processing and healing of their emotional wounds and psychological issues. And this belief felt like the tip of a remarkably massive iceberg of self-avoidance—one that spread pervasively throughout the spiritual world, somehow blocking our access to a more inclusive and integrated perspective. Ram Dass was a rare gem—a spiritual leader open to a more inclusive perspective, but many weren't.

I had to wonder: Were any spiritual teachers truly interested in the entirety of the human experience, or were they all looking for a way to sidestep their painful childhoods under the cloak of enlightenment? Where to find a spirituality that welcomed all of who we are, and all of what this is, into its arms?

The Weaver of My Heart

In the months after *Soulshaping* was re-published, my life was unfolding at quantum speed. I was selling windows full time, writing articles and original quotes far into the night, and doing numerous radio shows in between. I also continued to work on *Karmageddon* (my "labor of hate"), pumped out a series of inspirations for ABC'S *Good Morning America* website and other e-zines, went on a short book signing tour, and continued to grow in social media.

It was a wildly dynamic time, with so much compressed into each day—and yet I was overcome with delight. No one ever said that sacred purpose was going to make your life easier. In fact, it may do just the opposite, adding heaping new portions to your plate. What it does provide is the energizing satisfaction that comes with knowing that you are exactly where you belong on your life's journey. That satisfaction somehow compels and impels you, awakening deep reserves of energy you didn't know you had. Peace with path.

In the heart of the overwhelm, I continued to organically grow in the direction of a more integrative consciousness. Perhaps because everything was so compressed together, distinctions between compartments of self became more difficult to make. The extroverted salesman, the privacy-hungry author, and the media-friendly interviewee were all merging—albeit sloppily, but it was happening! The threads of my sacred purpose were simultaneously bleeding together.

My painful early-life issues around being highly visible, and vulnerable to criticism or diminishment, piggybacked onto the calling to bring my writing into the world on a larger scale. Every time my following suddenly leapt in numbers, I found myself fantasizing about hiding in my closet with a bag of Oreos. I even did once. And then, I would burrow into the healing of the hypervigilance and invite myself out a little further into that which frightened me. Similarly, the archetypal dance between my healer self and my warrior self continued to evolve, as my capacity to hold both ways of being concurrently became more fluid. I was slowly becoming more "one" after many years of being safely compartmentalized.

At some point, the call to write again intensified, waking me up in the night, demanding to be expressed. I could feel it in there, whispering incessantly in my inner ear, driven to take up more space. It was nearing the time to write another long book. But how? I was at my energetic limit. There were only so many hours in the day.

One night, I had a clear dream. In it, I was sitting in a house in the country, quietly writing the love story that I knew had to be told. I woke up with conviction—it was time to move to the country where I could get more fully lost in my call to write. I didn't need to look for signs outside of myself, for my next steps. They were inside me. Precise wisdom and direction born right from my own cells. I sold my Toronto home soon thereafter and purchased a new build in the country.

While waiting for the house to be built, a piece that had been nagging at me for some time came through me rapid-fire one autumn afternoon. "Apologies to the Divine Feminine (from a warrior in transition)" first went up as a Facebook note, and then went viral later that day, ultimately reaching millions. The message was obviously the next step that many of us were ready for, and a living reflection of my own internal shifts towards a more heartfelt, gender-inclusive, and surrendered way of being. As I explored my inner terrain and the spiritual community, it became unwaveringly clear that men had apologies to make before we could even begin to evolve our species. First things, first.

The piece was also inspired by my dynamic with my grandmother. I was particularly touched watching her—after my grandfather died—sitting endearingly in her little chair with the phone on one knee and a small birth-date book on her other knee, checking daily to see whose birthday it was and to give them a call. Ah, the days before texting. How heart-warming to hear an actual voice on the other end of the phone.

One day, in the flash of a moment, I saw the whole gender trip differ-ently. How my grandfather—off to the marketplace each day to claim his stake as a master salesman—had been elevated, while my grandmother, focusing on whether I was warm and ate enough, was seen as less signifi-cant. Through this new lens, her bravery and courage were remarkably obvious to me. Not that his path was easy, but there was something much harder and deeper and truer about hers. Because it involved all the intrica-cies and sensitivities of human relationships. We reward emotional armor because it allows us to "succeed" in a survivalist world, when we should be honoring those who have the courage to remain emotionally receptive and open on the battlefields of life.

After I moved into the new home, my creative life accelerated to the next level. With little to distract me, new language poured through me seam-lessly and ceaselessly. I scribed hundreds of new quotes for social media, and I began to edge into the writing of my relational tale: *An Uncommon Bond*. A passionate love story, the book was inspired by my profoundly soulful, transformative relationship with Rebecca.

At the same time, my ideas about spirituality continued to develop more solid roots. The daily phenomena of encountering thousands of fellow path-travelers through social media, was stoking the fire of my inquiry. As Facebook shifted from a platform that shared mundane details and prac-tical information, to one of more intimate revealings and explorations in consciousness—it became a kind of peephole into the array of pertinent, burning questions others were grappling with. I found myself feeling even more connected to humanity, and determined to wrestle with the questions of spiritual meaning that thread through our collective experience.

Fundamental to this humanization phase, was a shift in my perspective towards the so-called New Age world. I soon found myself startled at my prior adherence to ungrounded New Age aphorisms: "Everything happens for a reason!", "It's all Good", and "It's all a mirror." Once you see the depth of pain people are in, you can't help but see through superficial messages about transformation. The softee-toffee versions of reality no longer suffice.

Following many months of excruciating edits, we finally reached the end of the *Karmageddon* movie-making adventure. It was not a moment too soon.

The call to write *An Uncommon Bond* had fully seized me. Soon thereafter, a bountiful blessing walked through my door on Facebook. Susan Frybort, the woman I had waited for, for over five decades, entered my life. A brilliant poetess, she spun her magical word weaves while working as an overworked and underpaid retail store tailor in Indiana. The most rooted, compassionate, and integrated mystic I have ever known, she spoke more wisdom in one paragraph than hundreds of gurus and hyped-up thought leaders uttered in years. More evidence that it was all right here, in the bones of our being.

Our microcosms began to overlap on Facebook, forming interconnected threads. We shared sweet writings back and forth, like innocent schoolchildren passing notes. Soon they grew in depth, tenderness, intimate revealings, and real communication. It was not an ungrounding event like my first soul-deep love. It was rooting and rooted, the breath of love coursing right through my bones, themselves. Thread by thread, we were weaving an authentic relationship. We made plans to meet each other in person in Amish country—Shipshewana, Indiana. Earthy and pristine, it was the perfect place to come home to the beloved.

Shortly after Susan and I became involved, I was faced with the sudden death of my father. He had died as he had lived—isolated and anonymous. I immediately plummeted into a state of intense grief, challenged to make sense of our difficult relationship while still living an overwhelmed life. One thing came clear at this stage. When you lose your first parent, you realize that you are somewhat asleep on the path to awakening. It's a whole different world after they die. This is true whether you are close to them or not. The preparation work you do before they pass, may be the most important inner work you ever do.

Susan came to stay with me in Canada the following year. Our first six months revolved around our creative outpourings. I was finishing *An Uncommon Bond*, and she was readying her first poetry collection, *Hope is a Traveler*, for publication. Interestingly, many of the words she had written to me in our private correspondence found their way into both books—in hers, in the form of poems, and in mine, in the form of delicious love writings from Sarah to Lowen, the two main characters. Our private tender interweaving threads of affection were now unveiled for the world to see.

Soon after Susan arrived—it came clear this was a relationship that would stand the tests of time. This was not a fleeting romance—but would invite a solid foundation to build upon, and grow deeper roots over time. The apparent next step was to be married. It dawned on us both quietly and simply, and without fanfare. Shortly before both books came out, we married in a simple ceremony in downtown Toronto. A special and sacred day indeed.

After settling into the rhythm of married life, the universe struck a few more blows. God is funky sometimes. My beloved cat, Sophie, suddenly died. She was more than "just an animal" to me—but a dear presence who had entered my life at a point of particular intensity. This furry ball of affection comforted me through many of life's challenges. And she had become a dear friend to Susan. The next week, my mother suddenly died. Some months later, Susan's father also passed away, abruptly. I was again overcome with grief. But, this time, I found myself approaching it differently. Where I had found myself dissociating from some of the pain after my father's death, I was now propelled to stop dancing so fervidly with separation. To nestle deep into the heart of my bewilderment, lostness, and grief. To really be here with *all* of it—the devastating loss of two parents so quickly, the loss of my animal companion, Susan's own grief around her father—and at the same time, the blessed arrival of my beloved... all of it happening simultaneously. Shadow to light, and back again.

Fissures and Fault Lines

After the successful release of *An Uncommon Bond*, I was invited to a Non-Duality conference to present with a group of other authors. For simplicity's sake, let's define non-duality (or *Advaita*, in Sanskrit) as unity-consciousness, a state of being that reflects the non-separate nature of reality. Polarity is negated. You look out at the world and see everything as one unified field. Although reluctant to attend, I had begun writing this book, *Grounded Spirituality*, and I was curious to see if others' ideas of non-duality were similar to, or different from, the very embodied and enlivened experience of unity-consciousness I had deepened into. Were we having the same experience of presence, or were we inherently relating to something different?

Before the conference, I seized the opportunity to dig deep into an exploration of the non-dual spiritual community. I viewed online *satsangs* (a gathering of truth-seekers) with Advaita "masters," and browsed some of the core texts in the field.

Once more, I leaned into the possibility that most of my thoughts and feelings were distractions from my "true" nature. They weren't the real thing. They were reflections of my grasping, my misidentification, my inability to see beyond distraction. I even allowed myself to momentarily surrender to the teacher as knower. So much of this practice seemed to be dependent on the presence of a guru-knower, at the head of the satsang. Instead of rejecting his knowing, I embraced it. I engaged in a number of traditional non-dual inquiry methods. Sometimes I meditated on a singular question—"Who am I?"—for hours at time. I spent time contemplating the questions at the heart of their practice: Who is the watcher? What is the nature of the self? Why am I here? I sat in the car, in the house, in my favorite cafe, contemplating the self, and what was beyond the self. Sometimes I would sit outside, in front of my favorite tree, contemplating the tree until it was no longer a separate entity. It was intrinsic to a unified field of perception. Although these premises were reminiscent of perspectives I had already rejected, I was oddly drawn to them. I wasn't sure why.

And then, one afternoon, in the heart of yet another online satsang, I woke up, or, perhaps better worded, I woke down. The guru-in-chief was talking about the illusion of the self, and I began to feel tremors of anxiety surge through my body, as though my very humanness was being led to slaughter. Fear rose within me, and a storm of panic, like I was at risk of losing something essential, something that I could never again return to.

I suddenly sensed that what was being presented in his teaching and in so many of the other satsangs I had witnessed was little more than another self-negation practice. In truth, this wasn't non-duality—this was something very familiar to me from my previous experience. That is, the fragmented and over-development of a singular thread of consciousness. It all sounded noble—the plunge into the emptiness, the witnessing of the inner terrain, the masterful quest for my true nature—but there was something fundamental missing. The self was perpetually desacralized, as though God, the Universe, the Divine, made a mistake putting us in human form. A kind of personal violence—negate and kill the localized self in order to access the alleged 'true Self.' I couldn't feel my heart, I couldn't feel my toes, I couldn't feel my penis, I couldn't feel my passion for life. I felt like I was on a drug, one that nullified my very humanness. Was this an expanded consciousness or just a sequestered framework of perception? Advaita or avoida?

As I sat and listened, I inwardly flashed to images of Grandmother standing in the kitchen, preparing yet another nourishing meal for me so I could grow this self healthy and strong. I remembered Grandfather's delighted face as he entered the apartment and saw me, determined to give me all the love he could muster. To imagine that all of the decades of generational toil that brought me through—from the struggles of the ancestors to feed, shield, and nurture one generation after another, to the efforts made by my parents and grandparents to pass their love to their little Jeffrey—had been ill-conceived and illusory, a misidentified distraction from what really mattered, seemed entirely preposterous.

I then remembered all my years of overcoming, pushing beyond the hateful parameters of my childhood, trying to craft a better life for this self. I recalled many therapy sessions, countless hours spent trying to regain a sense of self after years torn asunder. I thought about the thousands of years it took for evolution to craft a finger, a toe, a functioning hand—all of the processes that brought us into being in this precise form. I thought of all those who fought and died to safeguard our right to exist, to combat attacks from malevolent marauders, to solidify rule-of-law and basic protections for each and every person. I thought of all the thousands and millions of years of intuitive knowing and innate intelligence that pass through the DNA—brilliance that traveled from one self to another. Through this lens, the suggestion that it was all foolhardy, and that the true self exists independent of our stories and personal identifications—in the selfless, barren emptiness—felt both ludicrous and entirely disrespectful.

The only one who can tell me that God made a mistake putting us in human form, was God herself.

I thought of Ramana Maharshi, the non-dual master who, once enlightened, went to the holy mountain Arunachala, and never came back to the world. Once there, a *sangha* (spiritual community) developed around him, catering to his every need. One has to wonder how authentic our experience of enlightenment is if it cannot engage with the world. Although he spoke often of self-enquiry as the principal means to remove ignorance and abide in Self-awareness, he was not referring to the individuated self, which he considered to be a fiction of mind. He was referring to a non-personal, absolute Self that is ever-present. Where yesterday, I imagined him a great being, today he looked like just another escapist, entirely incapable of weaving his wisdom with real life.

Is mastery patriarchy's self-evasion mask, the way that men bypass the messiness of reality under the guise of perfection? What would happen if they let go of their obsession with mastery, and allowed themselves to just be here, now, in the most inclusive sense, messiness, frayed edges, broken threads, and all?

The next afternoon, I fell back over my Bioenergetic breathing stool. I could feel the father wound that had re-opened around Bhagavan Das was newly festering, calling out for attention. It couldn't be resolved in my head—it demanded to come through the body. I went back over the stool and began to breathe into my constricted chest. At first, it was very difficult to find the breath, but then it came pummeling, hard and fast. And with it came an unstoppable wave of old memories and feelings skyrocketing to the surface. Tears poured down my face as I got on my knees and punched the nearby mattress with ferocity.

Despite hearing a determined inner voice cajoling me to retreat, I stayed there, moving deeper and further into feeling and expression. As I struck the futon, I remembered my father striking me hard as an adolescent. I remembered that knotted red fist landing on my temple, knocking me to the icy sidewalk on Bathurst Street in Toronto. Fuck that hurt. And then the unsaid words, words that I had been too terrified to express then, spat out of me pointedly, venomously: "I hate you Daddy, I fucking hate you..."

The outpouring built to a crescendo, as the uncoiled, spiraling rage and tongue-untied words blended into a tsunami of contempt. Clearly, none of it had gone anywhere, despite my efforts to invoke silence as a path. It was all waiting in my chest for its next opportunity for healing.

After the release, I lay sweaty and stunned on the floor for hours, waiting for my equanimity to return. Although terribly drained, I couldn't help but notice the meaningful difference between this enlivened emptiness, and the robotic emptiness I had felt meditating with the Advaita "masters." They were like two different worlds altogether. I actually felt closer to my "true nature" now, after one strong somatic release, than I had witnessing dozens of non-dual satsangs.

I got up and sat on the meditation cushion, seeing what would come of it. Various feelings kept floating back into awareness, each with the same essential message: "Stop running. Stop confusing self-avoidance with enlightenment. Just stop." And I got it. I really got it. Although my seeming equanimity was a momentary break from the world of feeling, it was simply too avoidant to be true.

There were fissures and fault lines all over my non-dual field, and they couldn't be meditated away. I could repress them, I could split off from them, I could label them illusory, but I couldn't untrue them. They were in my bones, after all. Like putting the proverbial cart before the horse, I had been putting a pseudo-unified framework of perception before the work needed to embody it. I couldn't know non-duality with so much work left to be done right here within the dualities.

In this way, my premature and unsustainable quest for non-duality was like a drug trip—a well-intended drug trip, to be sure... but still a drug trip. And like any drug trip, it actually postponed the work I needed to do within the dualities before I could taste from the unity tree for real. It was impossible to taste from the unity tree with a still toxic tongue. It was crystal clear by now that flat-lining, and floating into the eternal beyond, was never going to be my path home. After all, I didn't want to become adept at only one instrument—I wanted to become the entire symphony.

And yet, I was once again here for a reason. Like it or not, I still retained a part of me that wanted to bypass this difficult life trip. Some people are eager to get done with the messiness of being human. And sometimes, I was one of them. I wanted to forget my humanness, because I was in so much pain. The unhealed grief associated with the loss of my parents was simply too overwhelming. It flooded the inner regions of my consciousness. It kept me up at night. The pain was the portal that attracted me to another self-negating spirituality.

Of course, it's easy to understand why the state of being that arises when we disconnect from the messiness of being human could be mistakenly confused with a pure consciousness. There's no mud to slip on or mess to clean up. And there are few reminders of your unhealed aspects until it runs its course and you are brought back to earth by the mucky, and murky, nature of life and transformation.

Dissociation Highway

With these realizations in mind, I made my way to the conference. I wanted to more deeply understand what was motivating them—the omnipotent teachers and the eager students—to participate in something that was apparently not embodied, not inclusive, not heart-centered, not... unified. What was this Guru-as-knower stage show all about?

In a way, I felt like a kind of karmic spy, going undercover to find out what everyone was drawn to. Much to my surprise, there were a number of teachers who were leaning into a more grounded and integrative version of non-duality. Something with feeling. Something relational. Something deeply human.

And, yet, there were others who were teaching the traditional version of Advaita, startlingly devoid of humanness. I sat and watched as the all-knowing teacher took the stage stoically, eager to play his role as enlightened master, unruffled by the world. I wondered where he was coming from—the desire to be of service, financial benefit, delusion? I also watched the students, wondering what motivated them to sit before a teacher hour upon hour, or even year after year: Was it a genuine quest for meaning, the need to project God onto another, something to fill the existential emptiness of their lives, the search for the superhero parent they never had? What was igniting this magnetic pull?

Soon the shadow at the heart of the movement was clear in view. As I interacted with various teachers and students, it became quickly obvious to me that what was transpiring was more about transcendence addiction than spirituality. It had little to do with the horizontal or the heartfelt, such as human relationships and healthy self-development. Much of what I witnessed—both in the languaging and the energy of the discourse—was some kind of strangely discombobulated a-void-dance that was camouflaged as depthful inquiry. It was more of a cerebral and rarefied quest for meaning, than one rooted in the earthy and embodied pulse of human life.

It was clear to me that many of the participants weren't actually spiritual seekers—at least not in the inclusive way that I was coming to define spirituality. They were dissociationists—floating up and away from their God-given humanness. They were parceling off aspects of themselves—their feelings, their identities, their stories, their bodies—because they were in pain. Just like I had. They didn't know how to fix the self, so they abandoned it altogether, and covered up their desertion with a distorted story about a self with "no center." Yet in their flight from the centered self, they hadn't actually moved beyond victimhood and suffering. They had entrenched it. It was all still in there, momentarily hidden from view but covertly ruling their lives. As I had learned time and again: Pretending we are not fragmented, does not make us whole. As painful as it may be, if we truly seek non-separateness—we must come back into our body. We must tend to our fractures with precision and painstaking detail.

The Enrealed Life

After this foray into the realm of no-self, and no-selfers, I felt compelled to land back on earth. Something about this phase served as a kind of tipping—or perhaps better worded—grounding—point for my journey. It was now crystal clear. I couldn't evolve from the top-down. I could only evolve from the bottom-up—jumping into the full catastrophe feet first. It was time to fully inhabit myself again. And this time—there was no going back. It was clear that my self and I were together for the long haul. And the only option was to fully embrace it. So, I turned back to the oft-forgotten body to re-integrate it. This time, for goodish.

With this intention, I woke up each day with a more conscious effort to inhabit an *enrealed* life. When I wrote *Soulshaping*, I crafted the term "enrealment" without fully understanding what it meant. At the time, I was still a step back from a more inclusive way of being. I was circling the wagon of wholeness, not quite ready to embody the reality at the core.

Now I understood it more deeply. Not as a fully actualized way of being—because neither reality nor my consciousness are ever fixed and stationary—but as one that transforms and widens over time, continuously reaching out for more to include in its ever-expanding scope. What had begun as a quest for a detached and rarefied model of enlightenment had slowly become a quest for enrealment, an ass-roots philosophy that includes all aspects of the human experience in the equation: shadow and light, earth and sky, grocery list and unity consciousness, fresh mangoes and stale bread.

It's *all* real, all the time.

At its core, enrealment is about living within all threads of reality simultaneously, rather than only those realms that feel the most comfortable. It is experiential, enheartened, and embodied. Becoming really and truly human. Living in every direction while rooted in one's evolving humanness.

In the midst of finding home in my own skin, the coming years presented me with endless opportunities to cultivate enrealment. Overcoming a new obstacle, encountering a new boundary, stepping through a new threshold, doing something completely uncomfortable. So much turbulence, so many changes. It was about shedding one skin of self, and then embodying the next layer beneath—and this process seemed to have no end. There was no solid and stable landing platform. Every landing platform was only a launch pad that took me to the next: the next integration, the next grounding, the next opportunity for expansion. And my tumultuous life seemed to conjure them up naturally.

Of course, tumult was not unique in my life. It seemed to come with the territory. But what was unique was my response to it. Where before I would find parts of myself retreating from triggers and overwhelm, I now found myself entering right into the center of the cyclone—more and more able to hold to an enrealed consciousness.

For example, when a dear friend and I had yet another inexplicable falling out, I found myself able to hold the sadness and anger simultaneously. The last time we had parted, I had retreated from my anger altogether. Bypasser style. Similarly, I allowed myself to fully acknowledge my mistrust for a group of individuals I had grown close to. Not needing to focus on the light alone, I was able to step into a more realistic perspective on our relational dynamics. Rather than soften or re-frame my perspective, I took a straight and hard look—seeing things sharply as they actually were, and making the appropriate adjustments in personal boundaries. This was ultimately liberating not only for me—but for them as well.

The most effective laboratory for my enrealed expansion was my evolving relationship with Susan. Not unlike many couples, we had begun in the sweetest and most soulful place. From the very beginning, I felt like I was floating on a bed of light whenever I was with her. Pleasantly uneventful, like simply coming home. At the same time, it lacked a certain depth of shadow. Virtually no arguments, no tensions, no notable points of disagreement. Were we *really* that perfectly aligned?

Yes, we were. But not only with respect to the light—with respect to the shadow, too. It just took a little time to rear its transformative head. After a gentle easing into Canada, we were soon locking horns, as previously unseen issues rose fiercely into view. Trauma triggers, primal patterns, and reactive re-enactments riddled the domestic landscape, as the combination of living together and losing parents activated painful memories and patterns we had imagined resolved.

When the trigger-fest began, it was all we could do to stay in the same space. Startled by the intensity of our material, we found ourselves mutually confronted with those parts of us that still longed to flee and split-off in the face of hurt. Our inner children wanted out!

Yet, as the process unfolded, we gradually embraced a more integrated way of relating, one that insisted on a conscious working-through of the material that had emerged. It was no easy feat, as we had built no previous template to process this depth of emotional material and to healthily communicate in the heart of it.

With reverence for the painful experiences that had forged our triggers, we slowly, steadily, developed a language of co-creational relatedness that served us going forward. It was one thing to be soulmates—that was easy enough—but to also become "solemates," grounded together in practical reality, required a commitment to a whole other level of discourse and embodied awareness. Before we could weave the threads tighter, we needed to see them, raw and real, splayed out before us. With more parts in play, we were able to become more present to each other, and to all that is. The process was at times messy, graceless, and riddled with mistakes—but we were making it happen.

Grounded in the body of feeling and the primacy of the relational, my interface with the moment continued to change. There was a consolidation in the deep within, as my capacity to embrace *all that is* matured and strengthened.

Living a more enrealed life is like being loosely tethered to the ground. You aren't fixed, but you are solid. And from that solidity, you can handle whatever comes. Not just life's challenges and delights, but life's uneventful moments, too. Moments that were once dismissed as mundane or ordinary take on a whole new depth and dimension as you see the connection between all things and allow every thread of your existence to breathe the same air. You may still prefer certain threads, but none are denied their place in the sacred tapestry. Where you once separated out the threads, you are now inclined to live them as one full and rich experience.

Sacred Activism

The enrealing of my consciousness showed up, strong and clear, in my career as a writer. It was a disillusioning process. When it began, I found myself affixed to a childhood fantasy about being a published author. I remember walking into bookstores as a child, imagining myself the author of books for sale. This fantasy took root for many years, and, as I soon found out, prevented me from both seeing the publishing industry for what it was and from making decisions that would better serve my goals and purpose.

After several years of growing in social media, it became evident that there was no advantage to being published by anyone other than myself. Not because there aren't credible publishers, but because you have to do virtually all the work to bring your words to the world. There was a time when you had no other choice but to secure a deal. Social media didn't exist, so the publisher's distribution and publicity system was essential to sell content. This is no longer true. Nowadays, many publishers do very little to support and market an author's words. Authors are expected to be hands-on, working assertively especially through the world of online marketing. If you are someone who is not comfortable growing your name online, then you have little to lose by selling your rights to the industry. But if you are comfortable doing the groundwork to grow in social media, then it makes little sense to sell your rights. You can get yourself on many of the standard distribution lists all on your own, while earning far more profit per book.

With the priceless wisdom of experience, I signed a distribution contract and self-published my second book, *Ascending with Both Feet on the Ground*, on my own terms. And then, my third, *Love It Forward*, through my newly opened publishing company, Enrealment Press: an outlet with the core mission of sharing grounded, inclusive offerings with the world. *An Uncommon Bond* was my fourth published book. Around this time, I began publishing other authors, including my wife Susan, and activist-mystic Andrew Harvey.

As both the business and my social media support base grew, it became essential to summon my inner warrior more fully back into my daily life. He was a precious ally in dealing with publishing matters, especially when it came to issues with shrewd individuals. It's amazing who shows up—and in what seductive form—when you begin to succeed in your chosen profession. A whole cadre of posers, branders, sleek snake-oil salesman, and imitators roaming the Internet, looking for ways to make and/or keep themselves relevant. I needed firm boundaries, grittiness, and the presence of a fiercely benevolent warrior to manage all the bullshit that came with the territory.

Luckily, my warrior had never strayed too far. There was no question that I had needed to disengage from him at an earlier time, in order to create space to explore other ways of being. But it didn't serve me to stray too far. He had been a loyal servant in keeping me alive in the past, and he was ready to return with a newfound and aligned purpose. More essential than ever to my journey of unfolding, he was ready to do whatever it took to kick karmic ass and bring my enrealed voice more fully into the world.

In living an enrealed life, I made an enthralling discovery: many of those patterns that I had once referred to as "false identifications," ultimately proved to be fundamental to who I really am. It was like all the raw materials of my original self were now re-purposed for a more meaningful function. They were never false, in fact. They had just needed to find their rightful place in my wholly weave.

My sacred purpose began to expand beyond writing, and to move in the direction of sacred activism. The seed had been planted some years before, when a friend took her own life. One of the primary factors that contributed to her death was her immersion in what I now refer to as the "New Cage" Movement: those ungrounded and extreme New Age principles that—under the guise of liberation—end up imprisoning people in a limiting framework of perception. She had become ensnared in these dissociative principles, wanting so desperately to mute her pain and find an easier way. This would have been fine if she had simply utilized these techniques as a detachment tool, to pick up and put down again, but, instead, she descended further into their lair, and turned them into her way of functioning in the world. Unfortunately, these philosophies became weapons that turned against her.

When her old pain rose back into consciousness again (as it always will in its efforts to be seen and healed), she was now entirely ill-prepared to deal with it, having stopped her therapy sessions, floating away from reality in a pseudo enlightened-stupor. When reality again became too much to bear, she no longer had the tools or the support structure to manage it, and she ended her life shortly after. What she needed was more healing, not more self-negation techniques. Magic potions can kill people, especially when what they need is a rigorous healing process. Detachment is a tool—it's *not* a life.

This event was a rude awakening, and took my inquiry into the ungrounded spiritual community to the next level. It was time for my writing voice to embody a more pointed and direct, no bullshit form of truth-speak. For years, I had avoided my inner lawyer-activist, preferring instead to focus on gentler forms of contribution. This leaning reflected the work I had done to soften my own heart's edges after a conflict-ridden childhood, and in some ways, reflected my own unconscious buy-in to the entirely ungrounded belief that spirituality was necessarily tender and forgiving.

I remember the moment of decision clearly. My friend had taken her life, and a raging fire ignited within me. I longed to call out those teachings that had contributed to her death. I began to write a Facebook post, and then deleted it. Wrote it again. Deleted it. And then, I sat back and asked myself what I was afraid of. Clearly, something.

I heard many responses. The loudest one surprised me, "It's professional suicide. If you open this door, you will end up alienating yourself from the entire industry." I looked in the mirror, truly disappointed with myself. I thought I was more courageous than that. When I had left law, I chose against a profession that demanded I sift my words through a political filter. In choosing the writing path, I had chosen truthful expression.

I went in deeper, inviting all the feelings to percolate. After some time, only one inquiry remained: Who do you write for? The profession, or the people? Vested interests, or human liberation? Which path is yours?

The answer was easy. I could no longer stand by while these New Cage teachings literally destroyed people's lives. I wrote the post again. This time, without resistance. And I shared it. To my surprise—and may this be a helpful lesson to anyone retreating from their voice—my page began to rapidly grow thereafter. It seems I wasn't the only one eager to call out the spiritual game. There was a discussion waiting to happen.

In the coming months, my activist voice roared to life. With political shackles removed from my consciousness, he was fully permitted to see, and to say, things for what they were. It was no longer an inquiry into singular teachings—it was an inquiry into an entire system, one that often thrived on the backs of people's suffering in the name of spirituality.

There was an entire industry predicated on a perilous split between spirituality and humanness, that was intentionally perpetuating dissociative practices—both because many of the leaders in the field were themselves dissociated, and because the more dissociated one is, the easier they are to control and manipulate economically. When we don't have an integrated self, we are ripe for the picking by unconscionably capitalistic interests, who fill the void with their own self-serving versions of meaning. They seek out easy prey in those who no longer identify with their own story. For if you aren't centered in your own story, you are far more likely to take on someone else's.

The floodgates of clear seeing opened wide. I marveled at the degree of manipulation at work. A giant online world that positioned effective branders as awakened teachers. Imitative "Thought Leaders" who had few original thoughts, but merely reflected the appealing look that the industry sought to profit from. Treacherous valleys of pseudo-positivity and superficial shopping mall "poets" confusing art with artifice on Instagram. Pseudo-wisdom books scribed by ghost writers, and positively endorsed by authors' friends who had never even read them cover to cover. Unconscionable deals made with followers to write five-star reviews the day a book was released, in exchange for one benefit or another. And something I will never personally forget... a prominent 'spiritual' publisher who acknowledged to me that "publishing non-duality is like giving candy to a baby. The masses eat it up."

I understood their meaning: Pain-avoidant teachings are big business. The people will buy and consume any candy that feeds their addiction to disconnection. Those words stayed with me, stoking the fires of my inquiry. The deeper I looked, the more clarity I gained into the bullshit-shtick of the self-help/spiritual industry.

Another misguided trend that has gained momentum in recent years is the corporatized "soulebrity" (spiritual celebrity) movement. This is the West's God-projecting, image-obsessed variation of the Eastern guru trip. Just as the guru was often elevated as the one who knows, the soulebrity is imagined as the one who holds the key to spiritual success. There is one significant difference, though: where the Eastern guru trip was sometimes rooted in substantive teachings and philosophies, the soulebrity movement is focused more on the teacher's image and the flawlessly marketed presentation of a life well-lived, than on any qualitative offering. Any individual who is on the public stage, or a leader in their field, carries a certain responsibility in the message they transmit to their audience. In the soulebrity realm, the precious opportunity to bring forth a heartfelt message of real substance to a starving world—is often buried under the weight of personal ambition. When someone actually sits down to read a soulebrity's work, they quickly realize that their message is neither unique, nor rooted in any kind of dedicated inner work. They instead offer generic marketing constructs—a tasteless brew of popularized spirituality and narcissistic imaginings. Too many soulebrities, too little soul.

What disturbed me the most were those soulebrities and Hollywood stars who were using their platforms to repudiate the idea that our self-identifications are real. The fact is that most people don't have the luxury of pretending nothing is real. They need to get food on the table. They need to draw from every aspect of the self in order to get by. To deny the self entirely, and then to offer people little more than a float into nothingness, is erroneous and gravely irresponsible. Such a message could increase the suffering of trauma survivors or those struggling with fragmentation; and in extreme cases—lead them to their grave, well before their time. What would they do when their pain rises up in a feeding frenzy in the middle of the night, now with nothing to hang on to? Some might be able to take refuge in the witness, but many would be at risk. With no self to return to as a firm base, no feet grounded in the soil of lived experience, they would inevitably come crashing back to earth in the form of emotional distress and/or physical illness, as the sidestepped material re-emerges and ravages them over time. Just as it did with my friend who ended her life.

The message coming through my newly empowered writing voice was that we should not invite people so far away from the self that they no longer have anything, or anyone, to come home to. Better yet, let's make a point of reminding others that they do exist, and that they really do matter. It could be useful to see that there is something beyond the misidentified self, but it is also essential to be reminded that we each have a beautiful, authentic, unique self at our core. People need their self to be honored and healed, not denied. The survival of our species depends on our mutual regard for our own, and each other's, humanness.

Patriarchal Spirituality

At the bottom of so many of these philosophies is the skyprint of patriarchy. The wool had been pulled over our eyes. Men who were too unhealthily egoic to admit that they couldn't deal with their humanness, their feelings, their trauma, had to find a system that smoke-screened their avoidance. They found it. It was called Enlightenment. It was also called Spiritual Mastery. And it usually involved leaving the world, in one form or another. This way, these men could convince themselves that they had mastered the one true path. This way, they could conceal their confusion and fragmentation behind an all-knowing mask.

I saw it clear as day. From pain-avoidant New Cage teachings, to pseudo-superior spiritualities, to rules of discourse designed to suppress dissension, to sexual abuses of authority posing as awakened offerings, to a system-wide exclusion of the wisdom of the Divine Feminine, I saw the legacy of a man-based system that had spread its toxic tentacles everywhere. And it was riddled with contradiction: both self-negating and radically selfish, rarefied and not remotely realified, seemingly non-attached yet deeply invested in maintaining control over our consciousness. It wasn't weaponry they used to control us. It was the rituals of guru-worship, the dogmatic passing off of man-made "truths" as divine wisdom, the enforced distinction between "acceptable" and "unacceptable" spiritual practices, the disciplining approach to spiritual inquiry, the conditioned notion that someone other than us had all the answers we sought.

Everywhere I looked I saw a system that was created and controlled by men. And they weren't exactly the healthiest members of the brotherhood. They were deeply wounded men who had no interest in processing their issues or entering heart-first into the visceral world of feeling. Instead, they camouflaged their wounded egos and fear of the world beneath the cloak of enlightenment, in an effort to fool themselves and those who followed them. They wanted the benefits related to the claim of enlightenment without having to do the challenging work of emotional healing and ethical transformation.

It all felt like a hustle, a patriarchal landmine masquerading as a field of divine possibility. Evasion misrepresented as expansion.

I woke up one day, with a lengthy definition of patriarchal spirituality waiting to be written and shared on social media. It was a bold, imperfect statement, but it felt true, in its essence. People wrote me to angrily express their disagreement: "What you are describing is the way that the West has perverted the core texts", "Stop blaming the men for all of our problems." And of course, their favorite edict: "Spirituality does not include anger!" (except, their own ☺).

After that, I went to a spiritual bookstore, looking around at the books that had been written about spirituality and enlightenment. Almost all of the so-called classics had been written by Eastern men. I looked closely at the question of whether their original message was actually more embodied, more emotionally inclusive, more integrating than the way it was being interpreted in the West. And it wasn't. Almost all of the classics were speaking the same regurgitated, self-negating, emotionally dismissive vision of possibility for our spiritual lives. One that would serve us if we wanted to sidestep our humanity, but not if we wanted to engage it. The mad ones among us had been running the show.

I went outside, and sat in one of my favorite Toronto parks. Quakes of insight erupted. I flashed to images of various spiritual teachers I had encountered. In one way or another, nearly every one of them was leading us away from our hearts. Where were the spiritual models rooted in the bountiful wisdom of the Divine Feminine—relationship as path, heart as portal to the Godself, the emotional body as the breeding ground for the soul's emergence? Where were the models that didn't inherently adopt and build upon notions of spirituality put forth by the "saints" of yore, but, instead, began from scratch and explored entirely new frontiers? Where were the inclusive models, the embodied models, the models that would take us home, intact and tenderly intertwined? How could I contribute to their co-creation?

Arriving Full Circle (And Then Some)

As I stepped more fully into the shadowlight of reality, I accepted that the focus of my quest was misguided. In the same way as my quest for something called enlightenment became a quest for something I now call enrealment, my quest for a spiritual life had now become a full-on quest for *humanness*. That is, the *real* question was no longer, "What is spirituality?" The real question was, "What does it mean to truly be human?"

In many ways, my journey has been one of returning to the inclusive and embodied consciousness I knew as a child, one where the localized blended with the universal in a kind of wholly, holy weave. It is that, and it is something more. Most notably, there is a more thorough solidification in my capacity to be with—and within—the moment. It's like my innocent and un-self-conscious childhood experience of an open and integrated awareness, has finally merged with my adult self: a more stable and wiser consciousness, grown seasoned over time. A kind of informed innocence. But that doesn't mean I'm in a state of happily ever after. No, it's far more authentic than that. It's a state that threads right through the heart of the everything, light and shadow, and back again. Really, truly, fully, authentically, genuinely, comprehensively HUMAN.

Of course, I'd best not run the risk of overstating it, or I will end up no different from those mastery seekers I've critiqued. I am human, after all, and I will surely forget some of what I have come to know. That happens, often. Sometimes I wish I could place a bookmark in my lifeline in order to remember where I last left off on my learning curve. Just so I won't have to learn the same lesson, over and over again. But it doesn't work that way, does it? The book of life is not amenable to bookmarks. It is one where we continually lose our page and have to go back to find it. Back into the fires of re-realization, yet again.

As I look back on my journey, one crude but real generalization comes to me. We can either move toward separation, or we can move toward integration of our varied parts and aspects. Many I have known—and certainly myself at various times—have preferred to focus on singular ways of being, either because they imagined "perfection" on the path, or because they unconsciously feared bringing all of their parts into the light of awareness. Others still have worked to break down their internal blocks and defenses, and bring all of their aspects into one interlaced weave.

I am not sure which path is more difficult. One requires an exhausting repression of one's wholeness, and the other requires an enormous amount of integration work. However, I am fairly certain that the latter grants us more opportunity to live a fully expressed life.

Having said that, we have to be realistic about the pace of our human development. We may step into a unified field for a period of time, but sustainable transformation demands that we come back down into the dualities to both celebrate them and work them through. That is the nature of life—and maybe it's not something we are meant to overcome or reconcile. Maybe the goal is not so much for it all to be tied together in some perfect little package, but for all of it to be fully experienced. Perhaps duality is our actual gift in this life: the fuel, the gritty catalyzer that initiates expansion and necessitates transformation. Without it, we could never actually grow. We would just be trapped inside of a placid equilibrium. We need friction. We need dichotomy. We need polarity. In other words, it's not about trying to sidestep the jaggedness and grit—it's about settling into it. It is an intrinsic part of the human experience, and it is actually what helps us to evolve.

I had searched for my answers in the sky, but I actually found them in my battle-weary body, right down here on Mother Earth. In the heart of the madness, on the rockiest of trails, in the most imperfect of psyches, I have found a path to call my own. It isn't a pristine or peaceful path, nor one without obstacles, but it is truly mine.

In my mind's eye, I often travel back to that all too familiar lawn in suburban Toronto. The five-year-old version of me is lying on the grass. Thick head of brown hair, ruffled and messy. Blue plaid shirt with holes in the elbows. He looks at peace, marveling at the universe, in boyish delight. I look down at my 50-something body. Thick bare feet that traversed many paths. Face now etched with life's lines. I say to him, "Whoa! What a journey that was. You have no idea. And now—here we are. Here I AM." Not baffled as to my direction. Not desperate for answers. Just here. Living an embodied and purposeful life. Here.

PART TWO

HERE

NOTE TO READER:

The following chapters are based on dialogues between a Questioner and a Responder. It is a fictitious stream of conversation between myself— "JB"—and a questioner named "M" (Michael). JB reflects myself at this stage of my development. "M" is based on a tapestry of various seekers I have known and dialogued with, and is also a direct reflection of who I was at prior stages of my journey. I had considered writing a more 'objective' Q and A, one where the Questioner and Responder are de-personalized voices with little story revealed. But that form of dry, inhuman interaction felt incongruent with this book's embodied spiritual message. If I want my message to be felt on a deeply human level, it feels important to communicate it personally, in the heart of story. I have taken the liberty of engaging "M" in a deepening dialogue, one that invites us to cover a broad range of material over a series of regular sessions. I have also chosen to enhance the dialogues with various settings, and closing narratives that reflect my perspective on his process. It is my hope that the story comes alive in a way that reflects the message itself.

You will find Exercises dispersed throughout the dialogues, which the character Michael partakes in. These are hands-on exercises designed for you to try for yourself, if you wish to. In order to preserve the continuity of the Exercise, they will be presented in a pure form, without dialogue interspersed. This allows you to sample the exercises firsthand through your own direct experience, before assimilating the character's experience. Before participating in any of the exercises, please read the disclaimer on the copyright page (p.vi).

1 What is Grounded Spirituality?

I'm a dirt person. I trust the dirt.
I don't trust diamonds and gold.

—EARTHA KITT

I met Michael for the first time on an early autumn afternoon. The air was crisp, but the sun was sparkling brightly through the changing leaves. We met at one of my favorite Toronto cafes, right in the heart of the student annex. During my most challenging transformative years, it was one of my go-to spots. I would sip a cappuccino and gaze out the window, watching the people hurry by, while sifting through whatever enigma, issue, or relational pattern was up for me. Oh, the awakening path. It felt good to return, at this stage of my journey.

This meeting with Michael came upon me unexpectedly. I generally don't meet clients in cafes. But this request struck me. Over the past five years, I had delved deeper into my counseling practice. Online, Skype, through email, and in-person. A woman I worked extensively with over a period of 18 months through Skype— her name was Lydia—had found the sessions to be life-changing. She was an old childhood friend of Michael's, and had lived next-door to him for many years. She followed Michael's intensive spiritual quest through the decades—and recommended that he contact me. At first, he vehemently resisted the idea. He had read "parts of" Soulshaping and found it too "psychological" for his liking. Yet, Lydia made it clear that I was not a psychologist, "but a wise fellow path-traveler." Those words resonated in him, and he decided to give it a shot.

So, he emailed me.

After responding to his many scrutinizing questions and sarcastic retorts about the meaningless nature of counseling—I finally assured him that our work together didn't need to take a counseling approach. Instead, let's just meet in random places and chat together. Hear my perspective, decide for yourself. That did the trick. He softened his guard, and agreed to meet me.

I arrived a bit early, and sat down on the street side of the outdoor patio, sipping a hot chai. Bloor Street was noisy and full of life this afternoon. Michael arrived a few minutes later. I immediately knew it was him. I motioned him over, and he slowly made his way to the table. I felt an instant kindling of friendship—a warmth, a sense of brotherhood, like meeting an old comrade, and perhaps a bit like myself in earlier stages of life. Tall and lanky, short cut sandy-brown hair, late-30s, small round rimless glasses, white oxford button-down shirt perfectly tucked into plain khakis. And that "spiritual gazer" glint in his eyes. He felt both decidedly calm, and oddly close to the edge. It was soon into our initial dialogue that I knew this was going to be juicy.

As we met over the next months—I consistently recorded our dialogues. The following pages represent our progression. A journey from the sky... back down to earth... feet planted solidly, here.

Laying the Groundwork

M: Nice to meet you Mr. Brown, but I'm still not sure this is a good idea.

JB: Why is that?

M: Because I actually feel pretty comfortable with where I am on my path. I was realizing this on the subway ride over here. Yeah, there's a few issues, but who doesn't have issues? I'm not sure talking about them will make much of a difference.

JB: It's true that talking alone won't resolve everything, but it can help. When you emailed me, you seemed eager to sort some things through.

M: That's true. I'm not sure why I am feeling so resistant.

JB: How about we slow things down. What can I order you?

M: Nothing right now. Just give me a moment to gather my thoughts. I promised Lydia that I wouldn't retreat. She knows my patterns well.

JB: It's okay. I understand something about resistance from my own journey. It's there for a reason. Let's just sit together for now, okay? No one's marking our progress. We don't have to start in heavy.

Michael nodded, "yes." He looked like he wanted to cry, or perhaps bolt. He began to nervously play with the mala bead bracelet he was wearing under his shirt sleeve. He quickly closed his eyes, and I closed mine in response. I didn't want him to feel exposed so early in our meeting. I understood how perilous it can be to share our truths, particularly if we have reached a transformational tipping point. Sometimes the simplest sharing can evoke an epic paradigm shift. We sat quietly, for some time. Michael then began to speak sharply, rapidly, like he was firing up his strength to counteract his apprehensions. I opened my eyes to receive.

M: Okay, that's enough. Let's get to the meat of it. I want to hear your full-on perspective, if only so I can decide if I want to work with you. So don't pussy-foot around—give me the full load today. I'm here, because I'm seeking clarity. If you can provide some, I'll stick around. If not, no hard feelings. Sound good?

JB: My full-on perspective? That's not gonna be conveyed over one cup of coffee. It's far too nuanced. But I can give you a good overview. First, I want to understand you better, so I can have some context for my share. Can you tell me about your own path...

M: Can do. I've been traveling the world—both internally and externally—for what feels like lifetimes, and I'm not sure I'm any closer to clarity than I was at the beginning of this "search." I know that it's about living consciously, but, after decades of experimentation, I'm not even sure what that means. Sometimes I feel like I have nailed it, and then I come back to this persistent sense of confusion as to why I am here and what this life is really about. I don't want what I grew up with, but I am not quite sure where to step now. Truth be told, I feel as though I am back where I was at the beginning of my spiritual journey—knowing what I don't want, but not what I do want, 'cept this time I don't feel excited about the next exploration into consciousness.

JB: Got it. You've been on a quest, because you felt there was something more to this life than what you had been told and what you had experienced. Like many of us, you were wondering: what is the authentic *you*, and the real *this*? How do we locate the truth of who we are, and why we are here?

M: Yes, the who, the why, and something else—the where. Like *where* is the place I belong, the place that will feel like home and resolve my confusion.

Is it out there, up there, in here, or is it nowhere at all—is it just about finding peace in the meaninglessness of it all?

JB: Well, it's unlikely that we came into this birth with all these gifts, abilities, and longings if it's ALL meaningless, but let's talk about that later. Tell me a little about where you have been on your journey.

M: Been lots of places. Grew up in Indiana, in the US Midwest, in what seemed like a relatively normal—as in dysfunctional—family. I was the only child. Dad sold insurance, Mom worked at the high-school cafeteria. Both were devout Christians, dragging me off to their favorite Arena Church every Sunday, without fail. I would listen to the sermon and watch the ridiculous stage show and just knew there was something wrong. I mean, we're all sinners in need of redemption, really? Even children?

I had real issues with my father—he was sharp as a tack, but completely bereft emotionally. Kept himself shielded and protected, while my mother was more of a smothering nurturer. Very loving, but I don't think she ever got me. She just loved, because that was her role as a mom, but she had no capacity for an attuned connection. I grew up feeling pretty isolated, like no one truly saw me—and bored, like I just knew there had to be something more than this humdrum midwestern life.

Around the age of 16, I began having constant dreams about other possibilities. I was smoking a ton of pot, then later, hallucinogens, and they seemed to open a portal in my consciousness. I didn't really have language for any of it at the time—it felt like I was catching a glimpse of my past lives, and visions about how I would, or could, manifest in this lifetime. I'm still not sure if these dreams were rooted in something real—like a deeper knowing—or if they were just fantasies I employed to trip out of my unsatisfying adolescence. But it ushered me into consciousness studies, and I began to ravenously consume spiritual texts: Ramana Maharshi, Krishnamurti, *The Tibetan Book of Death and Dying*, Alan Watts—I loved Watts—and then I got really into the Transcendental Meditation (TM) movement in my first year of university. I mean, I was really into it, man. I spent more time yogic flying than studying, but somehow managed to finish a BA in Humanities. I had saved some money doing landscaping during the summers, and got on a plane the day after I graduated to go to India to find my path.

JB: What made you think India had all your answers?

M: Most of the spiritual texts I resonated with were written by Indian saints and gurus.

JB: All men, no doubt?

M: Yes, men.

JB: At that time, what were you questing for in India?

M: I didn't exactly know. I just wanted something more than the materialistic life I had grown up with in America. I wanted a spiritual life.

JB: And you believed that a spiritual life was necessarily non-material, I take it?

M: Yes, most definitely. Spirit, not form.

JB: And what did you find?

M: I thought I found everything, for a while. I traveled around India and Nepal, sat with great masters, became a vegetarian, explored Hinduism and Sikhism and Buddhism, and then lived for 18 months in meditative bliss in a high mountain Himalayan ashram, surrounded by waterfalls and deities and goats and some of the saintliest people I have ever met.

JB: Sounds fun. When you say, "meditative bliss," what do you mean by that? How would you describe the state you were in?

M: Pristine and pure, emptied of thought and worry, just inbreath, outbreath, inbreath, outbreath. And for once, real clarity. I felt like I had entered a kind of bubble, one that inoculated me from the madness of the world, and that allowed me to see the bullshit with a clear lens.

JB: Well, dude... it's easy to be inoculated from the madness of the world, when you've traded it for a prime perch on a mountaintop. Try doing it in the world itself, now that's something...

M: Right, and in a way, that's what I discovered. Although I still believe that what I found in India was much closer to the truth than anything I have found in the West. When I came back to America, I was 26, and I quickly realized that I had no idea how to hold to this awareness, here, in the heart of Western life. I moved back to my parents' house, just until I got my bearings and formed a plan. But I found being around them completely unbearable. I could see right through their masks and disguises, and try as I might, I couldn't get them to look deeper. They wouldn't even meditate, for God's sake. The shopping mall was their temple, and they weren't looking for a new place of worship. So I tried hard to accept them, and to not make my satisfaction dependent on their state of being.

JB: Yes, like if you have really arrived somewhere, why does someone else have to come along for the same ride? If it's real, it stands all on its own.

M: Exactly. So I tried that, kind of like testing my spiritual resolve. We would go out to eat at their favorite diner and I would try to remain in my center, even when the big sloppy veal parmigiana dinner was put down in front of my father. I would feel sickened as he slobbered it down, and then come back to my breath, and try not to judge, not to care, not to buy into whatever he was identifying with. I was beyond that. And then we would leave and go to the movies to see some Hollywood blockbuster and again, I would try to come back to the breath, and to remain unfazed by all the idiotic stimulation. Like, okay, this is their trip, and why can't I just love them as they are?

JB: How did you do?

M: Not so good. I moved to Berkeley after 6 weeks. I figured that it was okay for me to admit that this wasn't my vibe. That they were my parents but they weren't my people. And that maybe it was okay to accept that I needed to be around my tribe if I had any chance of holding to the awareness I had developed in India.

JB: Sure, its gotta be easier when we are around people of a like-spirited nature…

M: Yeah, exactly, although I still kind of resist this.

JB: Why is that?

M: Because I wonder if any of it's real, if you can't hold to it everywhere. I mean, isn't that the nature of mastery? Like if you are a master of something, you are always a master. It shouldn't matter who is near you.

JB: And being a master is essential, because…?

M: As the path to greater wisdom.

JB: *The* path, or *a* path?

M: Hmmm… not entirely sure.

JB: Okay, let's hold that inquiry for the moment. What happened after you moved to Berkeley?

M: Everything happened. Like, I mean EVERYTHING. It was the perfect place for me for a long time, because I could live in my Himalayan bubble and still have sex with lots of beautiful women and explore a range of spiritualities, and sensualities. Whereas my Himalayan state of being was a complete turn-off for midwestern women, it was a total turn-on for Bay Area women. I loved exploring the Tantric path...

JB: I bet you did. Which idea of the tantric path—the classically woven, emotionally vulnerable path of unifying connectiveness, or the one where people pretend that pseudo soul-gazing and technique-centered sex with strangers is actual intimacy?

M: Busted.

JB: Thought so. Then let's just call it sex. Not tantra.

M: Fair enough.

JB: When you weren't having juicy sex with beautiful women, how did you survive financially?

M: Simply. The first thing I realized when I got there was that the best way to protect the consciousness I had found in India was to take a job on the outskirts of society. I had gotten a job selling insurance from an old friend of my dad, and quit after three weeks. It wasn't a terrible job—it was just clear that if I took a traditional job, I would have to keep molding my consciousness to the traditional world, and I didn't want that. I wanted to protect and go deeper into the pure consciousness bubble I had experienced so fully in the Himalayas. I wanted that back. So I spent the next decade doing jobs that allowed me to stay a step back from society. I was a bike courier for six years in San Francisco, then I went in and out of a number of things… mountain-guiding, book-stacking at a neighborhood library. I even worked on the pot farms near Mendocino for two seasons. Whatever it took. Even though I was doing many things, I was always a minimalist. I didn't have a car, I would bike or take the subway everywhere. And I ate very little—never to excess—and rented a basic room in a community house full of spiritual seekers. I figured that if I kept my life simple, I would be less likely to get hooked into the matrix, and less likely to have to take a traditional job to pay for it.

JB: I understand. You chose to live a "step back" from the world in the belief that it would allow you to step closer to a purer consciousness.

M: Yes, exactly.

JB: And what did you do, when you weren't working?

M: I meditated for 2-3 hours per day. That is still the case.

JB: You're shitting me. You meditate for 2-3 hours a day, like now, in your daily life?

M: Yup, diligently. And proud of it. Back to my story—I also climbed Mt. Shasta regularly. I had a special relationship with that mountain. Once I hit a certain altitude, I would come back into contact with my elevated Himalayan consciousness. Sometimes I would stay up there for a week, losing all sense of conventional time, just being with the mountain. It was like heaven on earth. When I wasn't hiking, I was often meditating or studying spiritual texts. I wasn't an isolationist though—I developed a number of friendships with other seekers and attended many satsangs and spiritual retreats—but I always came back to my own company when I felt anxious or confused. I didn't lean too much on others, for fear that dependent connections would obstruct my spiritual focus.

JB: Did you do any psychotherapy or engage in any emotional release practices?

M: Hell no. I'm about spirituality—not psychology. I gravitated toward practices that kept me equanimous. You know, the middle way. I did do reiki sessions for awhile, and sometimes emotions and feelings would come up when I was on the table, but I didn't linger with them. I tended to see emotions and their related stories as a distraction from the spiritual consciousness I was cultivating.

JB: As many do in the 'spiritual' community.

M: Yes, but this proved to be quite a challenge in recent years. After about a decade in the Bay Area, my life took a swerve. I met a sweet li'l Canadian gal named Hannah. She ended up being my wife.

JB: I like her already.

M: We met at a 10-day silent meditation retreat in New Mexico. Even though we were instructed not to connect with anyone, we couldn't keep our eyes—and soon enough, our thighs—off each other. It was sexual, but it wasn't about physicality. I was drawn to her from a cosmic soul-level. And that was admittedly rare for me. As you already figured out, I tended to be relationship avoidant. Although she lived on the other side of the continent—in Fergus, Ontario—neither of us could bear to be apart after that first meeting. After spending a little over a year longing for each other, I made a bold move and re-located to Canada to be with her. I was scared shitless—it was a giant leap from my equanimous approach to life—but I had never felt such a deep knowing about anything or anyone before.

JB: I can surely relate. Love can turn everything upside down in an instant. Tell me more about your relationship with Hannah? What happened then?

M: At first, it was magical, like a coming home after centuries apart. For awhile, she was my oasis. Or my Himalayas. I felt a remarkable sense of peace in her presence. And then, it got progressively more challenging, as we had difficulty merging her worldly nature with my more transcendent nature. Actually, it was Hannah that characterized this phase as "reality bites." I saw it as progressively more unreal, as our connection became lost in practical issues and silly emotional triggers. Of course, I recognize that our vastly differing characterizations of our shared experience—reflect our vastly different views of a spiritual life. Mine is not tainted with worldly matters, while she sees spirituality everywhere, and in everything.

JB: Are you still together, Michael?

M: Yes, but hanging on by a thread, now six years later. We have worked through many things, but there are fundamental, perhaps never to be resolved differences, including a persistent conflict about whether we should have a child. She wants one, and I don't. We battle about this endlessly. I admit—I completely resist Hannah's call to emotional healing and couples counseling. She feels that the issues that come up between us must be resolved through some form of therapeutic process; and I feel that they will resolve themselves to the extent that we develop our spiritual muscle. It's not that I don't recognize that I have unexplored wounds and issues—everyone does!—it's just that I don't believe that digging into them is the way to transform them. I prefer to witness them, to rise above them, to use meditation and various spiritual practices as a means to move beyond issues, and gain true perspective. She believes in all of that in certain instances, but she also believes that some issues must be confronted more directly.

JB: What I hear you saying is that you both believe in making spiritual practice fundamental to your relationship life, but that you just have different ideas of spiritual practice. Yours is, like it was during your time on the West Coast, distinct from emotional life—and hers includes it.

M: Yes, in a nutshell, that's it. And this fundamental tension is no small thing—it continues to erode the connection.

JB: Because your practices are not actually softening the edges of your issues and triggers?

M: I guess. And because her therapeutic practices aren't softening hers. She claims that this is because they are relational triggers and we must work on them together, but I am not convinced. Well, actually sometimes, I do agree with her, but most of the time, I come back to my core belief that these triggers are trappings, one of the many ways that the world pulls us away from the pure consciousness that is our birthright. People spend their whole lives lost in their illusory stories, and they never experience any liberation from their suffering. Isn't it better that we empty ourselves of these illusions, so that we can finally know peace?

JB: Perhaps, but that begs the question: How does one truly empty oneself of them? If your way was so effective, the triggers wouldn't keep coming back in your marriage. I suspect Hannah also wants peace, but doesn't agree with you that the way to find it is exclusively through detachment practices. She wants to find it by jumping in—kind of like a Sufi—rather than by rising above, like a Buddhist. You know, Sufis and Buddhists don't always see eye to eye, or thigh to thigh ☺ for that matter, for very long. How do you explain your longevity? Not many couples can last six years when only one partner is willing to engage in therapeutic process. What holds you together?

M: Love, for sure.

JB: Just love? Because many couples with these issues don't make it. In the old days, sure, when people just assumed their traditional roles and obligations, but not in this new conscious relationship landscape. In this world, people don't stay together if they can't heal and grow together.

M: Fascinating. I think you're right. I am not being fully transparent with you. The other thing that holds us together is that every time we come close to ending, I inch a little closer to her way of being. Not just because I am afraid to lose her, but because I have this odd sense that she is somehow right. Although my core belief says otherwise...

JB: Or perhaps your defended belief says otherwise...

M: Possibly... Hannah does call me "Bubble Boy," because she feels I am hiding from my humanness inside a brainy bubble. But I'm not sure... The matrix is everywhere—isn't it better to separate ourselves from it? All I know for sure is that I feel confused about all of it, particularly the true nature of a spiritual life. Hannah reflects one way of understanding spirituality, and I reflect another. And there are three possibilities that I can see: I am either too defended to embrace hers, she is too defended to embrace mine, or there is a point of meeting that neither of us can yet see.

JB: What are you doing for work now, Michael?

M: Talk about the matrix. Coder for a high-end software company. I still can't believe it myself. From book-stacker to software developer. Yep, I sold out. Ending up joining the allegedly "real world." Nothing real about it, of course, but that's where the money is. The business expanded rapidly in the past few years, so we traded our small country home for a high-rise near the Toronto beaches. Contrary to what you might think, I am truly "in the real world." I'm not hiding out on some mountaintop. Yet I have limits on how far into normalcy I will go.

I suppose I am here in the hope that you can help me resolve all of this. I have been reading your writings on Facebook, and although I often disagree with them, I also get the vague sense that you may be onto something. Not sure what it is exactly. But, hey, I really do have nothing to lose. My marriage is crumbling. My job doesn't excite me. And, after all these years on the spiritual path, something still seems to be missing...

JB: You're right, Michael. You have nothing to lose. And perhaps "everything" to gain, if we can walk you back in the direction of a more inclusive way of being. If it's of any comfort to you, I've been where you are in many respects. I, too, reached a point in my life where I intuitively knew that there was more than mere survival and adaptation. And I, too, have struggled with the meaning of spirituality, the challenges of landing great love in real-time, the difficulties of finding gratifying work. Perhaps the only difference between us is that you looked for your answers beyond the world, and I—for whatever reason—looked for them within it. Right in the heart of it all.

M: I experience a strange resonance when you say that... "right in the heart of it all." Unexpected. And you are right—I don't trust the world to give me what I need. At the same time, I realize that the approach I have taken no longer serves me. I am floundering inside, and out. Something is off. Anyway, why am I talking so much about me? How did you just do that?

JB: Do what?

M: Get me to share all of that. I usually don't reveal so readily. I'm supposed to be listening to your spiel, and assessing if I want to move forward with your counseling. So, your turn...

JB: It's good to hear your story, Michael. I appreciate your honesty. It's a great place to dialogue from. Do you want something to drink before we continue?

M: Yes, I do. I got a feeling I'll need one. A double latte, to start.

JB: Let's order one for each of us.

Spiritual Beings Having a Human Experience

Michael again closed his eyes. He seemed to feel more comfortable with them closed. We sat in silence, waiting for the drinks to arrive. It was rare for me to find people I could sit in silence with. Michael appeared to be one of them. After the lattes arrived, his eyes popped open. He was ready for more conversation.

JB: So let's start with the basics. Let's talk about the word "spirituality"—a word you used often when talking about your life. We hear and use this word frequently, but we seldom take the time to clarify what it actually means. We seldom consider the possibility that it can be defined in many different ways, some of which are more supportive of human development and well-being, and others which are fundamentally incongruent with a truly sacred life. Based on your experience, how would you define this word?

M: I take it quite literally. Spirituality refers to the life of the spirit.

JB: And where is your humanness within that?

M: I see it as a kind of obstacle, or distraction from spiritual life. Like we are in a body for a reason, but the trick is to not take it too seriously. It's all about where you put your attention—into spirit, or into form. You will never find peace in form. It is too toxic, too contaminated with suffering and misidentification.

JB: Well, much of the mainstream world agrees with you. Even popular online and traditional dictionaries distinguish spiritual life from our embodied form, persistently defining spirituality as that which is not physical or worldly, that which is lacking in material form and substance, that which relates exclusively to the transcendent soul, that which is pure, divine, and heavenly-minded.

And much of the spiritual world agrees with you as well. In the way that it has often been characterized since time immemorial, 'spirituality' came to mean something that is distinct from our humanness, and especially from many of the messy and unpleasant aspects of our life experience. It has meant perpetual positivity. It has meant a pure, or absolute consciousness. It has meant squeaky clean premature forgiveness. It has meant repressed anger. It has meant the dissolution of the ego. It has meant painful feelings as an illusion. It has meant the bashing of our personal stories and legitimate victimhood. But it hasn't meant everything human. Only in those rare moments when you can 'transcend' the human experience, do you get to have a spiritual experience. But not here, not now, not in the heart of this embodied madness.

Simply put, our lived-in definition of 'spiritual' has meant the bypassing of the challenges of the human experience. They have been severed, abandoned, and transcended in the name of a 'higher,' or 'stiller,' or 'emptier,' or 'more evolved' path. Through this lens, spirituality is a shadowless and formless skyscape, one where the sun never stops shining and we float— peaceful, silent, and still—far above the messy complexity of the human experience. It has meant seeing God only when the sun is out. Love and light and everything nice. This, in a nutshell, is what I have come to realize about what we have been labeling as 'spirituality.'

M: Hmmm... Yes, but all of that is true. Not that spirituality can't include darkness—of course, that's part of it—but if we don't identify spirituality as something distinct from our messy lives, we are enmeshed, like Hannah and I, in the mundane. Stuck in a rut, man. Can't get the car out of the mud. Disagreeing all the time. Lost to the triggers. It fucking sucks. Better to rise above it.

Just as Michael finished his last sentence, a shirtless and scruffy homeless man ran across the street and approached our table, asking for change. Divine Timing? I reached into my pant pocket and handed him some quarters. He grabbed them quickly, and roared with delight before racing back across the street. I looked over at Michael and his eyes were closed again. Hmmm.

JB: Yes, but can you really rise above what you are? Is it rising above or is it turning a blind eye? And are you truly meant to? If you look at it honestly, this view does seem to suggest that God, Goddess, the Divine, or evolution, or whatever you believe brought us here, made a mistake putting us in human form. And I'm not arrogant enough to imagine that I can know that.

M: I see us as "spiritual beings having a human experience." Pierre Teilhard de Chardin said that. We're not denying our humanity—we are acknowledging that we are more than just human. That being human is only one aspect of our ultimate experience.

JB: It's not actually certain that Pierre said that, but even if he did, I disagree with his premise. This is the same kind of bifurcated thinking that is messing with your marriage and your life. It posits that we are something other than a human being—this thing he calls a spiritual being. But how can this be so? We don't exist independent of this human form. I understand why you resonate with this saying—it reminds you that you are actually a spiritual being, something we can easily lose sight of in the heart of our daily challenges. But what is missing is even more important. What is missing is this: *We are also human beings having a spiritual experience.* This version suggests that there may actually be no distinction between our spiritual life and our human life. Whereas the previous quote keeps them distinct, and at most, allows for the possibility that our humanness is a substratum of our spiritual life. This is the same critical mistake we have been making for centuries. We have been desacralizing the self, and imagining it something less than Sacred and Divine. This leads us in the wrong direction and, although it may provide momentary relief from the challenges of the human experience, it actually perpetuates the illusory divide, concretizing the idea that being human is necessarily sub-standard. This ultimately turns us away from the essential work we must do to make sacred our humanness. Same, same.

M: I'm listening, but I don't agree. You think that homeless guy wouldn't benefit from a more heightened perspective? Sure he would. If we try to find our spirituality in the heart of our humanness, we will always feel hungry.

Spiritreality

Michael got up to look for a restroom. When he came back, he had a glint in his eye. I sensed both a willingness to hear more, mixed with a hint of challenge—like a boxer putting on his gloves for the ring. Round two...

JB: Okay, try this on for size: Spirituality is reality.

M: Yes, it's the *ultimate* reality.

JB: No, I don't mean it that way. I mean that it is ALL aspects of reality, including those you shun. Both the form *and* the formless. The transcendent and the immanent—or material—world.

M: Okay, dude. So how does this actually translate into real-life?

JB: It means that your spirituality is not a hide-away from life's inherent challenges. It's not somewhere you go when the mundane tasks of the day are completed. It is not a foray into fantasy and fragmentation. It doesn't sidestep the uncomfortable, the muddled, the chaotic, the mortal. It's reality, in and of itself, in *all* its myriad forms. It is an inclusive consciousness, one that threads through every aspect of our lived experience. In other words, the more aware of and connected we are to every element of reality, the more spiritual our life is. Spiritreality. All one experience.

M: So, you are saying that I am, essentially, not living a spiritual life because I tend to prefer only particular states and stages?

JB: Yes, in a sense. Perhaps the better way to put it is that you have over-developed certain threads of consciousness—threads that are fundamental to the spiritual weave—but you have under-developed others. So you end up like a one-winged bird, flapping toward the sky, then crashing back to earth. Only part way home.

M: Hannah would agree with you. She often says that the seemingly unconscious guy sitting at the donut shop eating his chocolate dipped while watching the world go by is more spiritual than me, because he's more in reality.

JB: But it's ALL reality, so he's only "more spiritual"—if we can quantify it at all—if he is also holding a more expanded awareness at the same time. He may be, or he may also be a one-winged bird, just having developed the more material wing. In other words, he may be so identified with the practical realms that he doesn't see the bigger picture. So, he too may be tilted in one direction with respect to his consciousness. It all comes down to inclusivity—that is, how connected are we, moment to moment, to the everything. Which includes all threads of the weave.

Having said that, I do wonder if he may be, in a strange way, better positioned to construct an inclusive weave—and this strikes at the heart of my philosophy—because he is more grounded than you are in the here and now. Yes, you believe you are more present because you have tapped into something you call an "absolute" or "pure consciousness," but when one taps into that without, at the same time, developing a rooted consciousness—it is likely their experience of presence is fractured and unsustainable. Simply an avoidant presence—not an integrated one. Qualitatively different. In other words, perhaps you aren't as present as you think, Michael.

M: So, dude, you're trying to tell me I'm not in the moment? Fuck that!

He was now incredibly agitated. He stood up, as though to leave, or to move his body. It was hard to tell. Perhaps I was sharing too much too quickly. After a few moments, he sat back down and again began to play with his mala beads. This seemed to calm him.

JB: If you don't want to continue to dialogue after today, I totally understand. But you did ask for the full load.

M: I didn't think the full load would mean attacking my hard-earned presence.

JB: You are right, I apologize. I shouldn't have directed that comment at you. Let me just speak of my own experience. What I'm proposing is this: When we begin, solidly, on the earth plane, from and within the self, we have the foundation to move into a unified consciousness in a way that is more real, because we know where the self ends and unity begins. It's more genuine, and more sustainable. Yes, there may be no theoretical reason why someone can't connect in with an absolute consciousness first, before coming back to earth and integrating. But since many who turn to the absolute first do so because they are seeking to flee their troublesome experiences on the earth plane, it can become very difficult to come back and integrate. Perhaps it is better to begin with your feet on the ground before expanding into a more unified consciousness.

M: Most people that are trapped in the mundane, don't ever escape that consciousness, dude. They are so over-identified with form, with separation. You know that's true. Just look around… they're everywhere. I don't want to be like them, man. That's not my destiny.

Michael looked out at the street. I joined him. We watched as all manner of human hurried past: urban bike couriers, fresh-faced university students, colorful bohemians, construction workers on a lunch break, a yogi racing to class, a dark-suited businessman talking hurriedly into his smart phone. It was all here.

JB: Yes, but that's not because they can't escape the mundane. That's because we haven't shown them how. Part of the reason people remain so constricted is that society has developed in ways that keep us locked into our tight little boxes so we can be better exploited energetically and economically. As a result, our organic impulse to expand from and through the self has been stifled. This is my work, to find a way to invite humanity beyond a limiting consciousness, without denying the veracity, and *reality*, of their daily experience and divine selfhood. Because, although it may not all be preferred, it's *all* real—that's the point. And there is no point in pulling them out of one limiting consciousness—what you might call the matrix—only to invite them into another—the place you identify as true spirituality—because I see that too as a matrix, if it's not integrated with its other wing. On their own, both wings are lost. They have to function in relation to one another.

M: That's not what I am hearing from you. I hear you saying that those who are more fully immersed in the world, are actually more spiritual.

Sorry man, but that pisses me off.

JB: No need to apologize, your anger is welcome here. Just to be clear... what I am saying is that we would benefit from expanding our definition of spirituality, to include an embracing of all aspects of reality: the form and the formless, the seen and the unseen. A universal and localized lens, our emotional debris and psychological issues, practical challenges and Eastern practices, because it's all infused with spirit, and it is all part of the holy, wholly weave. There can be no inclusive experience of presence if we are not here, for all of it.

Let me ask you, do you think that there isn't spirit in everything? Do you feel that it is only in those stages and states that comfort or uplift you? What about the spirit that courses through your individuated self? Is that not as spiritual, as the spirit that flows through your consciousness in a meditative state?

M: When I enter that meditative state, I am perceiving another reality, one that feels more aligned with spirit.

JB: I beg to differ. What you're describing is not more aligned with spirit, Michael. You just have not yet learned how to find the spirit that threads through your embodied, daily experience. Spirit abounds. It is everywhere. It's *all* God, or Divinity, or sacredness, or whatever you choose to call it. Think of it as the *path of entirety*. With great reverence for the everything, you welcome everything into consciousness. Nothing real gets thrown out—everything comes along for the ride.

In other words, you see the world through every available frame of reference. And you also experience and explore the self in its entirety. You are here for all of *this*, and all of *you*. Your experience of reality—or the spiritual landscape—both reflects and is indistinguishable from a depthful experience of your own humanness. You own and inhabit every aspect of the self—even those parts that you are longing to heal or transform—both as a reflection of divinity, and as your blessed lens on reality. It took untold centuries to develop the self, with all its pathways of perception and uniquely individuated physical properties, and it is not to be denied its place at the sacred banquet table. And that surely includes those elements and aspects of the human experience that are frequently shunned by the ungrounded spirituality communities: your ego structures, your feelings and emotions, your personal story and identifications, your body itself. They are not sub-spiritual fragments—they are the very lens through which you know reality. All elements are fundamental to a truly spiritual life.

M: Man, that's a lot of stuff for me to digest at one time. I'm starting to feel a little tired. I'm still open to listening, but I might need another latte to keep me sharp. How about I grab you one too?

JB: Sure, I'll have another. Make it an espresso actually. And how about we drink and walk?

M: Yeah, let's do that.

Self-Avoidant Realization

We got our drinks and began walking the busy streets. We had been talking for some time, and this train didn't show any sign of slowing down. The sun was still high in the sky, as we made our way west along Bloor Street. Turning the corner north at Christie Street, we nearly stumbled into a groaning homeless man wrapped in a blanket of newspapers. I noticed Michael wince. Then he stopped and said:

M: So, I hear you dude, but I don't want to be here for all of it. It's way too difficult down here. So much needless wounding and suffering. I actually want my spirituality to be my escape, my refuge from this mad world—not a deeper penetration of it.

I nodded to myself. Just what I had suspected in our previous encounter with a homeless man—Michael was seeking to escape. His own words confirmed it.

JB: Then call that refuge, call that escape, but don't call it spirituality, Michael. Don't call it unity consciousness. Don't mislead yourself or others by feigning enlightenment when all you have done is flee your earthly challenges. Detachment is a tool—it's not a life.

M: Most of me wants to scream, but I can admit that some part of me resonates with what you are saying. A small part. For example, I've noticed that on many of my meditations, I'll feel nice and peaceful for a while. The world feels like it is in perfect order, kind and benevolent. Then, I'll leave the meditation hall, and listen to a demanding voicemail from my boss. And I'll want to hurl the phone through a window! What's with that? Are any of these practices capable of being sustained in this mad world?

JB: Sure, if you integrate them with grounding exercises, practices that honor and assimilate your selfhood into the equation. Look, the way that you are using your meditations is like taking a perpetual vacation—you are vacating your humanness. You are using it to get out of here, not to get *into* here.

Michael grimaced and began to walk. For someone who had been sitting for years, he sure could move quickly. I eventually caught up with him, at the next streetlight.

JB: In my experience, it's one thing to find your "center" while detaching from the world. It's a whole other experience to find it at the heart of the world. And at the heart of the self in the world. I often left the world to find my "self." This was an essential step, because I was not yet self-connected enough to find my center in the heart of society. I was too soft, too traumatized. But then I came to realize that if I couldn't hold to my center in the world, then I didn't have much of a center. If all it took was a few days in the marketplace, on urban streets, dealing with humanity, before I had to run back to the woods to find myself… then what had I found? A very fragile, hollow center.

And so the work continued, this time in the world itself. No easy feat, because of my trauma history and the often sedated ways of society, but the truest work I have ever done. Because now I can sit in the middle of hell, and continue to feel my core. Because now I can stand amid the fires of distraction, and sustain my focus. It's one thing to find our center while we are hiding from the world. It's quite another to find it in the everything. Because the holy and wholly grail is YOU, unstoppably solid in the heart of the madness.

M: Yes, but I am seeking self-realization when I meditate. I employ the watcher—a witness observer consciousness—so I can watch the localized self in action and distance myself from it. I observe the monkey mind, continually coming back to the breath until he quiets down and I can reconnect to the bigger picture.

JB: Have you considered the possibility that you may actually be seeking self-avoidant realization? True self-realization is a depthful internal process that integrates our humanness with our spiritual quest. Self-avoidant realization flees the self in search of an allegedly absolute consciousness that is bereft of feeling and non-individuated. You see this in the meditation practices of many avid seekers. They approach them in a limited way. Not in a complete way—not in a way that makes no distinction between the "bigger picture" and the "smaller picture." They continually restrict their inside experience to certain states of consciousness—for example, that of the witness—which is essentially a mind function. Or that of the one who comes back to the breath when the "monkey mind" arises. They are not using the watcher, or the breath, or their meditation practice to lend credence to and embrace the textures and voices of feeling, that arise from the deep within. Instead, they are using these techniques to nullify and distinguish themselves from these feelings. They limit their experience of the inner to those pathways that support their intention: to rise above their humanity. Meditation can quickly become medication, if it is not coupled with deep emotional work.

I remember doing a weekend workshop with a popular meditation teacher. I enjoyed listening to his sweet and funny stories about the spiritual path. At the same time, I was startled by the energetic gap between his calm voice, and the intense rage in his eyes. If ever there was a man who needed to smash a mattress with a baseball bat, it was him. I learned a lot from that workshop, but none of it had to do with meditation. If we are engaging in spiritual practice to avoid our undigested feelings, it won't get us very far. Everything depends on where we are moving from.

M: If you deny people their detachment practices you may destroy them. I know many people who would commit suicide without them.

JB: I totally agree. Healthy detachment practices provide us with an opportunity to breathe, to rest, to integrate, and to take a break from the challenges of earthly life. They provide us with necessary distance and perspective on where we have been and how we identify ourselves. They serve as a forum for the exploration of other ways of being. And yes, for some, they are actually a lifesaver, allowing trauma survivors to heal from unbearable experiences on the earth plane. Without them, many of us would have gone mad or killed ourselves. But the trick is to not stay out there too long. On a pogo stick to the stars, people float off to outer space and lose contact with Mother Earth, to such an extent that they can't find their way back. By turning away from old wounds, they have shackled themselves to their unresolveds. Often, reality brings them back to earth with a harsh and deadly thud. But not always.

M: Life has knocked me back on my ass a few times. But I don't opt to stay there very long. I resume my practice, and soon enough, I'm elevated again.

JB: The bottom line is that sustainable growth demands that we come back down into our bodies and work with what lives inside of us. I can't begin to tell you how many people I have known who fled the world for what they labeled as "pure consciousness," and yet they never found a way to bring it into balance with their daily lives. Their everyday lives remained as muddied as their meditation practice is "pure." It's one thing to realize that there is an expanded field, it is quite another to do the individual work to align our self-hood with it. This is the real work of our lives. We can only do that work by dropping back into our bodies, our identities, our heretofore buried shadows, and weaving our localized self with our vastest imaginings.

M: Woah. I know I asked for the full load, but I think this qualifies as an over-load! I may need a breather to mull these ideas over. I'm not running away. I just need to sit with this for a bit.

JB: I get it. Let me know if you decide to take this further.

The Transcendence Bypass

Michael shook my hand, and quickly crossed the street. I was a little taken aback by his abrupt departure, but I understood. He had moved through his life in a radically different way. This was no easy download for him. Before we could take it to the next level, he had to make a decision—deep within—as to whether he wanted to continue the conversation. It might end up being more than an engaging conversation. It could change his life. So far he was just testing the waters. Now he had to decide whether to dive in.

I decided to forego the subway and walk the long way home. As I walked, I felt a tinge of sadness. I hadn't expected to like this man so much, so quickly. For someone with a very detached way of moving in the world, Michael was remarkably human. In the course of a single afternoon, I became alive to his path, his struggles, his confusion. Reminiscent of my own path, in many ways.

Early the next morning, I awoke to a "ding." A text from Michael:

> Hey Man. You got me thinking lots last night. Didn't sleep a wink. I have some questions for you. When can we meet?

Apparently, he was ready for more. We agreed to resume at our original meeting place: the café in the annex. When I arrived, he was already there, latte in hand. We began walking, amidst the whizzing cars, honking horns and bustling passerbys on the morning commute. Michael picked up where we left off:

M: So, as I was laying in bed last night, restless as hell, I began thinking. You said that it's all about integrating what is down here. But what if you realize that "down here" is madness? What if you opt to transcend the bullshit, and go higher… move beyond?

JB: You mean trance-end. That's what it comes down to. You are trying to get out of one trance, by floating into another. But it doesn't work. Because you can't trance-end by just going into a different kind of trance. You trance-end by coming into reality, in all its forms. That includes the human form and all that comes with it. Which, like it or not, is where we find ourselves now. *Transcend nothing, include everything.* That's my motto.

M: I feel more home when I move beyond my human form, dude. In that space between form and formless—that's where my true home lies. It's warm, and blissful, and I feel nourished. And I don't want to leave that. I want to stay out there. I mean, don't you think that homeless guy would be better off transcending his shitty little life? Embodying his own divinity, so he's not just merely a weak lowly man encaged by his dire life circumstances. He needs to recognize he is much more than that…

JB: It's not certain that transcending his circumstances would help him. Perhaps facing them would. The fact is that many people do stay "out there."

This tendency even has a name. Author John Welwood coined the term "spiritual bypass" in 1984, to describe turning to spirituality in an effort to rise above personal challenges and difficult emotions. Spirit becomes a crutch rather than the expression of a natural unfolding. Meditation—when used to disconnect from or "rise above" our earthly challenges is only one example of this. Another includes reliance on simplistic New Age affirmations. I tried that for awhile. And many seekers bypass by spending their lives analyzing spiritual texts, or looking to gurus and hyped-up soulebrities for their answers, or actually imagining themselves shamans, high priestesses, and a whole gamut of esteemed positions on the spiritual hierarchy. Some even go so far as to change their names to 'spiritual' names, donning the garb and manner of East Indians, ignoring the fact that there is nothing any more spiritual about Eastern names or practices than Western ones. Am I less spiritual because I am named Jeff Brown, than if I changed my name to Je-free Sivananda Brown. Of course not.

M: You know, I never really thought about it that way. Now that you mention it—I can see there are some ways I have bypassed. During one phase on the West Coast, I began to call myself "Nothing." I even asked my friends to call me that. Not as an act of self-hatred, but to represent the insignificance of my history and my story.

JB: Well, Mr. Nothing, that actually is a form of self-hatred. Self-denial, at the least.

M: And I did sit before many a guru, trying to cleanse myself of my human bullshit by basking in their spiritual light. The truth is that it was a bit addictive. Every time my life became intense, I raced to the guru and all my stress would dissolve. But as I am reluctantly realizing with Hannah, it didn't really get to the root of the problem. It provided some relief, but very little resolution. You nailed it, dude. I don't believe that all of what I have engaged in spiritually is a bypass… but I have, at various times, been a spiritual bypasser.

JB: Me too, Michael. Big time. In a world of pain, it's an ongoing temptation. Interestingly, as a result of my own personal development, I seldom refer to this tendency as the "spiritual bypass," or at least the way it is intended. Because I believe that actually perpetuates the problem by labeling these forms of avoidance "spiritual." As I mentioned earlier, spirituality actually means reality—broadly and inclusively defined—and those that bypass reality, cannot be said to be turning to spirituality. If anything, they are turning *away from* spirituality—rising above the spiritual landscape in an effort to negate wearisome aspects of reality.

Having said that, if we re-frame the meaning of the term to communicate the idea that the "spiritual bypass," means that they are bypassing spirituality with their actions, then it works. But I think the term is now too entrenched for that re-characterization to take root. And so, I prefer to call it "The Transcendence Bypass." By 'transcendence' I am not referring to moving beyond the perceived limits of ordinary experience—which is a healthy form of transcendence. I am referring to something more avoidant. Transcendence addiction has become synonymous with spirituality in the West, sadly. Let me find my definition of "Transcendence Bypass," in my phone. Ahh, here we go:

> The tendency to bypass reality through 'transcendent' means: a rising above, a 'heightened' quest, an ungrounded flight of fancy. Common amongst those who identify themselves as "spiritual," the transcendence bypasser has abandoned healthy detachment, floating off into the dissociative abyss until reality brings them back to the ground. The great irony is that transcendence bypassers are actually the ones most controlled by earthly matters. Their addiction to the above is driven by their unresolved issues down below. They have actually trance-ended nothing. It's all still waiting for them here on Mother Earth.

M: But it feels so damn good out there.

JB: Yes, but it doesn't work—at least not for long. If it did, I would be doing it all day long. Like a one- winged bird, the transcendence bypasser comes crashing back to earth when the truth hits the fan. Because we aren't birds, watching the earth from afar. We are humans, standing resolutely in the heart of form. Our expansion is not waiting for us in the sky—it's waiting within, where Authenticity Avenue meets Reality Road, on the Highways of Wholeness. Grace is not something that pours down from the heavens—it's something that rises up from within us.

M: The "transcendence bypass" brings the whole concept up a notch. Man, you're good.

JB: Thank you. And not to be difficult, but it actually brings it down a notch. You see, there ain't no above. Above is part of the lie. It may be deeper or truer, but it's never "above." Because you can't actually rise above or transcend the self. It goes everywhere you go. You can clarify it, you can integrate it, you can expand it, but you can't transcend it. I personally have no interest in the dream of "heaven on earth," any more than I am interested in "heightened consciousness," or calling great human achievements "out of this world." These are just further examples of how we have adopted the belief that everything wondrous originates outside of our human form. I don't agree. There is nothing up there, waiting for us. It begins, and it ends with us. This precious humanness. Let's empower that. It's all in our hands.

What all these bypass frameworks have in common—whether we label them "up there," or "out there," or whatever, is the tendency to limit our understanding of spirituality to preferred pathways of perception. Self-avoidance models masquerading as models of enlightenment, they are more the "Woo Earth," than anything forward moving and evolutionary.

M: I like the idea of a Woo Earth.

JB: It can be fun. And it's fine, perhaps even necessary to visit from time to time. But it's not our place of residence. It's definitely messy business being human, yet, I see no concrete evidence that a mistake was made, putting us in this form. There has got to be an intrinsic purpose to it. In fact, I have discovered that there is. Let's not give up on being here for all of it, just yet.

Bones of your Being

M: I see all kinds of evidence that a mistake was made, but I'm willing to give you the benefit of a doubt for a moment… that somehow you found a secret to life. So, how then does one embrace your broadly defined lens on spirituality—that is, that the most spiritual awareness is the one that holds a tether to all threads of reality—in this mad world? How does it work? Is there a technique? Where does one begin?

JB: With the ground. The dirt. The roots of your being—your human-ness—rooted firmly and unwaveringly on Mother Earth. Stop looking for answers in the sky for the moment. Start right down here, on the planet you were born on. That's where the chaotic magnificence truly lives. In the *messence* of lived experience.

M: The dirt? Seriously? That doesn't feel very spiritual at all! I've had more of my share of shit in this life already.

JB: Life is a dirt path, buddy—not a cosmic chemtrail. That's why creation gave you toes, and not wings.

M: I thought you said it was both—the transcendent, and the immanent?

JB: Yes, but the "one" begins and ends with your feet and your roots. And this brings me to the crux of my philosophy. You asked for the full load. This sums it up. I call it "Grounded Spirituality." Let me explain...

M: Uh-oh. Here we go...

JB: Grounded Spirituality is an all-encompassing experience of spiritual-ity that is rooted in, and threads throughout, all aspects of our humanity and earthly experience. We begin and end our spiritual quest within the ground of our being—our embodied humanness—as both interpreter of experience and as our individuated portal to divinity. We don't look out-side our human form for spirituality, we look deeper within name and form, cultivating a more refined understanding of the divine reflection that exists right in the heart of our selfhood. We honor its sacred qualities and transformative properties, celebrating it as the perfectly constructed laboratory of expansion that it is. With our feet rooted firmly on Mother Earth, and in daily life, we become grounded in reality in all its identifiable forms. We expand outward, and inward, from there.

In essence, Grounded and Spirituality are synonyms. They both mean reality. The more deeply grounded you are in your body and selfhood, the more your fully you are here. The more fully you are here, the more spiritual your experience. It is from the depths of your being that you have the greatest access to the everything. What this means, in concrete terms, is that we stop stepping away from the uncomfortable elements of our humanness, and we fully incorporate and live deeper within the often-maligned self, understanding and appreciating that the more developed the self is the more profound our connection to the spiritual realms. Rather than identifying the self as the enemy of the sacred, we recognize that it is indistinguishable from it, and we embrace, honor, and live through every aspect of the self. Your selfhood: the thing you can truly stand in. The only thing that is truly yours. And the only way you can connect with the world at large and sense, feel, penetrate, this awake universe.

M: Wow, that was quite a download. You had me mesmerized there. But I must admit that I am feeling a tremendous amount of resistance to this "lens on reality." It's like you are turning my entire world-view upside down. My body, my stories, my aspects, have all been characterized as unreal for decades. They are delusions and illusions, all based on a misconstrued self-identity. As human beings, we have forgotten who we are. We think we are this bag of bones—when really we are the essence of divinity. What you are presenting is like trying to learn a new religion, before I have truly accepted that the one I have been practicing is misguided. I can only take in your message a little at a time...

JB: I understand—I am inviting you and others toward a radical shift in perspective. If ungrounded seekers choose to embrace this, they will no longer see the body as "unspiritual." They will see it as their Temple of Truth. They won't flee their shadow—they will embrace it as a great teacher. They won't deny their stories—they will go deeper inside them to uncover their ultimate meaning. They won't disparage the ego's function—they will learn to understand and honor its profound significance, and recognize how it reflects the soul's journey. They won't reference their feelings as illusions—they will see them as a trail back to source. They won't characterize their emotional life as inferior to their spiritual life—they will work to understand their inherent synergy. They won't shame the quest for a healthy self-concept—they will revere its role in protecting and growing the self. They won't deny the significance of our basic, worldly needs—they will see their efforts to meet them as one way they express their love for their self. They won't dismiss the value of psycho-therapeutic process on their spiritual path—they will see it as an essential aspect of the self-realization journey. They won't discredit relationship on the path to awakening—they will see it as a fundamental necessity.

With this perspective, you will find miracles right here, in the bones of your being. The miracle of birth. The miracle of selfhood. The miracle of love. Miracles coursing through your veins.

Michael looked down and began fiddling with his cell phone. He looked quite uncomfortable, like a deer in the headlights. Radically exposed.

M: That's a lot to absorb. To be honest... I feel like running away right now.

JB: I appreciate your honesty Michael. Where are you feeling that?

M: In my body, I guess—in those bones of my being. I am definitely aware of thoughts that are telling me to run, but sense that they are coming from my body. I actually feel nauseous and a bit dizzy. Suddenly very tired. Can we end this now?

JB: As you wish. But first a question: Why do you feel you are having this response at this precise moment in our dialogue?

M: Not sure, maybe because I didn't sleep enough? Is it fatigue talking?

JB: That's certainly possible. Any other possibilities drift into awareness?

M: Yes, I am feeling some sadness rising into awareness. I feel an urge to check-out, to create another fantasy version of this moment to hide in. The reality you are speaking of does not feel very pleasant. Not one bit.

JB: I know. It can feel like a harsh awakening. But that's just the first step. There is much more. This dance between truth and fantasy, real and feigned, cuts to the heart of our greatest struggle on this planet: the struggle to be genuinely here. Everywhere I look, I see people who don't want to be here. They don't want to die, exactly, but they don't want to be here, in the raw uncovered reality of existence. And it's not only apparent in their addictive tendencies, it's apparent in very normalized ways: *self-distractive* (and yes, of course, self-destructive) tendencies, shallowing of breath and perspective, perpetual positivity, the transcendence bypass, to give some examples. There are billions of ways to hide from the moment. I often wonder what has to happen before we can co-create a world that invites us to be here?

And how can we construct that world if we have already left it? Where is the bridge *back* to here?

M: Man, this is a lot to take in at once, especially if we have been living fantastically and "in transit," so to speak, for a long time.

JB: Yes, it is a lot. I know from my own painful journey—the descent back down to earth is not an easy trek, particularly because the return to the real often begins with an encounter with our buried wounds. It demands that we bravely face our dragons head-on. It implores us to find the Godself in the darkest of places.

But escapism isn't a walk in the park either. It takes a great deal of energy to remain constantly in-flight. Exhausting. What we need now are techniques that take us deeper into each aspect of the self, so that we stop flying away. Because these techniques have been underdeveloped in society at large, seekers and trauma-survivors have often had no choice but to turn away from themselves, in order to find meaning. There has been no other choice. To go deeper into the pained self with few models for working it through to transformation would have only created more suffering. And even those with the intention of developing a self-honoring spiritual model have had to deal with a spiritual world determined to convince us that our liberation exists outside of the world of feelings, relationship, and the "toxic body beast." These perspectives have been passed down generationally and continue to plague the spiritual landscape.

M: Not just in spirituality, but in religion too. I went through it with my dad. He wasn't a spiritual guy, by any means, but whenever he would be asked to deal with his feelings, he would always say, "Let's just leave that where Jesus flung it." He wouldn't answer the question directly, no matter what was at stake. And all the men—and some of the women—in his church would say the same thing. Pretty easy to pass the buck to a dead man.

JB: Yes, just kind of like passing the buck to a dead guru. Pretty safe, because he can't reveal his humanness and disappoint you. But ultimately ungratifying.

M: True dat. So, how do we make our way back down here? Can you give me a first step?

JB: Yes, I can. Are you open to a basic exercise?

M: Is it going to make me feel more nauseous? Because right now I feel I might hurl.

JB: It may even quell your nausea. But, it's your choice. If you feel you've had enough, we can call it a day.

M: No, no. You piqued my curiosity. Let's try the exercise...

I quickly crossed the street, heading for a small neighborhood park on Albany Street. I motioned for Michael to join me. I wanted to move swiftly before he changed his mind. I knew the perfect exercise for the moment: the grounding technique I had learned from Bioenergetics Co-founder Alexander Lowen.

When we arrived, I asked Michael to take off his socks and shoes, and stand before me. When he was ready, I took him through the exercise.

EXERCISE 1
ALEXANDER LOWEN'S BASIC VIBRATORY AND GROUNDING EXERCISE

Stand with feet about 10" apart, toes slightly turned in so as to stretch some of the muscles of the buttocks. Bend forward and touch the ground with the fingers of both hands. The knees should be slightly bent. No weight should be on the hands; all the body weight is in the feet. Let the head drop as much as possible.

Breathe through your mouth easily and deeply. Make sure to keep breathing. Forget about breathing through your nose for the time being.

Let the weight of your body go forward so that it is on the balls of the feet. The heels can be slightly raised.

Straighten the knees slowly until the hamstring muscles are stretched and you feel vibrations in your legs. Do not lock your knees backward as this immobilizes the legs. Hold the position for about one minute.

Once Michael assumed the grounding position, I added a little more instruction:

JB: Feel free to remain in the position for longer, if it serves you. Be particularly connected to your feet. Feel them to the extent that you can as they make contact with the Earth. Feel into the whole of your body, as you surrender to your breath. Sometimes the vibration will begin to excavate old memories and feelings. Be with whatever it is. If there are feelings that arise, give them permission to be fully felt and experienced. There is no judgment here.

Michael stayed in the position for closer to ten minutes. I attempted to stop him a few times—concerned that it would be too much too soon—but he ignored me and carried on. Something was clearly afoot. ☺ *When he was finally done, he got down on his knees and closed his eyes.*

JB: When you're ready, I invite you to share your experience. How did that feel?

M: Honestly, terrifying. At first, I felt a strong resistance and a kind of darkness, like the way you feel when it's about to storm. Things got grey, and I felt myself, again, wanting to hide. I began to have visions of myself meditating, perhaps in an effort to restore my equilibrium. Yes, that's it. I felt like I wanted something to soothe myself, or else I would just make up an excuse and stop. And then I heard myself say, "Come back into this experience."

JB: This is very common when people do this exercise. It appears simple, but it is actually quite impactful. Many of us have a tendency to be up there, there, there. The purpose of this exercise is to come down here, here, here. This exercise can be challenging, especially if we are not used to being in our feet and our bodies. We *know* we have feet, but actually feeling them making contact with the earth is a different thing. Where do you imagine that voice was coming from, Michael?

M: I want to say, "my ego," but right now I'm not even sure what that means. Not entirely sure…

JB: What happened next?

M: I felt a little faint, and then a kind of vibration moving from my feet, up my legs, into my tight hips, into my belly, where I began to feel pain and a sudden urge to cry. Again, the resistance arose and a voice inside told me to stop wasting my time… But I kept at it, breathing even stronger… and then memories flashed before me, as if they were riding on the wave of my breath.

JB: They were… and being released in the opening of the age-old tensions. Contractions that you have sustained in an unconscious effort to contain the feelings you don't want to assimilate.

M: Yes, that feels true… right after that happened, I felt a strong need to sob, but I wasn't ready. That's when I stopped. You are right. This exercise is fucking intense.

JB: I commend you for staying with it, my friend. You were down there a long time. No sense pushing yourself so hard that you end up retreating forever.

M: Interesting though, the nausea has left me. I feel somewhat settled actually.

JB: Great. Let's leave it here for now, and meet again after you have integrated some of these ideas and experiences, to see where they land.

M: Okay, this was a helluva meeting. You gave me a lot to digest. Let me give this a few days to process. I'll text you when I'm ready to meet again.

As I took the streetcar home, I noticed the vivid and vibrant spectrum of life… the rays of sunlight shining through the windows… a homeless man sleeping on a park bench, looking strangely content… an Asian woman arguing with her lover on the sidewalk. Life's ever-woven mysteries manifest in human form. I felt fully present for all of it, rooted in the bones of my being. And, at the same time, connected to a 'beyond' that was simultaneously unseen and showing its face to the world. I thought back to my own spiritual path, my own circuitous routes to bring me to this moment in time. As with Michael, it had started off with so much raw unbridled emotion, before the world shut me down. Unlike Michael, I had chosen to fight my way back to feeling. That was my choice, my path. His was to be decided, on his terms. It's like this for all of us. We are all confronted with the same question: How fully and deeply will I live? And then we decide, with every breath. With every step. Plain and simple — Life is not for the faint of soul. Few people actually want to be here for the full human experience. But when we can open to all of it — we also open to a vitality and a richness that no fantasy can ever parallel. What choice would Michael make, now?

2 The Art of Enrealment

To my surprise, three weeks went by and I didn't hear from him. I felt a hint of concern that maybe I had pushed him too hard, but I had an odd faith that he could handle it. His years of focus on his spiritual path belied a very strong and willful man.

Then, one morning while I was enjoying a turmeric latte on Queen West—I felt my phone buzz.

A text from Michael:

> Hey dude, it's Michael. Did the exercise a few more times. I want to talk to you. Name the time and place.

We set up a hike in High Park, one of Toronto's many beautiful refuges, nestled in the heart of a bustling city. Walking in nature would be the perfect grounding medicine. It was a beautiful fall day—autumn's touch splattering the leaves with a rainbow spectrum of vivid colors.

When we saw each other again—we didn't bother with any small-talk. Obviously, the last exercise had affected him, and he wanted to get to the meat of it. We sat down at a picnic table and he immediately began to share:

M: So, dude, I want to share my experience of the exercise and what came up afterwards. I had a shitload of feelings and reactions arise. You got to me, man. Enough that I even did the exercise a few more times on my own.

JB: Great, must have been a busy few weeks. Do tell…

M: Okay, after doing the exercise, I found myself shaking. It wasn't a severe shaking, but it was still intense. And there was like a vortex of energy moving through my belly. And a reservoir of feelings, mostly tears and anger. I assume it was old anger, but I couldn't really identify where it was coming from. What strikes me as strange is that I have done a position similar to that in yoga for years—Uttanasana—without having any emotional response to it. Don't know why this hit me so differently. But, dude, it really rocked me.

JB: I could tell you the difference. This was a body practice with a direct invitation for your feelings and expression to arise. You gave permission. Much comes down to intention, and how we create the conditions to excavate buried emotions. It doesn't mean they necessarily will arise, but it means that there is a safe container if they are ready to. This seldom happens in yoga class.

M: I find yoga to provide a very safe space. But, anyways, that's beside the point. Each time I did the exercise, I kept coming into contact with the feelings and their related anxieties. Not just raw feelings, but memories, too. Like shit I haven't thought about in ages. An image of my dad sobbing into his hands when he found out his sister was killed in a car accident. I never thought about that before—I was only three at the time. An image of wailing in my crib as a two-year-old, with my teen cousin babysitter ignoring me, and fearing that my parents would never return. I felt like I was right back there, experiencing all the sensations. While conceding that the feelings are real, giving them so much attention seemed to take me further away from the bigger picture. I felt completely unenlightened, trapped inside my pain. I felt like I was that little bawling infant again. Like I've barely matured at all. Lost and alone. Unable to find the light switch. Honestly, it sucked. So, that's part of the reason why I wanted to meet you today. Just to say—what the fuck, dude? We're just getting started and I am already going backwards.

JB: Yes, that could be jarring. But, look, part of the reason why it "sucks" is because you aren't accustomed to connecting with those feelings. You haven't delved into your shadow. The feelings have not been part of your spiritual practice and so, when they arise, you are overwhelmed by them. Through your narrow lens on reality, you don't see any way to go there while still remaining connected with what you call the bigger picture, what some call "an enlightened consciousness." But I assure you, my friend—there's light at the end of the feeling-tunnel. You need more time with your feelings, more process around them, before they can reveal their connection to the greater picture.

M: But, enlightenment is my highest aspiration.

JB: I totally get that, but just like with the word 'spiritual,' it all depends on how we define a term. Although it has been broadly defined in the consciousness literature, enlightenment is often interpreted as a rarefied and transcendent state of being that is detached from our everyday concerns—one that is focused on the 'light,' first and foremost. It is not integrative of the emotional body and our personal shadow. It is dismissive of them. This fragmented idea of enlightenment comes in many forms. For some—let's refer to them as "bliss-trippers"—enlightenment is a 'trip the light fantastic' joyous state, one where they float above earthly challenges. For others—let's call them "head-trippers"—enlightenment is a cerebral construct, one where the moment is experienced exclusively through the intellect, safely detached from the world of feeling. And often coursing through all of them is a version of enlightenment that defiantly dissociates from everything that is the self—as though the self, it-self, is necessarily unenlightened. By detaching from the "self-centered" dualities, by disconnecting from and flattening the personality, by witnessing rather than jumping into the pain, one allegedly nestles into a vaster field of awareness. In all of these states, one feels the barbs of daily struggle less acutely, not because they aren't actually occurring, but because they have been sidestepped, or more accurately worded, relegated to secondary points of focus. The enlightened sit on their perches above the fray, while the allegedly 'unconscious' chase their tails down below.

M: Yes, that's the point, man! Remaining in a state of being that is "above the fray" is actually more real than being locked in the prison of our feelings. What you are describing—feelings, emotions, stories—are momentary blips on a screen. They are not of our true self. Our feelings are merely fragments of imperfection. In reality, we are the background that holds this fleeting phenomena. THAT is the true self. The identification with our feelings is what separates us from our inherent perfection of "being." My aim in this lifetime is to return to that inherent perfection—and live it. That's why I'm here.

JB: Yes, but what would give you the idea that feelings are separate from that inherent perfection? Separate from your flawless background "self"? Why can't they be wholly included within it, complementary brushstrokes on your canvas of being? By contrast, what I call Grounded Spirituality begins with the concept of "Enrealment," a kitschy but pragmatic term that celebrates authenticity and inclusivity in all its myriad forms.

M: Enrealment. Did you make that up? How do you think up this shit?

JB: At its core is the idea that a more evolved, or evolving, consciousness is not all about the light (as en-light-enment implies) but is about becoming more real, more genuinely here in all respects. Again, spirituality IS reality. It is about living in all aspects of reality simultaneously rather than only those realms that feel the most manageable. We are not just the light, or the mind, or the emptiness, or eternal positivity. We are the everything. It's all God, even the dust that falls off our awakening hearts. What is enlighten-ment, Michael, if not intimacy with all that is real?

M: You seem to be talking about a wider perspective, that includes form and formless, equally. In that way, I won't be doomed to be stuck in my dense unresolved emotions forever, right? When those feelings and memo-ries arose from childhood, I found myself plummeting into a wave of fear, especially the fear that I would get pulled into them and never get out.

JB: Right, it's not about staying stuck. It's about living from a broader point of access, and becoming unstuck. Take heart, the more you take time to process your feelings and emotions—the more they will shift and change. Feelings are fluid and ever-morphing. In their true nature, they aren't thick, stationary, dense, concrete. As you saw in the initial exercise, transcending them doesn't make them go away. It just locks them inside your body—held within muscular tensions and habits of movement—and gives them more power, as they lie hidden inside and rule your life. They become like a sleeping dragon, and when they finally awaken, they ROARR. That could be quite overwhelming, Michael. I get it. But it is possible to thaw them out and enliven them, granting them the space they need to move, and to integrate with our other threads of consciousness. Waking the feeling dragon is not the end of the story…

M: Okay, tell me what's next then...

Ascending with Both Feet on the Ground

His eyes were scoping me out with a sort of cautious curiosity. In those last moments of dialogue, he had worked through his concern about being entrapped in the world of feelings. Yes. He was ready to hear about Enrealment. We got up and headed for the trail along Grenadier Pond.

JB: Can I tell you what it means to be an enrealed individual?

M: Go for it.

JB: An enrealed human-being has a wider energetic girth. She recognizes that sustainable transformation requires a turning toward all elements of reality, and not a turning away from them. Her consciousness may be focused on a single realm at times, but all the other gateways are ajar, accessible, and close at heart. He is alive to his feelings and attuned to his psycho-emotional state. He is aware of and actively works on his unresolved patterns and issues. She is relationally connective. She is aware of her sociological context, her ancestral roots, the family of humans that support her. Her feet are firmly grounded on the earth plane, while at the same time being attuned to subtler intangible states of awareness. He feels connected to his body temple—both its open and closed places. He is healthily boundaried but not closed off—fluid, not fixed. He is aware of the world around him, including the natural world. She is conscious of her localized reality and aware of her practical needs and responsibilities—things to do, obligations, commitments to honor—and yet is also aware of her place in the vaster field. She sees the bigger picture, not from a bird's eye view, but from the depths of her being. She sees spirituality everywhere.

M: That's a lot to hold at one time, dude.

JB: Yes it is. It's a process, Michael. An ongoing "real-eyes-ation" journey. With a little more real each day.

Michael stopped and gazed at the pond pensively. He went quiet for a few minutes, before turning toward me and speaking his mind.

M: One thing I have come to realize with certainty—particularly after losing a dear friend to cancer—is that we are only here for the blink of an eye. At least in this incarnation. As I listen to your ideas, I am left wondering if what you are expressing is remotely feasible, given how little time we have in our daily lives to do anything other than eat, work, shit, sleep? What you are proposing is that we work on so many levels at one time, it's hard to imagine that we could do anything else.

JB: Well, I suspect that if we become better at honoring our time and avoiding distractions, many of us will be startled to find that we have an abundance of time to be here. We have just enough time to come into our wholeness. After all, it is our natural inclination to grow in every direction. Having said that, I do recognize that I have a particular bias, something I came to realize early in life. At a young age, I reached the conclusion that if I could have just one day (or preferably one week), where I felt like I was fully and wholly present in this lifetime—like here in each and every regard—that I would be willing to work and strive my entire life for that. I became acutely aware around the age of 16, that this was going to be the lifetime where I would actualize myself in every respect possible, even if it meant that I suffered repeatedly along the way. That could even mean I would delay all contentment until just before the end. I was prepared for that sacrifice. I knew I could just opt for something less complete, like a strategy or a philosophy that would bring me relative satisfaction in my life, as many do… but I didn't want that. I didn't want an easier substitute gratification path, I wanted the whole enchilada. The enreal deal.

M: That's commendable. I wish I could say the same. But we just don't have time for that! Especially in this super-stimulated world. Life is too overwhelming, too draining, too rapid. Better to focus on the highest prize while we still can. Keep our gaze pointed at the mountaintop, lest we stay stuck in the valleys below.

JB: Let me express this another way. Is it fair to say that you would prefer your experience on the mountaintop to be sustainable, rather than just an occasional visit?

M: Of course.

JB: Great. As I see it, there are two ways to do that. One is the way you have been doing it. You touch that place, and then you come back to the world and lose your connection to it. You do this, over and over, for years, decades, maybe lifetimes... ever frustrated when you have to fall back into a more worldly consciousness.

M: You nailed it. That is what it's like, a sort of re-entry trauma when I have to come back down from that pristine consciousness and confront the world.

JB: Right, because you are—as I said when we first met—bifurcating your consciousness. Either heightened or human, or, in your words, Mountaintop or valleys. It doesn't work. How about if you try it a different way—the enrealed way—and work hard to integrate the above with the below, so that your visit to the mountaintop is sustainable, and you don't have to keep falling off the peak to attend to your blind spots. A truly spiritual life is about something more than bouncing back and forth between ways of being, like a relief-seeking missile. It's about integrating our various aspects into one multifaceted way of being.

M: It's clear that we just have different ideas of integration. For me, integration means sustaining that higher "bird's eye view" by lingering above the world, untouched by it. Being here, but not being affected and pulled around by all of life's highs and lows. Maintaining a serene equilibrium. This is the art form I practice. If I keep at it, if I keep diligently refining my higher state, I believe that I will integrate this vantage point as a permanent way of being. That's what it means to enlighten your consciousness.

JB: Good luck with that. Your disconnection from the world *will* become permanent, Michael. But only when you die. It's not possible when you are alive. That's not actually what we are here for. If we were meant to be disconnected from the world, we would be angels or etheric beings. You are trying to kill the self, before its time. It's a kind of pseudo-spiritual suicide and it doesn't actually work, because you are still of the world, like it or not. As it is, you are like a penthouse with no ground floor—a perfect recipe for disaster, or, at the least, a fleeting state of being. How about if you learn how to arrive at the mountaintop, not as a flight of fancy that inevitably falls back to earth, but as the organic next step in your own development? Think of it as the difference between seeing the top of the mountain on a pogo stick, or arriving there by going step by steady step up each rock, until you reach the peak.

M: But how does this actually happen? It sounds nice in theory...

JB: At the heart of enrealment is the vision of a person ascending with both feet on the ground. For a moment, let's lean into the vision—imagine yourself literally ascending while you keep both feet sturdily on the ground. Not ascending as in floating above, but ascending as in moving into a more expansive perspective, originating from your solid roots. Instead of moving into reality from the sky down, you move into it from the ground up. And, it is not enough for your feet to simply skim the ground. The authentic life begins with your feet securely fastened on Mother Earth. That is, you begin by deeply grounding your consciousness on the earth plane. You grow down, to grow up. With your soles firmly planted, your Soul has a leg to stand on in its efforts to evolve.

If we don't ascend with both feet on the ground, reality will always slam us back down to earth. This is the nature of karmic gravity. From a stable foundation emerges a natural and sustainable movement upward and outward. Instead of settling for the occasional peak experience, you are now capable of maintaining a more truly expansive way of being. Your experience of the moment is no longer fragmented, or reactive in its origins, but arises through a stable and integrated structure. You are really *here*. You have harmoniously integrated your bird's eye view with your localized lens, from the ground up. Now tell me—how is this not spiritual?

Masterybation

He was quiet for quite awhile, still looking out at the placid pond. His eyes belied a look of peering into the vista I opened up for him. I could sense I had activated a new realm of possibility. But expert level spiritual sophistication doesn't surrender easily. I also knew that. With a knitted brow and concentrated thought, he finally answered:

M: It's not spiritual, because it's not masterful. I was trained in the art of mastery. I don't want to be a "Jack of all trades, master of none." You find your particular spiritual practice, and you go deeper into it, perfecting it until you touch a pure consciousness. It is mastery that opens the gate. When we don't maintain a one-pointed focus, we disperse our precious energies in many disparate directions. It's sloppy.

JB: I'm not opposed to mastery, if what we are mastering is fundamental to our time on earth. But I am opposed to mastery that is a persistent, and determined effort to bypass reality. That's not mastery. That's little more than *masterybation*. Basically, you are using spirituality to satisfy yourself, in some odd and isolated way. It's like a porn addiction. It's no substitute for the real thing. In fact, it's the furthest thing from real intimacy, as you exist in an isolated sphere. Again, we come back to intention. Are you mastering a practice, or a path, because you have a deep calling to it—that is, it's one of your personally encoded portals to divinity, like the calling to heal the sick, or to become a parent... or are you mastering it as an escape hatch? It all comes down to this: do you want mastery, or do you want reality?

M: There is a third option, dude. Mastering something because it provides a clear highway into a more expanded consciousness, something difficult to achieve in this bullshit world. It gives me direct access, and it also gives me faith and hope there is something more.

I have a question for you, bro. Do you believe in past lives? You see, I believe I have been through this incarnation numerous times. I have already lived out the emotional bodies. I have probably even spent a whole past life sitting in a shrink's office processing my feelings. No wonder I'm so averse to them. Been there, done that. I truly believe my "calling"—as you mentioned—in this lifetime is about the bigger picture. It's not about the human hamster wheel. I don't know about you, but this is my last lifetime. I'm sure of it.

JB: Spoken like a true transcendence bypasser. A transcendence bypasser's proclivity to not integrate their feelings is so pervasive that they have actually formed a whole past lives story to justify their resistance. The truth is I can't tell you if there are past lives, or not. I prefer not to theorize or speculate. That's a head-trip. I go by what I know in my bones. And, what I can tell you for certain: Enrealment IS the way off the human hamster wheel. It is our destiny as human beings. The one-threaded consciousness called 'enlightenment' that you are referring to as the ultimate goal—is NOT actually the ultimate. It doesn't even begin to fulfill our purpose as to why we are here. What if... the whole point is to actually fulfill your unique blueprint of a whole human being in this lifetime—incorporating the ALL of you—and that's what frees you from any need to come back again?

M: So you are saying that the way out of *samsara* (the cycle of death and rebirth), as the Buddhists believe, is to go up the mountain and then come back again.

JB: Exactly. The Mountain is easy. It's what you do next that matters. If you just stay up there, without coming back and weaving this clarified consciousness with other elements of your reality, then you, again, end up highly developed in one regard, while underdeveloped in another regard. You end up on a one-way street home. But human beings are meant to be a multi-laned highway, with myriad exits and entry points. And, of course, this has been the intention of many in the spiritual community for centuries, particularly men. They have conveniently characterized 'spirituality' as little more than the perfecting of a single-threaded consciousness. Individuals become effective at one state or practice—skilled witnessers, expert medita-tors, head-tripping masterminds, Olympic champions of story reframe and premature forgiveness—and they deem that limited state 'spiritual.' Yet, it isn't truly spiritual or truly whole—because they have failed to develop many other aspects. They have developed one thread, at the expense of the others. But it's not the wholly weave.

It is my belief that mastery, in most cases, is little more than patriarchy's self-avoidant mask. I suspect it began with men who didn't want to deal with their feelings, but couldn't admit it so they had to portray their avoidance mechanisms as enlightenment. To them, being a "Jack of all trades, master of none", is a grave failure. To me, it can be a more awakening state, closer to an inclusive spiritual consciousness because more threads are active and alive: Jack of all trades, master of the "One." What would happen to men if they accepted that there is no final place to arrive at, but, instead, an endless not knowing to deepen into and explore? They might just find a deeper, and more persistent sense of satisfaction with this blessed life. Not rarefied, but realified—available to and within all. We are not striving to become perfect. We are striving to become real, to show up for our life in every respect, flaws and all. Be real now.

M: In his writings, Integral Theory founder Ken Wilber has said that it is entirely possible for someone to be well-developed along one developmental line, and not on another. So, for example, one could be very advanced spiritually, and simultaneously underdeveloped in other ways, including psychological maturity. Nothing wrong with that.

JB: The two are not actually separate. They are two sides of the same coin. Psychological and spiritual maturation are synonymous. The state of our psyche is a direct reflection of the stage of our soul on its journey through time. Yes, if you again define spirituality as something distinct from our humanness, one can make an argument like this. But I can't, because I believe that our humanness and our spirituality are moving along the same developmental line.

If your goal is to be here, I mean to really BE HERE, you must weave all aspects of reality, into one aligned and intricate tapestry—including those threads you most determinedly shun and resist. You can't mature within one thread, without maturing in the others. There must be a fundamental maturation across all elements of the human landscape. Think of it as a kind of conscious in-threading of elements and aspects, so that we are not approaching the spiritual field as distinct segments, each with their own level of evolution. Instead, every aspect weaves with the others, elevating, and deepening all of them, into a more inclusive consciousness. Again, the wholly weave.

M: But maybe they belong separate and distinct. Maybe it's not about mixing the aspects—but actually distilling them.

JB: That's the 'single-threaded consciousness' game right there. Pick the thread that feels good, zap the others. That way one can claim to be "spiritually evolved," without having to do any of the work to heal their wounds or change their behavior. Don't buy it. It's more of a desperate reach for God than an eye-to-eye meeting with the Divine.

I remember when I first tasted from the unity tree as an eager young bypasser. Compared to what I had known before, it felt magnificently complete. But it was only the beginning. It was only after I fell from my perch that the real work began. Once the soles of my feet hit the dirt, what

I had once called unity was revealed as a small fragment of possibility. Not because what I had seen was false, but because it was limited—in its scope, and endurability—by its lack of integration with my humanness. With new eyes, the gate opened to a much vaster and richer terrain. Simply put, the more deeply and truly we grow in our self-hood, the more deeply we penetrate and sustain a unified field of consciousness. It's a whole different universe when we absorb it with every cell. Then it's not just about height—it's also about depth, breadth, and an ever-widening lens on reality. In other words, if you want to live a more spiritual life, live a more human life. Be more truly madly deeply human.

M: This feels too conceptual. I need a more concrete understanding. My brain is maxed out. I think it's time for me to go.

JB: I have just the antidote for conceptual. Let me give you another exercise to try at home. Do it soon, and report your experience when we meet again. I call this "The Enrealment Walking Meditation."

M: I'll try it.

EXERCISE 2
THE ENREALMENT WALKING MEDITATION

There are two parts to this exercise. First, do a general sitting meditation of your choice. Spend at least thirty minutes engaged in it. When you are done, go for a walk in your neighborhood, alone, for at least thirty more minutes. While you are walking, pay close attention to both what you feel and what you see. Ponder these questions:

How connected do you feel to yourself?
Are you feeling any emotions? What are they?
Can you feel your body, your breath, your feet making contact with the ground?
How connected do you feel to landscapes, buildings, and vehicles?
To other people that you see?
Do you feel connected to them or distinct from them?
Do you feel connected to the "oneness" field?
Are you aware of your practical responsibilities, duties, and obligations?

*As you walk, would you describe yourself as cerebral, emotional, or
equanimous?*
What is your present state?
What thoughts and feelings are entering your consciousness as you walk?
Allow yourself to be with them.

The next day, do this exercise in a different way. Spend 30 minutes doing the
Bioenergetic Vibratory and Grounding practice. Do not meditate. Do not use any
control methods or mechanisms. Have no quest for equanimity, and make no efforts
to focus your mind. This practice is a mind-free immersion into the body. While
doing this, remember to give yourself permission to invite your feelings and any
expressions to the surface.

And then, go on the same walk and ask yourself all the same questions. Note the
differences between this walk, and your previous walk.

JB: So, after you try this exercise, we can reconvene. Sound good?

M: Hmmm, let me just get through this exercise. I'll let you know. I remember what happened last time.

*With that, we shook hands and parted ways. After his first exercise, it was no
wonder he might be uncertain about a follow-up meeting. I wondered if it would
take him another three weeks to call me back. Funny how challenging it can be
for someone living up on a supposedly spiritual perch, to suddenly re-orient their
lens back on earth. And live from the ground up. How did we get so disconnected
from our most natural state?*

*On the way back to the subway, I took a detour through my favorite part of the
park—the outdoor zoo. Something about watching bison, llamas and peacock move
about always brought me back into my animal body. As I stopped to marvel at them,
I breathed into my own aliveness—my open and closed places, my points of access
and pathways of resistance, the degree to which I could, and could not, truly feel
the moment. It is one thing to talk about being here for all of it. That's easy enough.
It is quite another to actually FEEL here for all of it. That's when real life begins.*

3 Truth is the Gateway to the Moment

Heaven knows we need never be ashamed of our
tears, for they are rain upon the blinding dust of
earth, overlying our hard hearts. I was better after I
had cried, than before—more sorry, more aware of
my own ingratitude, more gentle.

— CHARLES DICKENS

Quite unexpectedly, he contacted me soon after. Not three weeks—but three days. We met at Trinity Bellwoods Park on Queen West—one of the most vibrant parts of Toronto. I enjoyed meeting Michael in different areas of the city. It gave us a chance to be exposed to the energies of varied environments, while discussing a multifaceted consciousness. The perfect synergy.

I grabbed a cappuccino and sat down on a bench near the park's entrance. Moments later, Michael sat down gruffly, without a hello. He had a coffee and a few packets of sugar in his hand. As he dumped a load into the cup, his movements felt very controlled and contained. Like he was restraining himself. And he seemed determined to not look directly at me. I knew it would take some probing to uncover what was seething beneath the surface.

JB: Good to see you, Michael. I'm eager to hear about your experience with the exercises.

To my surprise, he didn't hesitate and jumped right in.

M: So, exercise number one—meditate for a half hour. Then walk. I went into my special sanctuary—it's all my own. Hannah doesn't dare enter it. Dim lighting—just a few salt lamps. An altar with photos of my teachers throughout the years, special trinkets I collected, a rock from the Himalayas, a crystal from Peru, my worn-out meditation cushion… you get the idea. So I did the meditation exercise I normally do each morning. Watching my breath—counting my mala beads. And then I walked to work, mulling over the inquiries you had suggested. The walk was the same as always. I experienced myself as both separate from everyone and everything around me—as though inside of a pristine consciousness bubble of my own—and, simultaneously, tapped into the sense that we were all part of the same field of consciousness.

JB: Did you feel connected to them in a personal sense?

M: Hmmm. No, more impersonally. This was not an inter-relational state. It was a state of pure inner peace. I had everything I needed right here, within me, and yet I was an extension of everyone else.

JB: And your body? How did you experience your body on your walk?

M: Again, somewhat impersonally. I felt strongly connected to my breath, my feet touching the ground, and yet my body felt very serene. As it usually does after meditation.

JB: And, how did the world look to you?

M: To be honest, I didn't notice much of it. When I meditate, it's about entering the within. Spirit. It's not about giving attention to the world.

JB: I find it interesting that what you often call spirit, or spirituality, is something with so little feeling to it. Whenever I am alive to spirit, I am vividly aware of the world around me, and full of robust feeling.

M: I think you have made that point already.

JB: You are right. No need to interject my own commentary. Is there anything else you want to add about the first walk?

M: Basically, it was the same-old same-old walk I do every day. Not much new to report.

JB: Okay, so what about the second exercise—the grounding and release practice before going for the walk?

M: Now this one was a bugger. First, it was incredibly agitating to do the grounding exercise. Harder than the first time. I had to stop and start a few times before I could go through with it. I would fall forward and deepen my breath, and then find myself feeling intensely fatigued. So I would stop. And one time I started coughing and choking uncontrollably. Don't know what that was all about.

JB: I can give you a hint. Our body is like a record of our existence. It holds all the imprints we have experienced—the joys, the pains, the scars, the traumas. So, when you are opening to your body, you are also opening to the feelings that are embedded within it. Those feelings you haven't fully processed are often the ones that come up first, seeking release and resolution.

M: But coughing and choking uncontrollably? What does that have to do with emotions? Maybe it was hay-fever.

JB: Lots. Repressed feelings show up in many different somatised forms. Disease, habits, patterns of movement, certain tics, twitches, and mannerisms. The list goes on. So, if for example, you repressed grief, sadness, and unsaid words in your throat and chest, this exercise could stimulate those buried emotions in the form of an intense cough, or choking sensation. Remember, you are waking up your sleeping dragon. First thing he does is spit and roar.

The body is a universe in and of itself. Built with innate intelligence and vigilant in its own protection. Constantly finding ways to contain painful feelings and emotions so that we can subsist.

M: Well, I mustered up the courage to face my spitting dragon and pushed myself through the entire exercise. It was not easy. I had to use every motivational thinking technique I could, and yet, at the same time, I felt progressively more angry. It was like the energy that was coursing through my body was drawing in every old remnant of anger, like a magnet.

JB: And what happened when you took it to the streets?

M: I was hit by a burst of boiling rage. Soon I wasn't just walking—I was storming around like a madman. In my usual meditations, I glide a step above the world. With this, I felt completely enmeshed in the world. Everything felt like arrows piercing me. The sun felt blinding and oppressive. The bird songs felt screechy. I felt angry at the street noises, the people driving by, you for making me do this. I would walk past people's houses and feel like kicking their perfectly placed garbage cans into the streets. Perhaps because I was in touch with my own anger, I experienced everything around me as aggressive. And then I began longing for the quiet, still, more placid world I experience when meditating. I wanted my filters back. I wanted to slow down reality again. So, I went back to my sanctuary and meditated, like I always do. Then I felt better.

JB: That sounds like a control mechanism, a way to circumvent getting carried away by the world.

M: Sure, it is, but it's a wise one. If you move too fast, then you lose contact with your center. And once you lose contact with your center, they've got you.

JB: Sometimes, but not always. Sometimes getting carried away by the world is what we need to energize us and invite us into new experiences. Like jumping into a wild ocean and being tossed around by the waves. It wakes you up. We can't always be in control—we also have to go involuntary at times, to bravely jump into the heart of the world.

M: Those who jump into the world get snared by it. That's what happened to those people in the houses and businesses I passed. They got ensnared and ended up living unconscious lives, selling out for money and the illusion of security. Thinking the world is 'it.' But it's not it.

JB: All of them?

M: Most of them.

JB: Is it possible that many of them have willfully made the choice to join the world because it serves their goals, helps them to create the base they need to grow to the next level? Many have kids they want to take care of, partners they want sheltered and warm in the winter. These are the people who built the structures, fought the wars, constructed the roads you walk on. Not sure you would feel safe enough to get lost in your meditation practice if they didn't work hard and pay their taxes—the taxes that fund emergency services, that provide protective structures, that ensure that even the iconoclastic hippies get some kind of a pension. Isn't it ironic that you only get to safely bypass the world, because of all the things others do to make it a relatively safe and stable place? Everyone plays their part.

M: Yes, but they don't do any of that consciously.

JB: Conscious or not, they are worthy of your respect. And I am not sure they are any less conscious than you are. They have developed many skill sets and threads of awareness that you haven't.

M: You have no idea what my skills are.

JB: Sounds like your irritation is pointing you back in your own direction. What happened to you all those years ago? Why have you pitted yourself against the world? Because it's imperfect? That can't be it. We are all on the collective wheel, sharing this imperfect context, marching together through time. Why no compassion for those who may be caught in challenging circumstances? Why no gratitude for all they contribute? Why us versus them? After all, you do claim to believe in a unified field of consciousness.

M: Listen dude, I don't want to hear any more about my anger. You're taking me down a dark path. All these years I devoted to conscious evolution—and now, I'm backtracking! Fuck this. I knew it was a mistake to meet with you. Should never have listened to Lydia about meeting you—she's an airy-fairy loon anyways.

With that, he hurled his coffee on the ground, and stormed off through the park.

The conversation had clearly triggered him. I stayed calm and continued on with steady sips of my cappuccino, letting his anger roll throughout my body. There was a time in my life when I would recoil in the face of anger, but no longer. As long as there was no threat of violence, vigorous anger was welcome in my world. A perfect part of the human landscape.

I stood up and began to meander through the park toward home. As I walked, I thought of Michael's walking meditation. While he experienced the world as harsh and invasive, I found it a poignant blend of all realities — the turbulent, the beautiful, and the ever-unfolding in-between. It was all here, and so was I.

This would probably be the last I saw of him. I hope he learned something from our talks — that could be watered within his consciousness, like a seed, perhaps sprouting at the ripe time, given the right conditions.

The Power of Then

As I reached Dundas Avenue — at the north end of the park, someone shouted my name. Much to my surprise, it was Michael. He hadn't fled altogether — he was just cooling off. He motioned me to sit down on the grass and continue our talk. We sat down together, under a large wide-trunked aspen.

M: Sorry, I took off. I'm a mess right now. I haven't felt like this since I was a kid. A whole tsunami of emotions are flooding me.

JB: It's entirely understandable. The way you have organized reality is being challenged. You are bringing feelings to the surface that you have barricaded off from awareness for decades.

M: To be honest, these last days have been bloody hell. I've been so agitated. My morning meditations just aren't cutting it for me. It's like the light has gone off. Whatever you unleashed in me... well, it finally reached a pinnacle last night. I'm almost too embarrassed to tell you, but I exploded on Hannah and threw a vase against the wall. It shattered in a thousand pieces. She was in shock. I've never done anything like that before. In fact, I've seldom even raised my voice in our decade together.

JB: Wow. And then what happened?

M: I thought she would be angry—but instead she reached out to me. I crumpled in her arms. She held me... and I cried like I hadn't cried with her before. Then, something amazing happened. We went into the bedroom and made the sweetest love. To be honest, we haven't had any intimacy the past six months. Our love life has been pretty dead. Robotic. But this was delicious. I woke up feeling refreshed, and the whole world looked different.

JB: This is incredible progress, my friend.

M: Progress?

JB: And it's just the beginning...

M: Wait, there's more? I don't see that there is any point in digging up the source of my anger. It has little do with presence. Do I really have to go there?

JB: Yes, you do. Because that part of you that longs to be united—the part of you that is compelled to return to our dialogues, won't satisfy its longing if you don't bring every part to the surface. Simply put, the problem is not the feelings themselves. The problem is our inability to feel them fully, to burrow so deep within them that we come through the other side. We have not been taught how to do that in a survivalist world where emotions were dangerous and associated with destructive anger and great suffering. We may not be quite ready yet, but the ultimate answer is to invite them all into consciousness—nothing gets buried in an enrealed world—and to convert them into the lessons at their core. Like good little students of life, we jump inside of our own hearts with a little elbow grease, shaping a newer and truer lens from the ashes of our suffering.

M: Again, I feel like we are backtracking. All these years I devoted to conscious evolution—and now you're taking me back into the muck, the elementary, the ugly base chakra path. Survival and instinct-driven, cruel, animal-like tendencies that start wars, where we battle our own flesh and blood. Madness! Into the world of samsara. Rehashing the long ago. No thank you. I'm done with that. The present moment is pristine. It's the only moment that is real.

JB: On the contrary. It has EVERYTHING to do with being in the now. There is no present moment if aspects of our consciousness are still trapped amid unresolved emotional rubble. Your consciousness is still back there. I call this the "Power of Then": the effect that the unhealed past has on our current consciousness. Although the physical body travels forward chronologically, one's emotional consciousness always remains at any point of departure. To move forward in life, we have to walk back down the path and heal the wounds and memories that plague us. We can pretend they aren't there, we can witness them from afar, but our experience of the *now* is only as genuine as our relationship to the *then*. If we sidestep the unhealed emotional body, if we pretend that all that we feel is an illusion, our experience of the moment will be fragmented and half-hearted. And the material will come back to haunt us, one way or the other. True presence is a whole being experience, one that includes everything we left behind on the path.

M: Dude, going back into the cesspool of repressed emotions only inhibits our growth.

JB: At their heart, repressed emotions are unactualized spiritual lessons. Until we go back down the path and claim them, they are still in their holding locker, growing in intensity, blocking our capacity for authentic presence. And they don't just obstruct the path—the congealed remnants of our stuff actually eat us alive from the inside out, turning against us in the form of illness and even death.

Right after I said this, Michael lay down on the grass and went quiet. I worried that I had gone too far. But instead, when he spoke his voice sounded vulnerable.

M: Geez, I wonder if that's why Brad died of cancer. He had a traumatic, abusive childhood. And yet he always kept a smile on his face. Always the "giver," the good guy, that never got angry. So much locked inside.

JB: Who was Brad?

M: My very best friend. College buddy. We traveled together. The Himalayas. Morocco. Portugal. Tripping the world fantastic in search of the meaning of life. God, I miss him.

JB: Not all physical disease is caused by repressed emotions, but some certainly is. When we flee the shadow, we flee ourselves. It's not all light in there, of that we can be sure. And the shadow that we fled with all our might, doesn't go away. It waits around the next bend to trip us up, reminding us that it wants to be seen. Not because it wants us to suffer, but because it wants us to heal. Because it wants us to grow. Our shadows aren't the enemy. Repression is. And if we repress for too long, some form of sickness will often ensue. Because we are burying something that is alive, and, one way or the other, it will find its way to the surface. Quick fix, long suffering. Long fix, authentic transformation.

M: Long fix, authentic transformation… that resonates. I admit that most of my life I have been seeking the quick spiritual fix. That sudden break-through moment where Enlightenment descends upon me once and for all, and my consciousness is irreversibly changed. Then I glide through life, a step above the world. Never to stumble into my mind-traps and patterns again. That's what I've been waiting on.

JB: Well, wait on through this life, and your next. That's not the way it works, my friend. Real change takes time, persistence, fierce determina-tion, and due diligence. By working through our old material, we both create space inside for presence to enter, and we mature in our capacity to be here. The masters of dissociation will try to convince us that we are "in the moment" when we bypass our pain, but I can assure you that they are sadly mistaken. You can't truly be here while you are nullifying essential aspects of your consciousness. If you don't deal with those unconscious aspects, you cannot fully open the doorway to the Divine. The mystery begins with your history.

M: Clever, dude.

JB: If you were one of the very few who remained intact throughout your entire childhood and youth, you may find that 'then' and 'now' remain integrated. But if you are like most of us, some piece of you was left behind on the journey. That's certainly been true for me. And if we really want to live, we have to go back down the path and re-claim it.

M: But my feelings and emotions are rooted in illusion. Why give them so much attention? That only fuels and emboldens them. Keep your eyes pointed on the still backdrop, beneath the feelings. Emotions are blips on a screen. Fleeting waves in the ocean. Passing clouds in the sky.

JB: No, Michael, they aren't. True, not all of our feelings are perfect reflec-tions of reality. We worry about things that we don't need to worry about. We get lost in beliefs, stories, and patterns that make peace impossible. I spent years doing that. But the answer is not to run away from them in their entirety. The answer is to reach a stage where you can distinguish between those feelings that require attention and healing, and those that do not. Throwing all of them out with the bathwater will not lead you anywhere good. The feel is for real.

M: But some of my wounds are crippling, man. I don't want to get within a thousand miles of them.

JB: Then you risk ending up like Brad.

M: Ouch.

JB: Look, it's up to you—it's always up to you. You can deny, repress, distort, and bury your unresolved wounds all you want. You can re-frame them, pseudo-positivity them, detach from them, bypass them. You can re-name yourself, hide away in a monastery, turn your story around. And you can spend all your money on superficial healing practices and hocus-pocus practitioners. But it won't mean a damn thing, if you don't do the deeper work to excavate and heal your primary wounds. The material is still there, right where you left it, subconsciously ruling your life and con-trolling your choices. This is the nature of unhealed material—it is alive, and one way or the other, it will manifest itself in your lived experience. It will language your inner narrative. It will obstruct your path and limit your possibilities. It lives everywhere that you live. And so you have to decide—excavate it and bring it into consciousness where it can be worked through and integrated; or repress it and watch it rule your life. It's one of the hardest truths we have to face: If we don't deal with our stuff, it deals with us. There is no way around this. Choose.

M: It is true that I have seen many of my most disciplined meditation teachers leave us early. Some from illness, and many from suicide. We always imagined that their early departure was a function of their state of enlightenment—they had evolved to the level of Brahman and were needed elsewhere. But deep inside, I'm not so sure.

JB: Yes, I have known many as well, particularly those who take their own lives. And they are not killing themselves because they have better things to do on the other side. They are killing themselves because the pain they are seeking to flee through their meditation addiction, is unwilling to die. They touch their limited version of pure consciousness—what I might call a momentarily effective transcendence bypass—and they cling to it like an addict clings to cocaine. It's karmic crack, but with far less feeling. They have confused pathways of relief with transformation. Then their stuff reappears when they least expect it, and they no longer have any tools to deal with it. They have so thoroughly abandoned the self, that there is no one, and nothing, left to save them. They have abandoned their humanness. So they decide to kill the self, once and for all. That's the great tragedy and the great irony of the transcendence bypass sales pitch. Those who practice it, spend their lives talking about the *now*, while still being ruled by the *then*. It is only through a growing interface with our real-life experiences and challenges that we can evolve toward a deeper spiritual life.

M: I don't know about that. My most poignant and complete enlightenment moments happened when I was severed from those aspects. When I was resting in the ocean of wholeness, right beneath and beyond the feelings. THAT is me. THAT is here.

JB: Again, it depends on how we define enlightenment. It's my view that what you are calling enlightenment is the same state of capped consciousness that many others reference. You are referring to a fixed or absolute state, rather than a relative, fluid, or awakening state. And you are right—once you remove your multifaceted humanness from the equation, the place you can go in your consciousness is somewhat fixed or capped, like a building with a rigid ceiling. It's when you try to enlighten, or in my word, *enreal*, your consciousness while remaining connected to all your aspects, that you recognize that there is no fixed state called "enlightenment." Through that lens, you see how brilliantly complex and unlimited our awakening possibilities are. So many as yet underdeveloped parts, so many weaves and sensations, and ways of touching the moment, so many kaleidoscopes of meaning. So many dormant resources, capacities and abilities. We are multi-potentialites. Once there, you quickly give up on the real illusion—the illusion of an absolute, awakened state—and you jump back into life. You actually find life itself is not fixed. It's fluid, forever morphing, metamorphosing. How could enlightenment ever be contrary to the natural flow of life? Isn't it all about being in sync with the flow of life? Isn't *that* oneness?

M: Well, Hannah would agree with you. She is constantly telling me that my path is a one trick pony. How utterly boring, she says! But I value that reliability in my practice, and I can't imagine life without entering a meditative state every day. Meditation is the road to the Kingdom of God.

JB: I have to meet Hannah one day. Wise woman. Grounded, enheartened women are our future. And, I don't have any issue with entering into a meditative state, as long as it is inclusive of all aspects of our consciousness. But I don't feel that traditional meditation is necessarily the most effective way to arrive there. Meditation—like any spiritual practice—can be something that works for us and is helpful for a time; or it can be something that is dissociative and destructive. It's no accident that you reference a "Kingdom," Michael. You were conditioned by the patriarchy to believe that the most complete spiritual experience leads to something masculine. What about the Queendom? What about the wisdom of the feminine? What about a consciousness that bridges both? The truth is that some of us come to a meditative state through dancing, crying, walking in nature, nursing an infant, riding a motorcycle, making love. And some of us do not identify a "meditative state" as the only heights, or the depths of the human experience. Some prefer to lose themselves in a dualistic consciousness—and there they find their Godself. Some prefer to dance between the ethers...

M: So how do we find it? What's your way in, man?

JB: These days, just about anything is my way in. Of course, I have some personal favorites. My general experience has been that deep emotional release and discharge is the most effective at inviting people into a naturally meditative state. Along my path, many suggested that I was wasting my time getting lost in my material. It was egoic, self-centered, narcissistic. Some said that I needed to simply forgive the past, let it go, focus on the light. Others contended that the trick to spiritual transformation is to bypass my ancestral material, to see my personal issues and memories as distinct from my ultimate transformation. Your view, as well. But where is the grist that transforms us, if not in our daily lives? What does it mean to love the world, if your heart is filled with unresolved anger? Once we clear our tensions and emotional debris, meditation is not just a practice—it actually becomes a way of being. I know that when I was emotionally blocked or stressed, I could sit on the cushion forever, without connecting to a unified awareness and without finding a sustainable peace. Yes, I could calm down, gain some perspective, but I couldn't reach a place of profound awakening, at least not in the limited period of time I had available. It was an endless struggle, often a very agitating experience. Yet when I focused my energy on embodied emotional release—that is, excavating and expressing my feelings—I would often arrive at a meditative state right after it came to an end. It was that simple. Clear the emotional channel, and peace enters...

M: Hmmm...

JB: It's akin to what you shared, in your lovemaking with Hannah last night. I believe that came from a clearing. It had been building in you for years, maybe decades. You finally emoted by throwing the vase. You cleared the build-up. You opened the dam. And something beautiful arose. It doesn't always have to look that extreme. Again, it's presently more intense for you, as those emotions have been accumulating over time. But, it gave you a glimpse of possibility. Once you do the excavating and clearing... how sweet it can be.

M: Sweet it was...

JB: You see, this principle doesn't only apply to the pain-body. It applies to the joy-body too. When we block the emotional body in any respect, we block our capacity for all forms of deep feeling. Opening our hearts to joy, celebrating the wonder of life, also opens the gate to divinity. The challenge for most of us, is that we either can't yet open that way, or we can't sustain the opening, because there is still so much unresolved debris in the way. It's a *paindemic* everywhere we look, and it doesn't get better when we seek to transcend it.

M: It definitely opened my pain-body. But I'm not swayed yet. What is missing from your dialectic is an understanding of the truth I seek. In my experience, there is a point of truth that I and other seekers are questing for. It's the difference between the fragmented world of form, and the seamless world of spirit. So, when I pull away from the world it's not because I hate it, it's because I recognize that I can't arrive at an experience of absolute truth if I am distracted by it.

JB: For now, let's put aside the question of whether absolute truth even exists in a relative universe. I too recognize the value of truth in this incarnation. Truth *is* the gateway to the moment. That is, the gateway to the now opens when we are able to fully embody that which is truth. But I am defining truth differently than you. Not as an absolute form, but as a direct reflection of our subjective experience. That is, the truth of our feelings, the truth of our intuition, the truth of our callings, the truth of our daily challenges and delights, the truth of our physical pains and discomforts. In other words, I am more interested in the state of the perceiver, than the perception itself. If we are emotionally fractured, so is our perception. Many people talk about being in the now, without deeply understanding what that means. They're not awake. It's their pain that's awake. What someone who is asleep experiences as the moment—is very different from a soul that is growing into its fullness and living as authentically and inclusively as possible. It all comes down to truth—truth or consequences.

M: Wasn't that a TV show in your day?

JB: Yes, one of my childhood favorites. And, not so old, youngster... ☺

M: Touché.

JB: Let me put it this way... if we have chopped off the ego, we have chopped up our awareness. If we have bypassed our story, we have bypassed the moment. I know from experience: what a "bypasser" calls "the moment"— is entirely different from the experience of someone in a more integrated state. You can't touch anything that approximates pure truth, if you are not embodying all of the elements that contribute to who you are. If you are looking through a shattered lens, if you are fragmented, or splintered—so is your experience of the moment. And even when you clarify your lens, I still suspect that there is no final destination. There is not the permanent irrevocable moment of Enlightenment that you have been waiting for. It is more like spirals of awakening that transmute into a kaleidoscope of richer color and texture; as we evolve into greater spectrums of consciousness, each one more complex, nuanced, and intricate than the one before. Just like there can be no awakening without emotional health, without relational integrity, without a healthy ego, without a strong sense of self, without a deep honoring of story and selfhood—there can be no truth without owning all that you are. You are trying to get to the truth, while sidestepping what is truly you.

M: If I understand, you are saying that I cannot know truth if I am a muddled mess.

JB: You can know truths in bits and pieces, but it will be limited in scope and breadth by the inner constraints of your undigested material. It's like over-eating a heavy meal that doesn't get digested. You just end up blocked and sluggish. If you are wanting to arrive at something you call pure, or absolute consciousness, then you would have to be healed, developed, and integrated in all regards. I do not believe that we are at a stage of human development where that has happened for any of us. Yes, there have been messengers who eloquently share a thread of the strand, but none of them can communicate the whole picture, because none of them have actualized and integrated every facet of the human experience. We're just not there yet. We have so much more to evolve into.

M: Do you think we will ever arrive there?

JB: It may never happen. There may never be an arrival point. Perhaps the more we grow and evolve—the more truth does too. It could be infinite, forever expanding beyond the soulscape of our human evolution—always a step ahead of us.

M: Whoa, this is deep shit.

JB: The possibilities are manifold, Michael. Far more than your notion of the "Big E." At this stage, we really can't know what pure consciousness is, or if absolute consciousness truly exists. In the capped way that its been defined by those messengers, sure, but I am not convinced that they were able to access the whole picture. We want to believe they have, so we have a trail to follow, but that doesn't make it true. It's just Godjectification—the tendency to project God's knowing onto others. I can get behind the idea that we are Godseeds in the making, but I can't get behind the idea that any one of us has arrived at the entirety of God's wisdom. Will we? I don't know. I prefer to begin with the truth of where we are and move forward from there. Truth is the gateway to the moment.

Enfeelment

M: A lot of profound concepts here, Master Jeffji. My mind is churning, but I am not sure I am absorbing it directly. Part of me is relieved by that, because I actually don't like the way your exercises have been making me feel. Yet, I can also sense a part of me readying to go in a little deeper. It's the question you asked that keeps entering my awareness: Where is the bridge back to here? That sentence really struck me. *Where is the bridge back to here?* I have had my own answer for a very long time—the bridge is up there, out there, here and now—but now I feel my certainty fading, and a kind of reluctant curiosity pushing up against it. While I am feeling open, it might be good to dive in for more.

And then, right on cue, he checked out with a long, pseudo-calm soliloquy about the spiritual need for a psychological death. I knew that this was part of his bridging process — returning to the safe, familiar side of the river… before stepping back out, further into the rushing currents of a new way of being. Human nature. The key was for me to keep inviting him back into this new experience at a pace that he could assimilate. Too much too soon, he might run. Too little, and he won't realize what he is missing. A skillful art indeed.

After he finished his monologue, he looked directly at me with a blank expression — clearly waiting for me to pick up the ball. His willingness was endearing. My turn.

JB: Enough talk about the bridge back to here. Let's make it real. I am going to give you another feeling-based exercise that you can try before we next meet. One can only glimpse this perspective to the extent that they have embodied it. First, I would like to know how you normally meditate. How do you sit, and where is your focus…?

He demonstrated by putting himself in lotus position. After adjusting his body to obtain a picture-perfect full lotus, he closed his eyes and continued to speak:

M: My focus depends on the practice I am currently engaged in. Sometimes I do a *Samatha*, where I focus my mind on only one thing, for example, my beads, or a chant, sometimes an image of one of my gurus in my mind's eye. I let nothing else garner my attention. By excluding all else, I come deeper into the moment. At other times, I do a Vipassana, or insight-based practice. I use my breath as my focal point, noting the ways that the mind attempts to interfere, coming back to the breath, proceeding to note all other sensations and perceptions. In this way, I peel away the patterns of distraction, and gain insight into the true nature of reality.

JB: Great. Ready for something new? Try this every day until we next meet again.

EXERCISE 3
THE EXCAVATION MEDITATION

Sit on a chair, on the floor, or on a cushion, in whatever position feels most comfortable. While sitting, do not close your eyes, or focus your gaze directly ahead or above you. Instead, keep your eyes opened and focused downward, looking directly and with great curiosity at your body temple. Gaze at your body as you would a loved one.

Begin to make contact with your breath, inviting it into awareness, feeling it move through you. First, start with gentle breathing, as if you are gradually warming up. Then, invite your breath to move strongly and pointedly throughout your body, infusing your body with life-force, pushing into and beyond tightly held regions. If you feel resistance, do not hesitate or recoil. Breathe even stronger. If you feel emotions, do not merely watch them as they float past. Instead, immerse yourself in them. Deepen into feeling, inviting all held emotions and memories to be fully felt. Use the breath as an excavation tool. With your breath, purposefully dig deep. Your aim is to bring repressed material to the surface, where it can be released and re-integrated.

Allow this meditation to become a kind of visceral, physical landscape of feeling and sensation.

If there are tears, feel into and move them, to the extent that you can.

If there is anger, feel into and move it, to the extent that you can.

If there are words or sounds, express them fully.

If you find yourself turning toward your habitual meditation style that includes a focus on the sensations of the body—return to the breath and intensify it.

If you find yourself getting distracted by thoughts—return to the breath and intensify it.

If you find yourself wanting this exercise to end—return to the breath and intensify it.

Whatever arises, return to the breath and intensify it.

Your breath is your excavation tool and your guide.

Now you are not just watching the body as it contracts and expands—you are fully experiencing and inhabiting the body, feelings, emotions, sounds, sensations, textures, roars, all and everything.

Stay with this process until you have abandoned the Watcher and have become a full-bodied total Experiencer. Feeling, moving, expressing, and releasing as fully as you can.

He listened to me intently as I described the exercise in depth. Then he shot up to go, muttering something about what furniture he might throw at Hannah this time. I stood to join him, and we began to walk together back through the park. Not one to stop and see the sights, Michael moved like the wind. It was all my 55-year-old legs could do to keep pace with him. As we moved, I was entranced by a cornucopia of visual delight. Trinity Bellwoods was like a symphony today. There were children everywhere, happily playing—fully in the now, occupying their bodies and beingness simultaneously, inner and outer coalescing as one uninhibited movement. There was a fresh-faced a cappella group playfully singing whimsical folk songs, while a large gaggle of humans from every walk-of-life gathered around in common enjoyment. There were dog-walkers, chess players, elderly bocce ballers, and two competing softball teams, playfully hooting and jeering on the field. This place was alive!

Just before we reached the bench where we first met, a young goth kid on a skateboard came roaring past. I yelled out to him, "Hey Kid, what's your path to God?" To my surprise, the kid did a sharp 180 swerve, and grinded to a halt before us. "Serious question, man?" "Serious question." "I find it on the board when I find it at all. Sometimes, not so much, and other times, I hit the Z. You know, the zone, and I'm like at one with everything." "Then what happens?" "I wipe out, and start over."

By the time we stopped speaking, Michael was already exiting the scene. I could tell he was done for today. I asked him to wait a moment, while reaching into my bag. I quickly scribbled a note on a piece of paper, and told him to read it in his sanctuary before doing the exercise. We parted ways. The note said:

Do not try to become anything.

Do not make yourself into anything.

Do not be a meditator.

Do not become enlightened.

When you sit, let it be.

Grasp at nothing.

Resist nothing.

If you haven't wept deeply, you haven't begun to meditate.

—Ajahn Chah

4 The Non-Dual Duel

> A new spirituality is arising, one that upholds the
> self, the heart and the body. It is both a very ancient
> and very evolutionary spirituality. It is a spirituality
> that calls on us not to denigrate, transcend or reject
> who we are as a self, but rather to embody it and
> ennoble it in service of mankind and the Earth. It
> is a spirituality of freedom and of service, in other
> words, of authenticity and solidarity.
>
> —CHRIS SAADE

The next day, I got a text from Michael:

> Would like to meet again. But need a few weeks to complete
> big work project. Just want you to know, I'm not running
> away. Ready to commit to your process.

*His text prompted me to remember the initial stages of my own therapeutic process.
I had done a session, and then retreated. Did another session, and then wrote the
therapist that if I couldn't do this on my own, it wasn't relevant to me. The essence
of her response: "You were wounded in relationship. You have to heal in relationship." Busted. I went back the next week, and never looked back.*

*Michael and I met a few weeks later in Kensington Market, one of downtown
Toronto's oldest communities. The market is an edgy part of the city, where butch-
ers, head shops, and used clothiers sell their wares in a kind of timeless bubble.
When you walk down Baldwin Street, you are at once overwhelmed by the smell
of fish, coffee, and ganga; while a fascinating, ethnically diverse collection of
people walk, bike, and skateboard past. Long established as a mecca for creativity,
the place is like a human gallery, where every person that passes by is like living
art in motion.*

We met in Bellevue Square Park, at the south end of the market. When Michael arrived, he surprised me with a quick hug. It wasn't a bear hug, by any means, but it was a hug nonetheless. We sat down face-to-face at a picnic table.

JB: How did the exercise go, my friend?

M: Hopeless, honestly. But I did it… I pushed against my tendency to turn away from the feelings and memories, and to instead explore the dense material in front of me. And there was a lot of it. Then Hannah and I went for our Saturday date night to a vegetarian restaurant nearby, and I felt incredibly impatient with her. She wasn't doing anything unusual—just sharing the details of her day—but I couldn't seem to calm down and hear her. I was all riled up from the assignment. So we had a ridiculous argument about non-duality, and I had to abandon my Buddha Bowl, and go for a walk around the block to calm down. When I returned she had finished off my Buddha Bowl. Typical selfer.

JB: When you say "riled up," what exactly were you experiencing?

M: Lots of anger, agitation, some sadness. The meditation, particularly breathing into the tight places, began to flood me with memories and regrets. Things I had done wrong, or opportunities missed, or paths I hadn't explored because I was so busy trying not to walk any particular path. I've been so focused on trying to empty my consciousness of the world.

JB: Well, if you want to empty yourself of the world, you may first want to start by emptying yourself of any suppressed emotions that relate to your worldly experiences.

M: Ugh, I may have to agree with you now. The emotions hadn't gone anywhere. In fact, they were even more evident when I came back from my walk. Hannah brought up her desire to have a child, something I have long resisted, and that topic took me over the edge. Usually, I very calmly explain why I don't feel that we need to bring another child onto this dying planet, but this time, I reacted like a child myself, spewing all kinds of vitriol about her demanding nature, and how sickened I am by the idea of being roped to a kid for the rest of my life. I kept repeating, "I want liberation, not incarceration," over raw vegan cheesecake. Got some outraged looks from nearby diners. I became a six-year-old who needed a time-out.

JB: You've already had a 20 year time-out. What did she say about that?

M: She didn't, for awhile. She was stunned by my intensity, and just went quiet. On the walk home, she only said one thing, almost too quiet for me to hear. "Having a child would liberate me. It's part of why I'm here in this life." There it was—front and center before my face: the fundamental tension between us. She finds her meaning in the dualities, I find mine in the non-dual field. And then we just went to bed, in a stony silence. I reached toward her to make love, thinking we could re-create the passion from the other night. But she curtly replied, "Keep your dualistic dick out of my dualistic pussy," before rolling over.

JB: Ouch.

M: So much for my abandoning the quest for non-duality. All it leads to is more suffering... and less pussy.

JB: So, share more about what the term 'non-duality' means to you.

M: It means submerging my awareness in the unified nature of reality. Not fixating on the minutiae, not riding the choppy waves of samsara, but floating within the inherent perfection at their core. Finding the ocean of stillness beneath the ever-changing waves. It's essentially a non-separate state, one where you look out at the world and see everything as one, because your awareness is stationed in the undivided field—not on the passing phenomena.

JB: And in your view, Hannah doesn't connect with the unified nature of reality? Would you say that she is too affixed to the waves of samsara to see the bigger picture?

M: Exactly. She takes all the details of the human story so seriously—how she feels, how she sees herself, how we relate to each other, what we do each day. She thinks it all real, when I am certain that it isn't. I see it all as *maya*, a phenomenal play. What is real is the permanent, not the fleeting impermanent. I'm here for the eternal.

JB: Is it possible that she believes that it's all real—her lens, *and* yours—but that we still have far more work to do within the dualities. That we need to work with all the separate moving pieces, before we can truly, sustainably, be at one with the 'oneness'?

M: I don't think it's a question of belief. I think she is just caught in her patterns.

JB: She may be, but if those patterns reflect where we still are as a collective consciousness, then she is focused where the real work needs to be done: right at the heart of our underdeveloped dualistic consciousness. So many lessons to learn and steps to take before we can merge with a unified field. And without an intact self, our lens to wholeness is inherently distorted.

And, of course, there is always the question of whether we are built to live within a non-dual field at all. Perhaps we are here to learn how to live more deeply within the dualities without tripping out, as you do. Perhaps we are here to explore an ever-changing kaleidoscope of experiences, one point of access, then another and then another. And even if you view non-duality as the pinnacle of humanness, you must accept that we need fuel to propel our evolution. Without the magnificently imperfect self as our clay—in all its as yet unworked through forms—humanity stops dead in its evolutionary tracks. We need grist to feed the soul mill. Lots of it.

M: That sounds like a deeply unstable and unreliable form of consciousness.

JB: Quite the opposite, my friend. It requires a profound degree of internal stability—the kind that can withstand and willfully seek out an ever-fluid, perpetually shifting array of experiences. Instead of a blown-open crown chakra—it requires deep stable roots. A foundation that can withstand the intrinsic pressures of this human life. Without a stable fulcrum point of self, you can't steadily integrate a broad range of life experiences. You show up for life with a partial consciousness, like a building with missing floors.

I stood up to demonstrate what I meant. Methodically, I pointed at each main energy center of my body, working my way up from the soles of my feet to the top of my head. Each stop along the way was essential in forging a complete human being. There were no shortcuts. Miss one point along the way—and the whole human construct is imbalanced.

JB: In tangible terms, this means that you begin your expansion by healing and solidifying the root chakra—the quest for OM begins at home. You meet your basic needs and deal with your security issues. You tend to the practical aspects of daily life that, if left unattended, leave you feeling agitated. From the root, you move organically to the next chakra, then the next, then the next. Imagine each chakra as a stage or level that corresponds to a particular element of reality. If you don't heal, open, and strengthen each chakra, you cannot fully experience the thread of reality that accompanies it.

In essence, this is what it means to enreal your consciousness. As you develop a healthy egoic foundation and equally strengthen your chakras, you rise into fullness and make every part of yourself available to the moment. And it's not just a vertical movement—you actually expand in every direction: upward, downward, inward, sideways, through and through. Then, perhaps if you really do the work on all these levels, you no longer feel the need to touch a "transcendent" plane, because you experience the richness of being human, right down here in your daily life experience.

M: I personally find the whole idea of chakras annoyingly clichéd and unoriginal.

JB: Unoriginal, or triggering, because it links your spiritual journey to the state of your energetic body? To become whole, we need to include each and every chakra or energy center, however you label them. They are all of equal importance in the assembling of a complete human being.

Michael, what you gravitate toward is actually the more unstable path, because you are choosing not to work through and solidify the self before diving into the Ocean of Oneness. Your foundation is faulty. You're a flimsy container. Top-heavy. Unbalanced. Unable to truly integrate and come into harmony with this world. That's why you invariably drown and wilt under the pressures of your emotional body. You have jumped ship without the benefit of a life-preserver—the sturdy ego-self—to keep you afloat.

M: I've surpassed that. I am well-seasoned on the path, and, yes, instead of "working through" my emotions—I have grown beyond them. Again, you are bringing me backward into a constrained lens. It's like squeezing into clothing that is several sizes too small. I've outgrown this.

JB: Quite the opposite, from my perspective. What you are describing is actually only the preliminary steps on the consciousness journey. It's the newbie level. Someone who has newly opened their eyes to the possibility that there is more than the drudgery of their daily life. The detached version of unity that we experience when we are beginning to wake up. But you are neglecting the next stage: coming back down into your selfhood and integrating your awakening with your human form. You haven't truly surpassed anything, my friend.

M: Hey, dude, watch yourself. I've done my due diligence on the consciousness quest. I've endured much worldly discomfort… you think it was a walk in the park spending 14 days in silent meditation in a cave in the Himalayas? Fasting for days, enduring severe physical pains and discomforts. How dare you call me a newbie? You have nerve.

JB: I'm not disputing you've done your fair share of what is traditionally called spiritual work. But there is a key piece you have yet to realize. After the work, it's essential to come back down into our body and re-integrate the localized with the universal. The two go hand-in-hand, like partners in a swing dance. It's essential to our wholeness that the wings of Oneness soon grow feet. And when you come into integration as a spiritual being, you no longer characterize your experience in polarities: local or universal, transcendent or mundane. You just call it life.

M: You are giving duality way too much credit.

JB: That's part of bringing our consciousness into balance. Duality has been vilified for far too long. The poor EGO. The heavy-booted bypassers just keep crushing it under foot, without giving it any credit at all. The poor EMOTIONAL BODY. They keep crushing it under foot, without giving it any credit at all. The poor BODY TEMPLE. They keep crushing it under foot, without giving it any credit at all. The poor PERSONAL IDENTITY. They keep crushing it under foot, without giving it any credit at all. Not much left after all that crushing. If we keep chopping off all our parts, there won't be anyone left to transform. Where do we think spirituality lives, if not in the heart of our HUMANNESS?

Whether or not non-duality is the ultimate goal, what is clear is that we are all dualists at this stage of human development. I have yet to encounter a human who doesn't have hardcore work to do in the heart of separation consciousness. And it has been my experience that those who assume that they have evolved beyond it—like those who those call themselves "enlightened"—are actually the ones with the most work to do. Each duality is a beautiful bridge, a juicy web of transformation with textures and contours all its own. Let's show up for all of it, and call THAT spirituality.

Boundaries... Don't Leave Home Without them

M: One of my favorite spiritual teachers, Eckhart Tolle, wrote that we find our "true nature beyond name and form," in his book, *The Power of Now*.

JB: First of all, Tolle's birth name is Ulrich, not Eckhart. He found "name" and "form" relevant enough to make a name change. That aside, the philosophy at the heart of his quote—fundamental to centuries of transcendence bypass teachings—is not congruent with integrated or Grounded Spirituality. It's rooted in nothingness and it denies the very fabric, and inherent significance, of our selfhood. As noted before, Grounded Spirituality finds our true nature within name and form. It is here within form that we deepen and expand our capacity for non-separateness. It is within form that we align our selfhood with our God-hood. It is within form that we touch the formless. It is within name—our unique face of the Divine—that we find the nameless. Our humanness is the launching pad, the rocketship, and the destination.

M: That's all very poetic, but one cannot become empty if they keep affixing to the dualities.

JB: Before you can become empty, you have to become full. And that fullness does not happen by transcending the container. It happens by filling it with a healthy selfhood, one that is a dependable container for the full spectrum of life experience. And again, I am not convinced that anyone has accomplished this at this stage of human development. I believe we have much more work to do within the dualities—in the distinctions between shadow and light, right and wrong, healthy and unhealthy... so that, as a collective, our ultimate foray into a more unifying consciousness does not bypass the as yet unresolved dualities, but builds upon their healthy and organic transformation. And my suspicion is that once someone arrives at a healthy, vital, and robust somethingness, they will have no interest in jumping beyond this human form—they will be too busy living, learning, and loving within it, to bid it farewell. Yes, you may then enter into an awareness of a unified field of consciousness, but it will be a meaningfully different and more wholesome experience. Because you will be intact, and you will know where your self ends and the everything begins.

M: Sir, you're missing the whole point. There is not an ending or a beginning in a unified field!

JB: Sure there is. Limits are an intrinsic part of reality. Think of it in terms of human relationships. It's the difference between those love relationships that crash and burn after an intense initial merging, and those that sustain themselves and grow deeper roots over time. In the latter case, the individuals involved probably had a stronger and more mature sense of self to come home to. Without healthy boundaries, our forays into mysticism—alone or in relationship—are likely to fail. They are more in the form of an escape than a true arrival. For me, this alone is evidence that we are not built for 'Oneness' if we have not developed as individuals. It's premature. Merely wishful thinking. You may be tasting from the unity tree, but who is the taster? To truly taste from unity, we must first grow into a recognition of our individual significance. We must learn where we end and the other begins. Without a healthy ego and well-defined boundaries, our experience of all one is ALL NONE, because we have no "1" to come home to. Let's begin with all-1, before we worry about all-one.

M: That's some high-level math. But my spirituality is all about the eradication of personal boundaries.

JB: That's not true. Your spirituality is actually about boundarying yourself from the personal. You aren't inviting a seamless flow between the personal and the impersonal—you're limiting your spirituality to the impersonal alone. And this is the core problem. It's one thing to distinguish ourselves from limiting dualities, but quite another to eradicate, or cordon off, the distinct self altogether. When taken too far, the quest for "All-One" is just another escape from individual challenges and personal responsibility. The more deeply we grow in our individual spirituality, the more genuine our experience of unity. To let go of duality, we must first establish our separateness.

M: Hmmm…

JB: Don't buy into the message that equates boundarylessness with an advanced spiritual consciousness. It is anything but. There is a crucial difference between an experience of unity consciousness that emanates from a healthily boundaried self, and the unboundaried experience of Oneness that results from dissociating from the self. If you want a shot at unity consciousness, unify your self first. That's where the everything begins. Boundaries, boundaries, boundaries. Don't leave home without them.

A Healthy Container

It was beginning to rain and I was getting hungry. I asked Michael if he wanted to go grab a taco. He agreed. We stood up and began the fascinating walk up Augusta Avenue. As we walked, we just shot the shit, nothing serious. And then, he surprised me with an unexpected question.

M: I get that you have strong convictions on my form of spirituality, and I get that you trace some of it back to my unhealed childhood… but I wonder if your lens on spirituality may also relate to something unresolved in you. You seem to have the same bias against transcendence that I have against immanence. Is that because you have garnered more wisdom, or is some part of that rooted in your own history of pain and suffering? I'm not asking to be an asshole. I'm asking sincerely.

I was taken aback. Not because I hadn't asked myself this question, but because I had yet to form a definitive answer. Like Michael, I am a work in process. Not all the answers have been clearly developed.

JB: That's a great question, and one that I have asked myself. My instinct is that my perspective is primarily coming from many hard-earned years of exploration. I've done the transcendence bypass, and experienced the numbing that comes with it. I have discovered that the authentic way is to move into a spiritual consciousness from within humanhood itself. But I will consider your question more deeply in the coming weeks. I'm always open to seeing my blind spots.

M: That's encouraging. Makes me trust you more.

We arrived at a favorite taqueria and grabbed a table. After our burritos arrived, we got back to talking between bites.

M: You mention the ego a lot, but not in the way that I have been trained to think of it. My work over the last 20 years has been to dissolve the ego, not to strengthen it. When it rises into prominence, as it often does, I find it very difficult to gain access to the purest consciousness.

JB: It seems you bought into the ego-bashing that is intrinsic to the transcendence bypass movement. It's ironic, because what motivates the quest for non-duality is often the unresolved elements themselves. Denying the ego is egoic. Its denial is often motivated by the unhealthy aspects of ego itself. The diminishment of the emotional body is motivated by the unhealed emotional body. The suggestion that everything is an illusion is motivated by a fear of reality. And the belief that simply witnessing the pain-body nullifies it, is motivated by the pain-body run amok. Witnessing our pain doesn't dissipate it. It strengthens it. If you want to dissipate your pain, get inside it and work it through, until it is thoroughly mended. And when it is truly healed, it will both create a richer, fuller life, and reveal its essential nature—grist for the soul mill itself. The granules of glory that grow us closer to the Godself. How can we evolve without this fodder for our expansion; the soil of our lived-in experience? You have bought into a kind of nihilistic world view that desecrates everything that nourishes and grows us forward. How can you escape into a full life, while leaving the self in your dust? Ironically, in your flight from these characteristics, you merely concretize their significance.

M: I call bullshit, man. When my ego takes over, I can't even begin to heal from anything. It's like I am completely consumed and controlled by my emotions, my thoughts, my feelings, drives and desires. I call myself, "Ego-maniac." Filtered and veiled, out of touch. Now tell me—how can this be good?!

JB: Ego-Maniac. Sounds like the name of a band. Want to start one? I've always wanted to be a spirit rocker. But seriously, calm down, dude. I am well-aware that the ego can become disproportionately pervasive in our lives. That it can misrepresent the essential self and alienate us from our inherent divinity. But let's not throw the entire ego away. Let's start by making distinctions between the healthy and the unhealthy ego. Because

I'm not talking about the unbridled ego, the narcissistic ego, the unhealthy ego run wild. I am talking about the vital self-concept, the boundaried sense of self, the healthy ego that helps us to manage reality and honor our purpose. I'm talking about the egoic structures that allow you to adhere to your path, and take care of your needs. Without a healthy ego, we don't have the solidity to meet the world full-on.

M: Hannah agrees with your perspective. She often says that her therapeutic work has been about enlivening the ego, and that my spiritual work has been about killing it. No wonder we are in conflict.

JB: This is why so many spiritual seekers are confused. Western psychology professes valuing the self, while many threads of Eastern (and now, Western) spirituality desacralize the ego in its entirety and purport that dissolving the ego is fundamental to an enlightened path—rather than making the intelligent distinction between the healthy and unhealthy ego. So seekers end up lost in the middle, reluctant to imagine themselves magnificent, and, at the same time, immobilized by an underdeveloped self-concept. Talk about a mind(ful)-fuck. In many ways, too much ego or too little ego, leads us in the same direction: profound imbalance. The answer is to support each other in actualizing all that we are—not in a way that contributes to a narcissistic self-concept—but in a way that supports our movement toward wholeness. We have so many gifts inside, a treasure trove of wonder just waiting to be lived...

M: Even if you believe in a healthy ego, surely you agree with Wayne Dyer's famous acronym, Ego is "Edging God Out."

JB: No, Michael. I think it's misguided. The healthy ego is a seamless part of our whole human package. What tips the balance is when we mistake our ego for our entire self. When it is really meant to be an integrative landing pad for the much-more of us—for our sublime nature. A healthy ego is not the enemy of the sacred. It's the foundation that the sacred stands upon. The ego gives the sacred—form. It makes the unseen—seen. Rather than dissing it, what we need instead is to support the construction of a healthy, balanced ego. One that celebrates our intrinsic value, without imagining itself as "all that." One that honors the self, without a need to dishonor others. There's nothing Godless about that.

M: Leggo my ego!

JB: Cute. But don't diss the ego. Celebrate it. Take earnership of what you have built over time. A pat to the back, Michael! Congratulate yourself for all that you have overcome. Be willing to forge a new inner template that is self-honoring and healthily egoic. Well done, grower! The trailways of transformation are no easy walk. Giving yourself some credit won't erode your spiritual life—it will empower it.

Michael's angry expression quickly changed to a quality I hadn't quite seen before. A kind of contemplative tenderness. He closed his eyes. Something I had said had touched him. After a few minutes, he began to speak. Softly, from his heart...

M: Thank you. I actually feel moved by those words. They remind me that I didn't get much validation as a child, particularly from my father.

JB: That must have been painful. I can surely relate—mine was relationally challenged, too. He had a good heart, but he was too immersed in his complex world of past wounds to be truly present with me. I regret that I didn't get to spend more time with the authentic Albert. I often think to myself what if he had done more inner work, actually cleared out and healed his stuff. That would have made for an entirely different relationship. We could have really seen each other, met each other. And I think we would have really gotten along. We did have a lot in common—he loved to write and ponder spiritual matters. He too had a very vibrant sense of wonder. But we never got there. Heartbreaking to think about, actually. Perfect example of how our unprocessed wounds bleed their toxic energy on to others, when we don't or can't take responsibility for our material. It has real-life repercussions.

M: Yep. I get you. My father caused me a lot of pain and disappointment growing up, as well.

JB: Perhaps this is some of the reason why you gravitated toward a version of spirituality that is painless rather than painful. To avoid more disappointments.

M: Could be. I do know that I would find myself day-dreaming, and racing off to spiritual texts when he was around too much. I had tried for years to gain his favor, but to no avail. He just wanted to preach religious dogmas, and watch sports. He knew the name and alma mater of every single NFL player. He didn't want to address anything emotionally real. He never took an interest in my life. I often wondered what had happened to him. I do now know that he was sexually abused as a child. By his older brother. And that he never ever confronted him. Perhaps if he had, perhaps if he had done the emotional work you speak of, he would have been able to connect to me more genuinely.

JB: These are very vulnerable admissions to make, Michael. Thank you for entrusting me.

Michael closed his eyes again. His sadness was palpable. His long-held grief was close to the surface. I was sure I saw a small tear glisten in the corner of his eye. When he was ready, he began to share, eyes still closed:

M: Yes, Jeff, I can see how Dad confronting his own wounds would have changed the whole climate of our household. I can also see how it may have changed my entire spiritual trajectory. Drew me more into the world of feeling and emotion. But, instead, I didn't have a template for staying present and remaining open. It hurt too bloody much.

JB: Same here, my friend. It's the way that the patriarchy unconsciously perpetuates its own predicament. We don't get the love we need from our fathers, so we become just as emotionally armored as them, likely in order to avoid more disappointment and pain. Then we form safe spiritual philosophies and constructs that keep our feelings at bay, rather than healing ourselves, and humanity, by welcoming a spirituality—a God-full-ness— that embraces all that we are, and that finds comfort and expansion in the heart of connection. This is the way of the Divine Feminine: the earthy, fertile, feeling-based Mother Earth that we stand upon, the pulling together of all the threads of our humanness into one acutely sentient Godly weave. If only our fathers had known that, and developed healthier egos instead of thicker armor.

M: I don't completely agree with that. The ego actually IS the armor to our true nature. It is the shell, the veil. Your philosophy just gives it more substance. But it already has enough steam. It is what blocks us from our

God-self. It is separation. Why fuel that? Rather than focus on healing their egos, our fathers should have eradicated them altogether. Then you and I would have had happier childhoods.

JB: Happier? I doubt that. Perhaps less painful, but also left vital. Less colorful and richly nuanced, craziness and all. We would have been better off if they had supported their egos coming into a true and healthy balance. Not eradicated them. Is ego annihilation even possible?

M: I believe it is possible, and many Masters have paved the way.

JB: This question is fundamentally where we differ. To add more fuel to the duel, I am going to take it even further. Where you see the ego as an enemy—I see it as an ally. A beloved servant. It just needs to be put in its rightful place. I often imagine the Ego as the Soul's precious worker-bee, implementing and over-seeing the foundational tasks necessary to honor The Queen Bee. It doesn't run the whole hive—but it makes an essential contribution to the overall vitality of the hive. In the hive, the Ego has an essential function. It clears the debris and manages the world so that the Queen Bee—the Soul's light—can shine. The worker bees are essential to the Queen Bee fulfilling her purpose. Ego and Soul are both complimentary and completely reliant on one another.

From another angle, the Ego and the Soul are essentially mirror reflections of each other—on a developmental level. That is, there is little or no distinction between the stage we are at egoically, and the stage we are at spiritually. If you believe, as I do, that we come into each life with encoded lessons and callings, then wouldn't that mean that the current developmental state of the Ego reflects the current developmental stage of the Soul?

M: Hmmm… You know, in all of my decades of seeking and finding, I have never heard of a philosophy quite like this. Never. At the very least, it's fascinating to consider. In the way I understand it, you are essentially saying that our emotionally unevolved aspects, are a direct reflection of our spiritually unevolved aspects.

JB: Precisely. As I shared weeks ago, I make no distinction between emotional and spiritual transformation. You can't mature along one thread, without maturing along the other. Emotional maturity and spiritual maturity are synonymous. Those who keep them separate are not just perpetuating great suffering—they are initiating it.

The Authenticity-Personality

I could see he was taking in my words, letting them work and rumble within. I noticed his face looked slightly different than before—more flushed and full of life. Our dialogue was arousing him. Stimulating a new possibility—whether he was ready to admit it or not. We paid our bill at the taco joint and began walking back to the park. The air was now brisk. The trees were stark and skeleton-like. Winter was hovering near. When we arrived, we sat right down at the picnic table, and continued our dialogue.

M: In a way, what you call the unhealthy ego sounds an awful lot like 'personality,' something I have worked hard to extinguish.

JB: I beg to differ Michael. Your personality may reflect the unhealthy ego, but it may also reflect the natural adaptations and masks one must wear to function in the world. We must survive. Have some compassion for that. It's not the whole story. At the same time, our personality has the potential to be infused with life-force—reflecting our idiosyncratic nature, our soul's unique blueprint. When we are integrated and aligned, both inwardly and outwardly, our true personality can shine forth. Do you not believe that each soul has a unique quality, unique temperament, unique blueprint, that is manifest as the personality?

M: No, I don't. I believe that we get lost in our false identifications and imagine them real. We forget that they are adaptations, and not the real thing.

JB: What then is the real thing? How would one express their unique personhood if they were living from "the real thing"?

M: They would be more equanimous, less individuated. Less 'person' and more essence.

JB: Amorphous blobs. How boring. I guess that's what they mean by "persona non-grata." The personality is truly an unwelcome presence, caught in the trap of misidentification. So, there is no actual distinction to be made between individuals on an authentic level?

M: Not exactly. There would be differences, but they would be much less pronounced.

JB: Like the way many perpetual meditators manifest their personalities—somewhat robotically, with a uniform placid expression on their still face, but with slightly different spiritual personas. One wears mala beads, another wears a colorful scarf. ☺ Some like their meditation cushions soft, while others like them hard. One believes enlightenment is found through sex, the other through avoiding sex.

M: I think of it as equanimity, not automation. But yes, more rooted in the bigger picture. Less concerned with the fluctuations of the small self.

JB: So here we are again, my friend. Rather than you making sensible distinctions between ways of being that reflect who we are, versus those that are fractured, you sweep personality under the carpet and jump to the emptiness. This could be another device to bypass your own challenging fluctuations. Awakening happens in the heart of the self—not in the heart of the eternal emptiness.

Michael went quiet for a moment, his eyes rapidly scanning the park in search of something.

M: Look at that kid over there, the one playing by the tree. He tantrums and makes demands when he can't get his mother's attention. He tries to control her. He is clearly attached to his ever-fluctuating wants and needs. He takes it all so seriously, while what really matters—the state of serene equilibrium beyond fluctuation—is outside his awareness. I can't understand why Hannah wants to bring one of those monkey-minds into the world. Hell, I can barely deal with my own monkey mind.

JB: I see something entirely different. I see a kid with his own beautifully nuanced, vibrant, and colorful personality, fighting to be seen and heard so he can develop his own distinct personhood. A necessary and vital step as a human-being. I feel the intensity of his drive to actualize his various aspects, a force of nature that cannot be controlled or denied. I see a strongly present self, that is at the same time, an individuated reflection of essence, in a distinctly unique and magnificent shape, energized with its own intrinsic purpose.

M: Whoa. Okay, make me feel like an asshole.

JB: I understand the temptation to deny the veracity of the self in a harsh world, but I will remind you that there is a very real danger in denying the self. It's one thing to acknowledge that there are false selves, masks and disguises, but to not also acknowledge that there is a healthy self, a purposeful self, a magnificent and authentic self, is to potentially do grave harm, particularly to trauma survivors and those who struggle with a fragmented psyche. They have a big mountain to climb with healing and re-integrating. The last thing they need are teachings that take them further away from their individual selfhood. They need healthy self-love and self-regard.

And… I would take it a step further. As I have listened to you these last weeks, I have often flashed to images of the Holocaust.

M: The Holocaust? That's gnarly.

JB: Yes, it is, but there is a reason for it. I have been reflecting on this for weeks, and now I see it. In many ways, there is a stark similarity between your views, and the views espoused by the Nazis. I know this is not your intention, but the parallels are apparent to me.

M: Dude. I think you've lost it.

JB: Well, if it makes more sense to you, chalk it up to my sensitivity from my Jewish heritage. For example, I see real parallels between Nazi's Aryan Nation superiority trip, and the patriarchal enlightenment trip. Both emphasize mastery, perfection, an untarnished consciousness. Both are about being beyond the human condition. Both are impersonal and ruthlessly automated. The no-self trip denies the value of story, personal identifications, feelings, body, and self—in the same way as the Nazis desacralized the Jews and others. They ripped them from their homes and communities, rid them of their possessions and clothes, dissociated from their suffering, and then gassed millions of them, killing their embodied selves altogether. I get that your intention is different—that is, to rid yourself of the misidentified elements of the self. But because you, and many of your teachers, do not then provide a map for coming back into—or dare I say, *remaining within*—the body and integrating your newfound wisdom with your human story, it makes for glaring parallels to Nazism. You too are killing the self before its time to go. There's a sadism, and a deep-rooted hatred of the human form in it, if you look closely. It's on the same continuum with respect to its valuation of our humanness.

M: Holy shit, you're calling me a Nazi! Fuck, man, that's preposterous!

JB: I'm not calling you a Nazi. I recognize that you are not promoting such horrifying atrocities. But I am making a parallel between two philosophies that negate our humanhood. Theirs has a different intention, but the effects are not necessarily that different, particularly if your philosophy is embraced by trauma survivors who are then propelled to leave the world by their own hand... because they have been led to believe that their feelings and their stories are unreal, and their selves don't matter.

M: Okay, I'm not going to get defensive. Partly because I don't want to give you more evidence that I am hooked into my self, and partly because I have heard this from Hannah for years. She often says that there is a "Nazi-like rigidity" about the spiritual community I come from. That they are soft-voiced sadists, mocking the human condition from their airless mountain-top hideaways.

JB: I'm with Hannah—I have noticed the same. And not only that... During my excursions to Advaita retreats or satsangs in my spiritualized past, I would notice a particular air in some of the students and teachers. It wasn't always immediately visible, but there was a subtle tone of self-righteousness, hidden below a flat-lined, equanimous mask. When I observed or interacted with some of the participants, I continually confronted a certain degree of superiority or smugness, as though they alone held the key to an expanded consciousness. I noticed many were quick to assert their views, interjecting and correcting other people's perspectives with a militant rigidity.

M: Hmmm... I'm not going to deny that. I've been both the victim—and the perpetrator—in that regard.

JB: There was a particular code to language they deemed appropriate—akin to the spiritualized version of being "politically correct." I call it "S.C."

M: Another of your kitschy terms. Let me guess. Spiritually correct.

JB: Non-duality and Advaita philosophies are intended to be based on a space of neutrality. Yet I found that all too often the unhealthy ego was running the show. What an odd thing to seek egolessness from within the ego, itself. What a strange phenomenon, to be riddled with judgment while the whole premise of Advaita is non-judgment, allowance, and acceptance of "What is."

M: Again, dude, you sound just like Hannah. She often imitates the admittedly strange way some of them laugh, particularly when they describe the tragedies that befall humanity. Maybe you and Hannah should go on a date. And sing the praises of the human story, over a glass of scotch.

JB: Thanks for the offer. Already happily married.

M: Well, good for you. Didn't know that. I assume she's not a no-selfer?

JB: Got that right. She has a beautifully nuanced authenticity-personality, one that reflects her unique and multifaceted nature. Anyway, that's a chat for another time. Over scotch. For now, what I hear you saying is that you and those that share your perspective do not experience a distinct identifiable self. It's like this brand of spirituality doesn't know how to integrate their true selfhood, so they flee it altogether.

M: Again, there is no true self. There is only our true inner nature.

JB: There is only the self, even when it falls into patterns of misidentification. It is the only way you can connect with the world at large. Even when you are touching into your version of the formless emptiness, your sense of it is all arising through the self—it is your antennae, your conduit, your perceiver, your foundation for expansion. Your selfhood—broadly and inclusively defined—is your base to stand in, even in your efforts to reach beyond it. You may choose to neutralize aspects of it, but it cannot be bypassed. Not really. Not until death. One day, we will no longer be in this body on this earth. This can happen sooner, or it can happen later. But it will for sure happen. And then we won't need this vessel anymore. So, while you are here, don't squander the opportunity of being in a body. It's the gift of all gifts. We're only here for a moment. Don't waste it, Michael.

M: Okay, even if I accept that there is some merit to what you say, we give the self way too much credit...

JB: That's because it's the foundation for reality. The very idea that the self is not real, dishonors and desacralizes all that it took to reach this stage in human development. It is to suggest that God, or evolutionary processes, made an error developing this human form. You can't make that determination... but what you can do is work to develop this creation in a way that reflects its inherent magnificence. Fleeing the creation won't accomplish that. Enlivening and actualizing it will. Just think of the billions of cells that carry an intrinsic knowledge of their very specific life-affirming function: the muscles, tissues, and organs that function in perfect harmony, the marvel of birth. Oh, and let's not forget all that karmic and ancestral lineage that threads through us. All of this gift-wrapped in a brilliantly unique humanhood. Simply put, we are the course in miracles. We don't need to look outside of ourselves for that. It's staring at us in the mirror.

M: I can't dispute that there is something nourishing in your words.

JB: Through this lens, the suggestion that it was all foolhardy, and that the true self exists independent of our stories and personal identifications—in the selfless, barren emptiness—feels both entirely disrespectful and ludicrous. If there is a God, (s)he would no doubt be offended by your desperate need to de-personalize her most glorious marvel of creation. THE SELF. The only one who can tell me that God made a mistake putting us in human form, is God herself. And I haven't heard a peep.

A Weastern Consciousness

M: I still feel, on the whole, it is more evolved to withdraw from the muckiness of our dualistic aspects and reside in the great beyond—at least until it is safer for humans to come back down and work within the dualities. At this stage, it's just too brutal down here.

JB: Michael, can you be open to the possibility that your intensive spiritual work could all be to avoid and escape that underlying fact: that it is "too brutal" down here? Is it possible that this is a driving force behind your quest?

M: I feel it is much more complicated than that.

JB: How so?

M: Because I may have initially gone on the quest for that reason, but I have come to many realizations along the way that support this way of being. Through my lived experience. It's not all about avoidance. It's also about advancement. I have seen the light.

JB: Yes, and you have sidestepped the dark. You have already acknowledged that this is fundamental to your pattern.

M: True, I have made that admission.

JB: Back to your original statement—that it feels more evolved to pull out of the muckiness of our dualistic aspects... until it is safer for humans to drop back down and work within the dualities. How will humanity arrive there if we don't actively and intentionally heal our world?

M: Perhaps it's for some of us to do the work you describe... and for others, to do a different kind of work. Some get in the trenches and grunt it out. Others elevate their consciousness and pray for humanity.

JB: Yes, prayers are fine—but activism is just as essential. In one meditation movement, they have two-year pray-athons, hundreds of them praying for the well-being of humanity, while right outside the temple their fellow humans stand begging for a meal. Enough of these detached, emotionally safe versions of connection. Better to be a living prayer, and bring your benevolent intentions into grounded action. Better to spend five minutes feeding a homeless person than two years in meditation. Take to the streets and connect with lonely humans, offer a blanket to someone who is cold, hug the world. That's a much more effective way to co-create world peace. Meditation-in-action! Who doesn't need a hug?

M: Yes, but you speak often of purpose… perhaps some of us exist to get down and dirty in the world, while others exist to detach from the world and elevate their consciousness. Ever hear of the "hundredth monkey" phenomenon?

JB: Okay, Monkey-ji. To practice detachment and bring back some tools to humanity, sure, but not to remain out there, while the world burns. You are needed, we all are needed. Our purpose does not exist in isolation from humanity. You are missing the significance and meaning of the individual birth. The magnificent gifts, abilities, callings, offerings we are each here to bring forth to the world. Are they not true and worthy of acknowledgment and expression? Are we to ignore these unique gifts and find our purpose in an amorphous field of consciousness? Our combined gifts of expression form an intricate web of co-creation that ripples through the world. Each playing their part. THAT'S the hundredth monkey.

M: There's less pain, less war, less chaos, less destruction, in transcendence.

JB: No, just lots of repression, which ultimately means more pain and war. And even if we accept that transcendence is a more painless path, it also means a more joyless path. As we discussed earlier, you can't turn off the tap of feeling in only one regard. It's either all on, or it's off altogether. You can't have it both ways.

M: How then do you reconcile your belief in the magnificence of the individual self with the idea that we are "All-One"? I do find this perplexing.

JB: By accepting that both are true, both are fundamental to our experience of wholeness. We don't have to choose one awareness—we can integrate both. Yes, we are connected. Yes, we are all part of the oneness. And yet we are not the same. I am not another you. You are not another me. Every soul has a unique role to play in this dance of sacred imagination.

M: But how do we know of our true oneness, without getting lost in separation?

JB: That is the central question. How do we hold both: the transcendent and the immanent? This is what I call "the point of sacred balance." And it's the great art form of the human experience. If we go too far in either direction—transcending the self and swimming in unity, or affixing to the self with no awareness of our communal nature—we end up lost in translation. We ascend so high in the sky that we are no longer living a human life, or so crouched down within the self that we can no longer feel our connection to the everything. It's like spending your whole life looking up, or spending your whole life looking in the mirror. It's only half the picture. So, what then is the bridge between these polarities? What is the point of sacred balance where the bountiful rivers of selfhood meet the boundless oceans of essence? Until we find that bridge, we will just bounce back and forth between 'realities,' neither of them more or less real than the other. One thing I am sure of: If our version of All-Oneness is not built on a healthy regard for the rights, boundaries, and magnificence of the individual self, it's All-Nonsense.

M: Yes, but the philosophies that I delved into are tried, tested, and true for thousands of years. They have withstood the tests of time, and they still apply, even amidst our insane modern-day world. These are eternal teachings. Timeless wisdom...

JB: What if we sought a consciousness that bridges both truisms, rather than choosing between two points of focus ad nauseam. I call this "Weastern Consciousness"—the integrative bridging of the wisdom of the East and West. Rather than advocating for one way of being over another, we create a map that is inclusive and that honors the merits in each. We make a conscious effort—in our daily lives, in our spiritual practices—to find the point of merger between the wisdoms of the East and West. We bridge the Eastern quest for unity consciousness with the Western quest for self-development and emotional health. That is the appropriate blend of the two ways of being. Separate voices inextricably woven through a choir of unified light.

Our life's work, then, becomes to both swim in the vaster ocean, and to find our uniquely individuated place in the heart of it. To find that place where the individual droplet of meaning meets the oceans of essence. If you go too far in either direction, you are lost. Too much ocean, you drown. Too few drops of water, you die of thirst.

M: What would that actually look like in my daily life?

JB: Good question. You would work to bring all aspects of the human experience into your moment-to-moment awareness. In your daily life, you would spend more time—as Hannah often nudges you—embodying and working through your emotional material, while maintaining your thread of connection to the more expansive realms that you cherish. You seem to be grounded in many of the elements of the practical realms—excelling at your job, maintaining a high-functioning lifestyle, taking care of business—yet when it comes to the world of feeling, emotion, embodiment, and personal expression, your awareness is underdeveloped. I would actually suggest that you focus almost exclusively on embodying your selfhood, both to bring you into balance, and to give you a deepening taste of the difference between an experience of unity that flows from a healthily developed self versus a bypassed self.

M: No way, dude. I have too much to lose. I didn't do all this spiritual work for decades just to toss it away and bury myself in my psychological patterns. Nope.

JB: I get that. So, for now, just see if you can more fully integrate your emotional life into your daily travels. I do ultimately want to invite you toward the true non-dual field, one where you no longer see anything in polarized terms... but let's begin where you are.

M: Hmmmpf. Well, as I said, I'm not about to throw away my whole foundation and identify solely with the small self. But, I will do as you suggested. For this week, I will attempt to hold both polarities in my consciousness—the bigger picture, and my various feelings. It should be an interesting week...

JB: Interesting, to say the least. I look forward to hearing about it.

We got up from the table, and said goodbye. Michael walked south to Dundas to catch a streetcar, and I began the long trek home. As I walked, I reflected on my own path to embodiment. I particularly thought of my work with Lowen, where I came deeply into my feet, energized and alight, standing FOR something. What was Michael standing for, sitting still hour after hour, eyes closed, like his fellow neo-Advaita meditators, sleepy like goats? What could he be standing FOR, if there was no self to stand in? What was he grounding into? Nothing—the non-earth. Ground zero.

Despite our differences, I was truly enjoying my meetings with this no-selfer. Although he continued to return to his dissociative comfort zone, we were making real progress and trust was building. He had hugged me, and perhaps more significantly, called me by my first name during this meeting. In other words, my personhood now existed for him. This was significant, perhaps more significant than the ideas being exchanged. No matter how compelling my ideas might be, it would mean very little if he didn't feel a personal connection. We are wounded in relationship—we must heal in relationship. I looked forward to the next stages of our unfolding.

5 The Body Temple

> Your body hums to the present—and when you
> become aware of that, you feel the Present living
> within you. When the Present is embodied in that
> way, all sense of separation fades. The embodied
> Present is the lived Present.
>
> —PHILIP SHEPHERD

The next time Michael texted, I suggested that we do a yoga class together. I had been missing my yoga practice, and I was curious as to how energizing our bodies before speaking would impact our interface. He agreed.

We met at my favorite Toronto studio for a morning Vinyasa class. Not surprisingly, Michael and I had very different approaches to yoga class. He remained focused and rigid, diligently adhering to each of the asanas, in their perfect form, never once stepping off the mat. My practice was more fluid—allowing the free-flowing organic expression of my body, with little concern of technicalities. Doing some of the poses in their true form, while drifting off into my own imaginative practice in between. I noticed he gave me a few narrowed sidelong glares.

After class, we grabbed some coffees on Ossington Avenue, and headed down to the lake. On the way, we talked about the class.

JB: How was that for you?

M: I liked the pace of the class, but I did feel a little frustrated.

JB: Why frustrated?

M: Because my gnarly feelings were coming to the surface, particularly when we did the shoulder stand and downward dog sequences. That's not usual for me. I have been doing yoga for years and I have never gotten emotional on the mat. If anything, it helps me to subdue my emotions and to purify my body. And I also felt particularly triggered. Your style of yoga was annoying me. Dude, what were you doing over there? It's so sloppy. Mats are for doing yoga ON.

JB: Chillax. We have different styles. Did you expect it to be otherwise? You do yoga in the way it was first intended. To get away from the human shadow. It may come as a surprise to you, but many of the origins of yoga were premised on the spiritual bypass.

M: Here we go. I knew there was a hidden agenda to taking me to class. You're like the archetypal Zen teacher, putting me in different scenarios, just to make a point.

JB: Actually that was not my intention. But while we are on the subject. Yoga may appear as a positive "body-loving" practice—but much of it was founded on the idea that the body was a toxic chamber, contaminated by shadow emotions, that needed to be purified of its imperfections. In other words, it was premised on the same bifurcated, self-bashing version of unity, or non-duality, that you and I discussed. The purpose of the practice was to "purify" the shadow by opening, strengthening, and enlivening the body, as though our spiritual lives exist independent of the body and the emotions we hold. It wasn't intended as a whole-being integration tool. Again, this is the nature of patriarchal spirituality—the disconnect from the world of feeling, the assumption that our most awakened spiritual path is vertical and exists independent of our feelings, our relationships, and our body itself. Only through the discipline and mastery of the body could the student touch pure consciousness. It was about focus, not feeling. Of course, just because you are doing an 'embodiment' practice doesn't mean you are actually *in* your body.

M: Yoga as patriarchal spirituality? Pffff. Is there anything on the spiritual path you keep sacred? You're a killjoy. 'Patriarchy' is certainly not the feeling I get when I attend a yoga class of hot babes in tight clothes. It's positive energy and expression. Not patriarchal suppression.

JB: True, yoga classes serve a different purpose in our present-day society. But surface appearances can be deceptive. Take a look at the deeper origins. See where it stemmed from. It still carries some of these threads, even now. I'm not saying everything about yoga is amiss—it has supported me tremendously in my life. And it helps many to get fit and flexible, and to have some peace and solace in their busy lives. It's a welcome addition to Western life. But I am saying—*when used as a tool for spiritual development*—it's incomplete. Particularly if we define spirituality as I do: Spirituality as reality. As an inclusive experience. It's time for a new paradigm of yoga. Not rigid techniques applied from the outside-in, but a true listening from the inside-out. Not a practice that is limited to perfect asanas and contained emotions, but one that invites all that we are to the mat. Think of it as a perfect example of a Weastern consciousness. Instead of becoming adept at only one instrument—you become the entire symphony.

M: How would this look in a studio class, dude?

JB: I call it "Barking Dog Yoga."

M: Say what?

JB: A new system of yoga practice that invites students to use the asanas to open parts of the body and excavate repressed memories and emotions. Think of it as the complete yoga experience—encompassing not just the physical body, but the emotional body, too. Practitioners would be welcome to cry, or safely express a range of emotions, without judgment or discomfort. They would be encouraged to express sounds and words that come up in the process. In this way, it would be very similar to a Bioenergetics exercise class. You do the physical exercises, both because they are opening and strengthening, and because they are an opportunity to release and to heal what is held within the body. The asanas that were developed throughout the years do contain an intrinsic genius. The alchemy of the specific asanas, their sequence, and the extended time holding each posture, creates the ability to reach into deep, covert places in the body. Subtle areas we cannot normally access through general physical exercise and activity. The asanas are masterfully designed to access these unattended places, stimulating our subconscious, and the memories and emotions encoded in the tissues. And yet, it is incomplete. There is no follow-up. After being stimulated, our subconscious is not granted the space to express itself, and be integrated into the exercises. In this way, yoga falls short in reaching its potential as a spiritual tool.

It is lacking in the complimentary aspect: expression and integration of all that arises. This is the next step for yoga in the West, in my view. It is already beginning to happen with some yogis.

M: Sounds like going to a serene yoga class would now be akin to going to the circus. I don't want to hear people huffing and puffing and emoting. I go to class to relax. Get some peace amidst my busy day.

JB: Oh, it can be relaxing. Expressing your emotions is the deepest form of rest. The whole process has to be held in a safe container, and it would be essential for teachers to be trained in the art of holding space for deep feeling. Because this material can be very hot to touch into. As it is, without that training, many students are having their wounds rise to the surface on the mat, and there is no one there to support their journey. This alone can be re-traumatizing. Better we take yoga to the next level, and create a container that invites the feelings into awareness, and that supports their healthy expression. Classes could perhaps be labeled Barking Dog Yoga Level One (moderate degree of emotional healing process). Barking Dog Yoga Level Two (significant degree of emotional healing process). The higher the degree of process, the smaller the class, or the more teachers on hand to ensure that each student gets the proper amount of care. There could be gentler Intro classes for students who are not yet conscious of the material they are holding. Classes geared to anger release, grief work, all manner of expression and healing. The practice doesn't have to happen in a studio. It can also happen in your home practice, any time you feel called to it. Or in a body-centered psychotherapist's office. It's less effective to reach deep into the substance of your wounds by talking about them. That often just skims the surface. Adding in a physical component can take the whole process to the next level.

M: Barking Dog Yoga would surely help us to get rid of the ego that plagues the yoga industry. Instead of teachers and students walking around thinking they're so hip because they can out-asana everyone, they would be humbled by the fact that everyone—themselves included—is carrying wounds below their perfect ass and perfect posture.

JB: Exactamundo!

Waking Down

Right then, we arrived at the lake and sat down on a bench at the edge of the beach. It was an unusually warm November day in Toronto. With a knitted brow, Michael slowly stirred more cream into his coffee. He looked like he was pondering deeply. Then he said:

M: I had a difficult week.

JB: Is that part of the reason you were being testy about my yoga practice? What was difficult about it… do tell.

M: Well, as you know, I work for a high-end software company doing coding. Pretty abstract work, but I'm highly skilled at it. Much to my surprise, I was offered a far more lucrative position this week—heading the sales division in bringing our new cutting-edge app to the market. I had been the one to pitch the idea of creating the app to the team, and they liked my presentation so much, that they saw me in a different light… as a savvy salesman. Imagine that—me, a people person. Hah! It was so ironic, this all happened right after I had spent the weekend working with the integration exercise you suggested. I came into the office, already feeling a little agitated by my humanness that was plain in my face, and they presented the offer. I did my best to appear excited, but inside I was a complete fucking mess. I have been working almost in seclusion for years, and this was the last thing I expected.

JB: How did you experience this mess, as you call it?

M: My body began having a meltdown.

JB: The body speaks its truth.

M: Or it just freaks out. As soon as the day ended, I raced home and did a long, intense meditation. Almost two hours. I strived to transcend the body and enter a state of peace, so that I could accept the job offer and do it effectively.

JB: So, rather than embracing your body's inherent wisdom, you hyper-meditated to tame it.

M: Well, that's the idea—to train the body so that it doesn't undermine our goals.

JB: Oh, the old override the body routine again. Train and contain it to find peace. Can you be more precise as to how you experienced the actual meltdown? What precisely were you feeling? What was your body actually telling you?

Michael closed his eyes. He didn't say anything for a long time. When he finally did, I could barely hear him. His voice was unusually soft, almost a whisper:

M: When they presented the offer, I felt immediately sick to my stomach. I felt a knot in my throat, and my neck got progressively tighter. My left eye began twitching intermittently. And my feet started tapping, like they wanted to run me out of that room. I felt like darting back to my corner office, and locking the door behind me. It was all very uncomfortable and I wanted to turn off my body and come back into the moment.

JB: Thank you for sharing so in depth. Those are all very important responses to notice—they are actually cues and signals. You see, there is no distinction between an embodied life and a spiritual life. Grounded Spirituality is rooted in the body, rooted on Mother Earth. And not just superficially connected to the body—as many flat-lined "spiritual teachers" are—but deeply and intimately at one with it. Because you can't be in the 'now,' if you have severed your connection to the body. You are embodied essence. Turning off your awareness of the body will only take you further away from the moment.

M: I am not suggesting that one becomes unaware of the body—but instead, that a calm and peaceful physical state is your best shot at entering the moment. An agitated body is a distraction from true peace.

JB: A calm body is only real if you arrive at that peace organically, after moving through all the related feelings and sensations. But not if you willfully direct your body, as if it's an entity entirely separate from you. The body naturally falls into alignment as a consequence of deep honesty, truth-telling, and uncovering. In other words, it offers vital information about our path. It calms down and comes into alignment when you heed its advice. The transcendence bypass is like finding nuclear energy without a reactor. The body is the reactor. It's where the real alchemy happens. It is our transmitter of encoded information.

M: I see it as being akin to the mind—it needs containment. It calms down when I subdue its rantings. I can note the body's sensations, but I don't want to get lost in them. My path is peace.

JB: The more your consciousness is rooted in the body, the more connected you are to the here and now. And the more here you are, the more spiritual—or enrealed—you are. Being rooted within the body means that you are energetically fluid, with a harmonious flow between body and mind. See this book. It's my friend Philip Shepherd's masterpiece *Radical Wholeness*. He's also a Torontonian—worked for years to develop his ideas right over there, on Toronto Island. Cutting-edge material about the mind-body linkage. Let me read you an excerpt:

> Embodiment isn't about sitting in the head and paying attention to the part of you we call the body—it's about fully inhabiting the intelligence of the body and attuning to the world through it. It's about listening to the world through the body. It's about feeling the world through the breath. For our purposes, then, we might say that embodiment is a state in which your entire intelligence is experienced as a coherent unity attuned to the world. In that state any distinction between 'mind' and 'the body's energy' becomes meaningless.

In other words, it's not about removing the mind from the equation, as many patriarchal spiritualists have suggested—it's about bringing the mind into dialogue with the felt experience of the body. And, bringing the energies and wisdoms of the body—including the heart's wisdom, cellular wisdom, and the intuitive wisdom stored within the pelvic bowl—into alignment with each other. To the extent that your experience of your body is fragmented, your experience of the now is fragmented. This is as true for your body as it is for the selfhood it houses. Chop off or segregate any aspect of our humanity, and we limit our experience of this precious moment. You're either here—in every sense—or you aren't fully here. And presence is not to be found on the skyways of self-avoidance. Presence is to be found here, in our body temples, sole to soul, on Mother Earth.

M: That sounds like the furthest thing from inner peace. Surrendering to the body doesn't leave me peaceful. Controlling it, does.

JB: I prefer an authentic and integrated peace over a forced and divisive one. Let's see what Philip wrote about this topic:

> Inner peace is made even more challenging by the cultural fantasies that attach themselves to it. Inner peace can mean different things, but it often implies the ability to rise above the distractions and needs of the body and slip free of the concerns of the world—as though our state of consciousness ought not to be blemished by mundane matters; as though the idea of purity, which by definition excludes, is superior to wholeness; as though the issues of wholeness and integration were mere inconveniences that could be sidestepped rather than the work we are here to undertake. This, again, is the dream of the dissociated male principle within us: to cast off the immanence of embodiment like a smelly coat and strive towards the pure, transcendent realization of the self... Of course, an inclination to manage your way to peace is an inclination to divide the self—and where there is division, there cannot be peace.

M: I experience quite the contrary. Real presence is a state of awareness. It has little to do with the physical plane. It's a field of consciousness. Consciousness utilizes the body for its own purpose. The body is a vehicle, a conduit, for our greater awareness.

JB: Just consider this for a moment. What IF... the body is actually inseparable from what you call "consciousness." It is consciousness in-form. We can't exist solely as consciousness. Consciousness exists to take form—its movement is unstoppable. It doesn't come down INTO the body. The body IS consciousness.

M: This is trippy. You are giving me a mind-flip.

JB: Yes, rather than conceiving of the body as the vessel that transports us from one spiritual experience to another, we relate to the body as the embodiment of consciousness. It means honoring our physical form not simply as a 'vessel' for the soul, but as the embodiment of the soul. It is here where our real life is lived. It is here where our soul expresses its truths. It is here where our prayers are heard. Remember, at the heart of Grounded Spirituality is groundedness within body. We have to wake down the body, before we can wake up our awareness. Who needs higher, when we are already living right inside the God temple? Walk walk walkin' on heaven's floor…

M: Wake down the body? Say more.

JB: To wake down the body is to enliven it, in all regards. To open its lines. To melt through its armor and enable its sensitivity. To attune to and invite its advanced wisdom. To align the chakras, or energy centers. To regain its natural energetic fluidity. To heal and nourish the temple so that it can be fully dynamic. It's about enlivening the body so completely… that we come to know it as spirit incarnate.

M: What does it mean to be energetically fluid?

JB: Think of the way people move and inhabit their bodies. Some seem to be energetically aligned and flowing from head to toe. They emanate a vitality through and through. It's palpable. Like free-flowing rivers. Have you ever met someone like that?

M: Hmmm, now that I think about it... my late grandmother Louise. My mom's mother. She was a spitfire. It pulsed throughout her body. An eccentric with a wild passion for life. She was said to have led pole-dancing classes in her garage, and used to steal away on weekends and attend Kundalini yoga workshops. Pretty revolutionary for Indiana. When I was a kid, I used to love cozying up on her lap, and she would stroke my head, and my whole body would tingle from head to toe. I felt so peaceful near her. Serene, yet alive. Wish I had her around longer. She died suddenly when I was 19.

JB: Yes, I've encountered a few of those gems throughout my life too. Bio-energetics Co-founder Alexander Lowen was like that—vital like a mustang. Embodied human-beings have a gravity—an actual substance—to their presence. It is palpable and contagious. Their presence pulls on your inner gravity and catalyzes a waking down process. Then there are others, many others, who are only energized in certain ways. Perhaps they have a lot of energy coming off of their minds, while they are deadened in their bodies. Or they have a lot of sensual energy coursing through their hips, but their throat chakra is blocked. Perhaps even their heart is closed. Or, quite often you will encounter people who are clumsy and ungrounded. These are examples of a corrupted, or obstructed, fluidity. In other words, at some point along the way, they closed down some of their energetic lines—likely because it felt too painful to remain open and to develop them—and they began to live their lives through another portal, to compensate. Some energy centers are open, others are closed, and so their experience of the moment—and of *all* of life—is limited to the energetic realm they have over-developed. And, because they are deadened in certain aspects, they have a limited lens on reality. They perceive things as they are—either through the mind alone, or through the hips, or through the heart—but not through the eyes of an integrated beingness.

Unearthing the Body's Wisdom

M: I am compelled to understand more. I remember there was a time when I was very young, when, like Grandma, I felt very fluid energetically. I remember feeling like I was open and available to everything, until somewhere around the age of 8 or 9. I had a ton of energy. I was a firecracker. My mom and dad felt like I was too much to handle. Couldn't harness my energy at school. I wanted to be out living life, not reading about it. If I was a child in current times, I probably would have been hooked on some ADHD drugs.

JB: You said this shifted around age 8 or 9. What happened then... did the difficulties of life shut you down?

M: I am not really sure. I want to say that it was a conglomeration of factors that all culminated around that time, but that doesn't feel exactly right. I'm not sure I have access to that knowledge.

JB: I have an exercise I think will be helpful. It's a simple method that accesses your memories by going deeper into the body. Perhaps we can stimulate your memories by connecting with the body's intelligence. Would you like to try?

M: Nothing to lose.

JB: Well, actually, you might lose something you're better off without. Let's move over to the beach, and have you lie down on the sand. It's warm enough today to do this outside.

After Michael assumed his position, I began:

Stretch out your legs, and get comfortable. Now close your eyes, and get intimate with your breath. Feel it deeply, as it moves evenly throughout your mouth, throughout your nasal passages, throughout your throat, and then circulates throughout your entire body. Don't push it. Just let it gently and organically circulate. This exercise is not meant to be rigorous—but more of a gentle unfurling. Be with your breath openly and steadily, through the entire exercise. Let it roam quietly through you, like a flashlight in the dark, illuminating the path. When you feel deeply relaxed, lift your finger to let me know.

After a few minutes, it was clear he had relaxed into the breath. He lifted his finger. I continued:

Now we are going to take a walk back in time to that phase in your life. The time you were a pre-adolescent. Around age 8, 9, 10. Within, set the intention to re-connect with that time. When you are ready, tell me in general, what do you see or feel?

M: I see myself youthful and vibrant. I'm wearing a bright red shirt. My cheeks are pink. I'm running through the woods behind Grandma's house in Northern Indiana. There was this tree swing I made around this time… I tied a long rope around a towering branch. I would swing on it, and sail through the forest. I'm seeing myself happy and exuberant.

JB: This was a time of life where your body and your being were inseparable. You simply exuded one cohesive life-force—and there was no trying, no efforting, no witnessing—in order to be that. Would you say that was the case?

M: Yes. It was like that. I can remember it. It feels good.

JB: Now, in your awareness, move a bit forward in time from that point. Can you recall when you began to feel more separated from that, more divided. Describe that boy you see then.

M: I can see him. I see a prepubescent boy behind those same woods, but he suddenly looks very alone. Like a lone wolf. He looks troubled. He is kicking stones into the creek. His head is down—like he is working something out. Grappling with something.

JB: Do you have any sense of what you may be working out?

M: No, I don't.

JB: I am going to name some people, and some scenarios… I want you to pay close attention to the most subtle sensations of your body. Every tiny minute sensation is meaningful. Don't discount any of them… The finer the sensation—the more valuable the information. Tell me in detail what you can track in your body. And don't forget to remain attuned to your breath as you explore…

M: I will try.

JB: Think of your mother. Picture her face. Her scent. Her touch. What does your body tell you?

M: I feel relaxed.

JB: What does your belly tell you?

M: I feel a warmth there.

JB: Where?

M: Heat right below my belly button.

JB: Anything else?

M: I feel sadness, higher up. My solar plexus. I feel a longing to see her.

JB: Think of school…

M: I feel a coldness. A clamminess. An emptiness.

JB: Your dad...

M: Hmmm. I feel this blockage there. I can't feel. I feel nothing.

JB: Okay. Think of your dad in a new context. Tell me some rituals you had with him in daily life.

M: Well, he would sit by the fireplace each night and read the newspaper, and puff on his pipe. Sometimes he would let me take a puff too. As long as we didn't tell mom. I can still remember the taste and the scent.

JB: But then something happened around that time—to block or dam up those warm memories of him. Does your body agree?

M: Again, I feel nothing. I feel numb.

JB: Is there a moment where your dad broke your trust?

M: My mind is saying no. But my body—it is saying yes. I don't know how I know that. I just do.

JB: Where are you feeling that?

M: In my legs. And my arms. I feel like running, or punching.

JB: Very good. Anything more you can say about that?

M: I'm sensing it doesn't include only my dad.

JB: Are you seeing another person involved?

M: Yes.

JB: Who can it be?... Is it a friend...

M: No.

JB: Is it another relative?

M: I felt a flash of heat in my solar plexus when you said that.

JB: An uncle… An aunt?

M: Yes. It's my uncle. My dad's brother Russell. I see him now. He is standing atop my dad. There was an incident at Grandma's house—a very dramatic fist-fight between them. I'm not sure what provoked it. Something my dad said made Uncle Russell go ballistic. Russell had my father on the ground and was about to smash his head with a broken bottle of vodka. I screamed and ran to protect my father. Uncle Russell shoved me violently out of the way. I fell against the coffee table and lay there paralyzed for a few minutes. I remember feeling like I was going to lose Dad, and that I would die if he died. I began breathing heavily, hyperventilating. Then I started to hold my breath, in a desperate attempt to control it. I don't remember anything after that. Mom later told me I had a Reflex Anoxic seizure.

As soon as the words left his mouth, Michael's breath slowed to a grinding halt. His whole body clamped up, like he was in a vice-grip. Perhaps he was—the vice-grip of the past kept locked by unresolved trauma. It keeps pressing up against us, until we are finally ready to heal it.

On the Wings of the Breath

We sat in silence for a long time. Michael's breathing slowly deepened, and his body relaxed. He had been on quite a journey—a journey of remembrance. I moved in a little closer. He slowly opened his eyes.

JB: How you doing, my friend?

M: That was quite a ride. I can't believe I blocked that out for so long.

JB: Great work, Michael, great work. I noticed when you spoke of the seizure, your breath became very constricted. In that moment, decades ago, you made a conscious effort to shallow your breathing—so that you would never again feel that kind of pain. And that shallowing of breath didn't just stop there. It became a life-long pattern, a defense mechanism, to avoid the intensity of feelings when you breathe fully.

M: It's interesting you say this, because I do remember developing the habit of shallowing my breath and stifling my expression at an early age, particularly when my father was angry. They even took me to a doctor, because I would stop talking for long periods of time. I guess I learned how to shut myself down. I think I even learned techniques that would support that—turning my gaze away from people when I'm uncomfortable. Stretching my neck up high, when fear arises. I think it's my way of inhabiting my analytic mind, and turning away from the wild, unruly world of feeling.

JB: Excellent insight. And when we are in a survivalist interface with life's challenges—rather than a depthful embrace of them—we are limited in our capacity to be here. We constrict our inner resources. We are actually brilliantly designed with a wellspring of inner resources to adapt to life's challenges. We are designed to take on—and directly meet—this often gritty, difficult world. Not transcend it, except in the most horrifying circumstances, where our very survival or sanity depends on it. Our bodies compartmentalize in an effort to protect us, and often, those coping mechanisms become entrenched ways of being that limit our access to reality—to life, in all its forms—for years, decades, or, sadly, our entire lives. So, for example, by shallowing your breath, you shallow your life. Because if you don't breathe deeply, you can't live fully. When you tighten your belly, you restrict your ability to feel. The more armored your physical body, the more congested your consciousness. Similarly, for head-trippers. Safely sheltered up high, they can't feel into life. They *think* life rather than feel it. Think God—and (S)he remains at arm's length. Feel God, and you're dancing arm-in-arm, cheek-to-cheek. When we are open and fluid, we can avail ourselves of our whole spectrum of resources. Our bodies are not meant to be hiding places. They are meant to BE the expression of life-force itself.

M: I suspect I have been going through life without knowing what I am missing.

JB: You are beginning to see things more clearly. How do you feel now?

M: Different. Very different. I feel calmer, more at peace. Yet at the same time, my body is pulsing with energy. I feel electric. I think I need to take a walk. Hard to lie here with so much energy coursing through me.

JB: Let's go. Movement sparks transformation.

We got up and began to walk the Harbourfront path toward the city center. It was a mesmerizingly serene day. A good day to heal.

JB: Michael, I have a question. Is it possible that the profound intensity of that one traumatic event is still living itself out and shaping your perspective? Is it possible this traumatic incident catapulted you to look for peace outside of your body, on the spiritual path?

M: I suppose I can finally begin to consider that possibility.

Michael looked at me with a sincerity I had not seen before. His eyes were softer, his face transparent. He continued to speak.

M: It may be possible that I'm not the man I thought I was.

JB: Say more...

M: What if it all comes down to me just being a meek individual who doesn't have the courage to face his pain. What if there's nothing special about me? Maybe I just wanted peace, without my issues tearing me to pieces. What if I have just fooled myself all these years?

JB: These are some hard truths to look at. I admire the courage you are showing right now.

He stopped dead in his tracks, and just stood there, looking out over the lake, shaking his head. This was clearly a profound moment of realization on his journey.

M: Wow, it's like my whole path has been about calculatingly landing the "higher bliss," while strategically avoiding the "lower" wells of pain. Now that I look back at some of the techniques I sampled over the years... even when I did breathwork exercises, I was always careful not to activate my body. I did the exercises, while, on the inside, kept a tight rein of control over how far and deep I would go.

JB: Yes, because our breath is our greatest truth-revealer. It is like a shovel, it digs in deep and brings everything to the surface where it can be felt and seen. It breaks through the illusion of purity and catapults us into the messiness of the human experience—messiness that cannot morph into a more clarified form until it is fully and deeply felt. If you witness one of Stanislav Grof's Holotropic Breathwork sessions, you will watch dozens of people screaming, crying, releasing, shrieking, flailing… simply because they had permission to intensify the breath and plummet into their chaotic inner worlds. Made all the more chaotic by their self-protective decisions to block their energetic flow, necessary to manage the world.

M: Right now, messy feels like an understatement.

JB: One often forgets that "noticing the breath"—a common witness-observer practice in the meditative world—is a cerebral function, not a FELT experience. In Grof's work, he has reported—and I have personally experienced—great truths and wisdoms arising on the wings of the breath. Memories and words and feelings that are longing to be released… grief and anger set free, giving way to a joyous presence and visions of divine possibility, inklings of your purpose in this world. All of it unveiling itself through the deepening breath. It's all in there, waiting for its moment of liberation from behind the dams we have erected to protect us from reality.

I had a similar experience with Alexander Lowen. He was the truest spiritual practitioner I have ever known, because he had such a deep and courageous understanding of the relationship between transformation of the emotional body and the awakening of the spiritual, or what he might call, the "spirited body." During a session, I once said to him, "But Dr. Lowen, I can't feel my body." His reply changed my life: "What a perfect way to avoid reality. Are you ready to come back into reality, Jeff? Let's begin with the breath… Breathe yourself back to life… don't watch it. Breathe it." And I really got it—we don't transform by observing ourselves. We transform by embodying ourselves.

M: Perhaps this explains why I have had such a hard time finding my place in this world. It appears that I deadened, or blocked my access to my body.

JB: Exactly, and you can't come to know who you are, if you can't access the information that is held within the body. The purposes you are born to, the geography and particular places that feel like home, your unique relationship to the world, can only be known through the body. It's like trying to decide who you love through thinking alone—it's not possible. The analytic mind can help you to make pragmatic decisions… but it can't tell you what is intuitively known.

I have some clients who numb themselves with heavy food. Workaholism. Porn. Smoking pot. That's a common one these days. Although it can be a useful tool once in a while, it ultimately creates a smokescreen around our feelings, and expands our witnessing mind. And then there's many who actually deaden their feelings by using 'spiritual' practices.

M: I don't touch any of those lower things. Not since my college years. I am well-evolved beyond that kind of self-indulgent, low vibration behavior. They become a prison. I'm all about liberation.

JB: Ah, there's your resistance cropping up again. Hmmm, dare I say it. It could be that your austere and rigid avoidance of any of these "lower" things, IS your particular escape drug. Perhaps you do need to "indulge" the self for a while, to come into balance after years of depriving it. Think about it. Michael, it's not about "avoiding" anything. You are anything but free when you live your life in avoidance. You are actually imprisoned in a different way.

M: Imprisoned. Pfff. Freedom is my middle name.

JB: Real freedom emerges when we surrender to the fluid and integrated truth of the body. And in that state of inclusive awakening, we have access to all kinds of information about who we are, and why we are here. In Philip's words, "When energy does not flow, it cannot inform." The body is a masterpiece of intelligence, far ahead of our thinking minds. When we clear the channels of blocked debris, we can become even more alive to its precision. We can learn how to read its intricate wisdom. In a state of division, we cannot see our place in the world. In a state of integration, we can. The body recognizes when truth is owned, because it is the body that carries the knowledge of who you are and why you are here. Your mind may have an *idea* of who you are and why you are here, but you can only confirm it in the body itself. The body is the temple of truth. Not a temple that you visit, but one that you are.

M: I guess I have some re-acquainting to do with this suit of meat.

JB: Yes, you do, and it comes in a vibrant spectrum of cues, knowings, sensations, intuitions. For example, you know the energetic malaise, the depression, the disenchantment you experience when you don't express and live your truths? They are the body's way of signaling that you aren't aligned with your authenticity. You bury truth within the soma, and you suffer for it. On the other hand, you know those chills you get in your body when you recognize and express a long-buried truth. Like the sensations you got today, when you pierced together some early life memories. These are evidence of the ways that truths—truth of feelings, truth of wants, truth of directionality—are held and recognized within the body itself. A built-in authenticity-mometer, the body dulls when we are living falsely, and glows when we are true to path.

M: Actually, I once had a glimpse of what you are saying. I had a breathwork experience at an ashram in India, where we participated in a 3-day Kapalabhati practice. It was bloody intense. After a few hours, I began to cry, releasing layers of old grief and pain. On the second day, I began to feel as though I was standing outside, or actually, inside of myself, seeing myself in high-definition color. And I can't say I liked what I saw. I saw myself the way you are describing me: false, avoidant, defined by my mechanisms and unresolved issues. I remember that I lay in my tent all night, and just cried and cried. In the morning, I came very close to fleeing the ashram, but something told me to stay. About an hour into Kapalabhati that day, I came upon clear visions of the path I was here to walk—and it was remarkably different from the one I was walking. It was actually very relationally engaged—with a wife, and, dare I say it, children, and *seva* (selfless service)—in the world. In the vision, I appeared glowing and buoyant—probably more akin to what you call fluid and integrated. Afterwards, I asked the guru how to interpret the vision and he asked only one thing: "What does your gut say?" I said, "My gut says that I have been walking in someone else's shoes—not truly my own."

JB: Wow, this is a potent memory. Astonishing you even recalled your vision of having a child someday. This is big. What happened then?

M: You know what happened. I ignored my gut and went back to the patterns that were familiar to me. I guess I needed many more breakthroughs before I could step into real change. One three-day practice wasn't enough to overcome my patterns and resistances. And, sadly, seems like a couple more decades still haven't been enough time.

The Body Alive

We were still standing upright, but now it was different. Michael was looking square at me, something he had often managed to avoid doing. Even when we were sitting face-to-face, he had often looked off to the side, or down at his coffee. But now, he was fully present, in direct contact. He was standing several inches taller, shoulders broadened and opened. Our eyes locked for a moment.

JB: What a day. Now we are really getting somewhere. Only when we can move that debris and construct a bridge back to our bodies, can we get a clearer glimpse of our purpose in the world. We often look for our purpose "out there," outside of our body temple, when what we really need to do is heal, enliven, and integrate our relationship to our bodies. From there, our life path and purpose can reveal itself. It's incoded, not out-coded. It's in the bones of our being.

M: Are there any techniques to support this process?

JB: There sure are. Let's take this one step further. Literally. To reach a stage where you can fully experience the body as presence, it helps to enliven it, through movement. Not regimented "masterful" forms of movement—like marathon running—but more free-flowing, and imaginative movement. Michael, I feel you need some frenetic movement in your life. The kind where you surrender to the body wild and alive, in whatever ways it wants to experience itself. Where uncontained energy builds upon itself, and new pathways of expression are cultivated. For example, free-form dance, unrestrained sexuality, and expressive art forms. All effective armor-busters if you can allow yourself to fully unleash. Instead of seeking to perfect your movements, you allow the body to stretch beyond its habitual range of motion and embody a wider canvas of experience. This will excavate untold levels of emotional material contained within the tissues, and open up a fluid spectrum of expressive and experiential possibility. It's the difference between leading the body, and surrendering to the body alive. The latter creates more space inside, for life to be lived. Imagine a free-flowing river with many tributaries, as opposed to a stagnant, dammed river. This is what I am talking about.

M: The disciplined physical practice you mentioned, that used to be me. I was a very active mountain climber in my traveling years, and I used to religiously sprint 3 miles each day along the Beaches boardwalk, here in Toronto. I loved being physical, as long as being physical was a rigidly disciplined, willful activity, that pushed me to my limits. When Hannah wanted to go to transformational or ecstatic dance, I would always make excuses. I assumed it was because I didn't want to be around her hippie friends, but I can see now that I may have just been resisting what might emerge if I explored my body in a new and different way.

JB: Sounds like you didn't want to shake things up, literally and figuratively. But maybe now you are ready for a more dynamic, spontaneous, form of movement. It's time for you to try Barking Dog Yoga.

M: I'm ready to get my bark on.

JB: I'll tell you how it's done. But first, I want to read you something I wrote this morning, before leaving for the yoga studio. It frames today's conversation:

> I am tired of hearing what God is from head-tripping men. I am tired of hearing what God is from isolationists on a spiritual quest. I am tired of hearing what God is from lovers of detachment. I want to hear about a juicy God, a creative God, a relational God, a God that arises when we jump into life and stop playing it safe, watching it from afar like a passing train. It's time for the dancers to tell us what God is. It's time for the artists to tell us what God is. It's time for the lovers to tell us what God is. We are not here to watch God from afar. We are here to live God from the inside out.

EXERCISE 4
BARKING DOG YOGA PRACTICE

Find an area in your home where you feel safe and comfortable, with space to move. Lie on a mat on the floor. It is optimal to have a mattress or futon also nearby—but a couple of pillows can also suffice. Do this exercise in solitude.

Decide on the yoga practice you will use for the exercise. You can put on a yoga class video, if that will serve you, or do your own sequence of choice. It can be an intense practice, a gentle practice, or somewhere in between. Be sure to include postures that you tend to resist. Do what you feel will best serve your body opening in new ways.

Now set the intention for the class: To use the asanas as an excavation and integration tool. To feel into and express the emotions held in the body. It is not important if you complete the sequence—it is only important that you allow yourself to become more intimate with the material that you are holding within your body temple.

Now begin your practice. As you move into the asanas, invite yourself to feel into any emotions that are held within the body. No rising above them. No sidestepping. No cushioning. No bypassing. Feel your emotions deeply and fully and directly. Allow them to take whatever form they demand. If you feel moved to cry, cry. If you feel called to express anger, express it. If sounds or words come, express them. If joy, happiness and laughter bubble up—express with gleeful abandon. If any uncharacteristic actions arise—trust them. Howl at the moon, bark at the stars, whatever surprising shape takes form—flow with it and express it. If you feel like dancing, dance frenetically. Allow for the fullest range of feeling and organic expression possible. This is not the time for self-judgment, and no one is watching you.

While expressing, you can continue to deepen into the posture, if it brings more feeling to the surface. Or you can stop and attend to your feelings. Feel free to wander off the mat—there are no limits. If you feel called to move, move. If you feel anger or rage arising, feel free to hit and punch the mattress, futon, or pillows. Do not judge yourself. Anger is a healthy blazing fire that hungers to be discharged. The purpose of Barking Dog Yoga is to not to master the postures—it is to use the asanas as a depth charge for the awakening and healing of any unfinished memories and emotions that you are holding inside.

If, at any time, you feel like what is arising is simply too painful to manage on your own, immediately retreat from the process and seek therapeutic support. Activating the emotional body can bring up all manner of unexpected and overwhelming material, and must be approached with care.

Remember to leave space afterwards for integration of the experience. Before you go back out into the world, be sure to ground and center yourself. We don't want you barking at strangers. ☺

After we parted, I walked over to a nearby bench and sat facing the water. I was invigorated by today's meeting. It was a genuine breakthrough, and the electric ripples were palpable throughout my body, and even throughout the atmosphere itself. I had been concerned that more embodiment work would compel Michael to retreat... but, instead, he opened the door to his heart wider, making profound admissions about his early life. It was a marvelous sight to behold. A very real part of him was ready to transform.

At the same time, I could feel his resistance looming ever close. It wasn't as obvious as it had been in the beginning, when it came through in the form of verbal jousting... but it was still in there, tugging at the seams. I could subtly sense it, waiting patiently to rear up and impede his progress. That's the nature of the healing journey. The closer you get to the core material, the more sentries rise up to protect it. Today, they may be fast asleep. Tomorrow, they may come out all guns blazing.

It was almost sunset, and the red glow over the water was breathtaking. I breathed all of it in, allowing it to soak into my cells. And then, my own little wave of resistance took shape. Suddenly, I wanted a coffee, and felt an urgent need to get home. It had been an intense day of space-holding, while vicariously accompanying the journey. I wanted a time-out. In this way, I was no different from Michael. I could only take in the deep feeling for so long, before retreating into my mind, or looking for a subtle way to feel safe and cozy again. This seems to be intrinsic to the human condition. We spend our lives working toward these rare moments of deep feeling. And then retreating from them, only to begin the quest once again. I wondered: What will it take before we can all remain there—holding the magnificence safe and building it into a crescendo of delight? What will it take before we will all stop playing hide-and-seek with the Divine?

6 The Heart of the Matter

Michael texted me mid-week to arrange a time to meet on Sunday morning. We agreed to meet closer to his condo in the Beaches. He seemed to need that comfort this week. When I arrived, he was already there, waiting for me. He looked particularly haggard, like he had been tossed and turned in the waves of an emerging-sea. I moved to hug him, and he backed off, eager to get moving. We began to walk the boardwalk along the lake. It was an overcast late fall day, with a biting chill.

JB: How has your week been, Michael? So much transpired in our last session. You've had a lot to assimilate. What was your experience of the yoga exercise?

M: It was horrible. I did the exercise twice last weekend, and each time I found myself flooded with more emotional pain and more hideous memories. What I tapped into last meeting was only the tip of the iceberg.

JB: More like tip of the painberg.

M: Yup. And the week got worse as it went on. My monkey mind has been going berserk these past days. It's like everything is going up in flames all around me. I'm fucked. Hannah is threatening to leave me if I don't agree to have a child with her. And I began that new job I told you about and it's a nightmare. It was fine when I was working in veritable anonymity in my quiet corner office, but this job is forcing me to confront the fact that even my career was some kind of hideaway from my real purpose. I wasn't just hiding from the other employees—it seems I was hiding from myself, too.

JB: Uh-hmmm.

M: I detest technology, actually. Suddenly I can't believe I have worked here all these years. And, last night, to cap it off, my dad called me and we had a blow-out on the phone.

JB: Ouch.

M: Usually, we just talk superficially, but this time was different. This fire suddenly blazed up inside me, and I was compelled to ask him about the incident with his brother. But he wouldn't answer—his voice just trailed off. I went off on him about the way he represses and evades reality. And he hung up on me.

JB: Geesh, you're sounding like me. But that is an important breaking point. A fire arose within you, to finally confront this long-standing issue. That's a sacred fire. Real progress.

M: Doesn't feel much like progress. I feel like I am in the throes of a nervous breakdown. My energy is leaking in every direction. I've been trying to retain my still-point in the center of the madness, but it's near impossible. Even when I find some momentary inner peace during my meditations, my monkey mind hurls me back into madness. I feel like my chaotic mind is only amplifying the chaos around me.

JB: What if it's only a nervous breakdown if you don't allow the feelings that are trying to come to the surface, to move fluidly through you? That's what causes the breakdown—the resistance to what *is*, the stopping of the process before it has an opportunity to move toward realization and resolution. What if something beautiful is actually happening within you, something that wants to heal and move into full authenticity? What if this is not a nervous breakdown—but a nervous *break-through*—a profound emotional cleansing, a dissolution of the false structures that have ruled your life, a breaking through to a more authentic state of being?

M: Tell that to my monkey mind.

JB: Ready for another mind-flip? I have already alluded to this. What IF… it's not really about the mind at all? What if it's about the heart?

M: I know exactly where this is going. You're going to try to negate my meditation practice. Bro, don't even go there. If I give up this one point of peace and sanity in my day, I'm going to end up in a loony bin. No joke. That's how bad things have become.

JB: I am not suggesting you give up your meditation practice. I am simply bringing another perspective to your process. After all, it is such a fine line between meditating to get here, and meditating to get out of here. Or, perhaps better worded, whether a spiritual practice is effective—both with respect to technique and intentionality—depends entirely on which 'here' we want to experience. Do you want to be here for some of it, or all of it? It would serve us to define our terms, and our intentions, with great care.

Fundamental to accessing wholeness in the body temple is the opening and healing of the heart. And, fundamental to accessing peace in your life—is the clearing and mending of your heart. Not only because our capacity to feel is inextricably linked to our capacity to be here—what I call 'enheartened presence'—but also because the opening and healing of the heart calms and subdues the mind. This is part of what I was trying to illustrate for you with the Excavation Meditation and some of the other exercises.

M: Hold on a second. You are saying that my monkey mind, with its endlessly persistent chatter, can be calmed by working with the emotional body itself? I think you're wrong... that little bugger is the cause of my chaotic emotions!

JB: The primary cause of our unhappiness is not our thoughts. The monkey mind is not the source of our anxiety. It's a symptom of it. Forget the monkey mind. The mind is not the enemy—unhealed pain is. Men have been blaming the mind for their neuroses for centuries, while deftly avoiding that which sources its maladies—somatic constrictions, and unprocessed emotions stored in the body itself. It's like losing your keys somewhere in the house, and looking for them in the car. Useless, useless, useless. Until they stop blaming the mind—and recognize that its neuroses stem from the unresolved emotional body—there will be no liberation. Shifting out of unhappiness is not a cerebral process—that's just another ineffective band-aid. It is a visceral full-body experience. It's the "monkey heart" that's the issue: the state of inner turbulence and agitation that emanates from an unclear heart. The more repressed your emotional body, the more repetitive your thoughts. Flooded with unhealed emotions and unexpressed truths, the monkey heart jumps from tree-top to tree-top, emoting without ground-ing, dancing in its confusion. Often misinterpreted as a monkey mind, the monkey heart is reflected in repetitive thinking, perpetual anxiety, and negative imaginings. All of which are emanating from the emotional body.

M: That sounds like me. So, what's the panacea?

JB: To calm and clarify your mind, you have to heal your heart.

M: Woah. And may I ask: How?

JB: It's a process. First, you have to be willing to face it heart-on. You have to have a rare form of courage, and a true sincerity. Key ingredients. When you are sincere, you can't go wrong. You will find what you are looking for. Your body's innate intelligence will bring up everything you need to see. As was demonstrated in our last meeting when we took a walk back into your past. Your body led the way—and did so brilliantly, with a precise intelligence that is unparalleled by your mind. As an added support, you can employ some valuable heartfulness practices: emotional release, armor-melters, heart-openers. Like the exercises we have been exploring. Healing the feeling stops the mind from reeling.

M: I believe in a different approach. It's witnessing the mind that is the antidote. I have spent these past years trying to calm the monkey by strengthening my capacity to witness him. No longer believing that the mind is "me." I am bigger and greater than my mind. And I affirm that, by witnessing it from afar, rather than being enmeshed in the thoughts themselves. It's not just about watching—it's about breaking the ties of self-identification with thoughts and feelings. That is fatal to the mind. I watch him, and I choose not to feed him the bananas ☺ of self-identification, and he appears to go quiet.

JB: "Appears" is the operative term. As is clear from your web of issues, the monkey hasn't actually gone anywhere. Again, the over-emphasis on the watcher is fundamental to the bypassing nature of patriarchal spirituality: to sidestep the originating material that is held within the emotional and physical bodies. It's very safe to blame the mind for many of our problems, but working within the mind to transform the mind seldom works. You witness, you watch the monkey... and if you are effective at that game, he then appears to go away. Because you are strengthening the witness-observer and dissipating the full-bodied experiencer. And if you continue to employ those practices day and night, you can get quite good at it. But it comes at a terrible price. Because you have left the world of feeling behind.

M: I can't argue… my monkey continues to return. Annoying little fucker.

JB: That's because witnessing doesn't really transform us on a core level. The monkey returns, often with a vengeance, and drives you crazy again. Because the true source of unrest is found a floor deeper on the human elevator: the heart. The mind is a reflection of the heart. The mind is not an enemy, it is merely a mirror of our inner state of being—which originates deeper than the mind. Peace begins and ends within the world of feeling. The heart of the matter.

M: The mind is a reflection of the heart, huh? I feel like you're way out on a limb here. Absolutely every practice I have ever engaged in has asserted the value of calming our mind. Every guru. Every spiritual teacher. And not just current day, but timeless wisdom from across the ages. For anyone interested in spiritual evolution, this is common knowledge. It's imperative to calm the mind. This is what allows us to access the heart. It's not the other way around. And the only way to do that is through meditation techniques, witnessing, dis-identifying with our thoughts. The mind MUST be tamed. It must be stilled. If not, it controls our life.

JB: I don't disagree with the idea that the mind has to be calmed. I am merely saying that much of its state of uproar is caused by, and ultimately must be resolved within, the emotional body, itself. Otherwise it is not true and profound change. It's not some disembodied talking head that's the issue. That voice you hear in your head is there for a reason. It's not bad. It's not the enemy. It doesn't need to be TAMED. It is simply a reflection of the inner rumblings of your heart. It's the somatic constrictions and unresolved emotional holdings from the past that are the issue.

M: Look, dude, I'm just looking for a little peace of mind.

JB: Say what you will, the witness is, as we discussed weeks ago, primarily a cerebral function. It's not taking you away from your mind—it's taking you deeper inside it. And our human lives are not about "thinking" God. They are about "feeling" God. My friend, author Ondrea Levine says it this way: "There is no such thing as peace of mind. All peace is from the heart." The top-down method is seldom effective with respect to transforming your thoughts. The more work we do to clear our emotional debris and open our heart, the calmer and more amenable the mind becomes. Try healing from the bottom-up.

M: But when I strengthen my watcher, I feel peace. I am breaking the binding cords of identification with my small 's' self. The rampant thoughts, the emotional wounds, are disempowered when I rise above them as the Observer. And claim my rightful place as the big 'S' self, not the small 's' self.

JB: I hear ya, Mr. Big 'S' Self.

Michael was now talking much faster, clearly agitated. I could sense what was happening. He was needing to take another step backwards, toward the familiar ways that he had organized reality for decades, before he could make the next leap forward. I knew to be patient with him, and let him ride it out. Three steps forward, two steps back, is still progress.

JB: The real litmus test is in your daily life. And from what you have been sharing with me, things are not peaceful and rosy. With your techniques, you may feel a momentary relief, a break from your persistent agitation—but it is not a sustainable peace. It is not a true and authentic resolution. If it was, you wouldn't have to keep at it so often, and your life would be more congruent. Not necessarily easy—but congruent. You wouldn't have to continue to deal with the same repetitive thinking patterns and thought cycles. With the same life-issues and quandaries blaring in your face. Have you noticed your mind becoming strong… or weaker? I suspect it's the former. That's because you are using one part of the mind, to calm down another. But that is not true healing. It strengthens your analytic capacity, while delaying your transformation. Excessive analysis perpetuates emotional paralysis.

Bottom line is that you cannot heal and resolve your emotional material with your mind. Knowing our issues is not the same as healing our issues. Your emotional material does not evaporate because you watch it. I have known many who could watch and name their patterns and issues—as if they were scientists, researching their own consciousness—but nothing fundamentally changed, because they refused to come back down into their bodies and move their feelings through to transformation. It's safe up there, above the fray, witnessing the heartache without actually engaging it. Yes, you may be able to get so skilled at a witnessing consciousness that you can overpower your triggers. But that's not presence. Real presence comes through the open heart. The key to the transformation of challenging patterns and wounds is to heal them from the inside out. Not to analyze them, not to watch them like an astronomer staring at a faraway planet through a telescope, but to jump right into the heart of them, encouraging their expression and release, stitching them into new possibilities with the thread of love. You want to live a holy life? Heal your heart. That's the best meditation of all.

M: It seems as though you have not experienced the transcendent delights of a profoundly meditative state. You are on a mission to bash meditation and meditative states. Maybe you need to meditate on why. Maybe you need to look in the mirror and see why YOU are the one with so much resistance to meditation. What are you avoiding? There is something you are afraid of, some reason you cling to the world so tightly.

JB: It's not resistance—it's experience. I was a hyper-meditator for some time. Been there, done that. Meditation can be a wonderful way to connect with our center. Yet what matters the most is your life when you leave the cushion. As human beings, are we truly designed to engage in various techniques and meditation practices on a daily basis, just to keep negativity at bay? Isn't there a day where we finally need to *awaken to the act of living*? Where our lives on the cushion become a seamless expression of our lives in the world. Where all of life becomes a living meditation.

M: But I love the blissful state meditation brings…

JB: Yes, but when your heart is open and unfettered, many of life's happenings propel you into a natural state of meditation. For example, falling in love. Not ungrounded, frenetic love, but the real kind, the kind that settles into your belly as a deep knowing. Or when you hear shocking news—for instance, a loved one has suddenly died. Or joyful news—your god-child was just born. Notice how you may naturally sit and become still, to absorb it. Your mind goes quiet, as waves of energy reverberate through your body. Your energy is pulled right down into your heart. You are meeting life directly. This is true meditation. Meditation-in-action. And do you notice… it doesn't really engage the mind? I call this "mind-not-full meditation." Life itself will give you endless opportunities to practice it.

M: Speaking of living life to the fullest, can we go get some ice cream?

JB: Pretty cold day for ice cream, don't you think?

M: Maybe, but I've been craving a banana split all week.

JB: With a cherry on top. Let's do it.

Somatic Psychotherapies

We walked up to Queen Street—the main Beaches thoroughfare—to get some comfort food for Michael. I understood—sometimes ice cream really is the perfect antidote for life's demands. When we arrived, he ordered both of us splits, and we sat down inside to indulge, and talk.

M: You sound an awful lot like Hannah. She also disses my loyalty to meditative and other spiritual practices. But I have found that feeding the shadow, only expands it. Why give so much energy to that which causes suffering? Why enliven that which is dead? Jeff, don't you know the basic law of the universe: what we feed—multiplies. What we give attention to—grows. This isn't even spiritual. This is nature. Feed a seedling water and sunlight, it grows into a flourishing tree. Feed a dark shadow your attention, your energy, your validation—it over-shadows your whole life. This isn't healthy. Sometimes we've got to rise above the filth and grime. Not stoop down and play in the dirt. Embody a higher state of awareness. It's our divine nature. It's our birthright. Claim it. Ever hear the biblical quote, "Do not cast your pearls before swine..." Bingo!

JB: First, with respect to Hannah, are you sure that it's meditation she disses? Perhaps it's the avoidant intention behind your particular practice. I'm sure she would have a different perspective if you directed the same devoted and focused energy into your relationship, rather than your meditation cushion.

M: Snap! Can't deny that.

JB: Secondly, with respect to not playing in the dirt. It's true, if we see our pain as parasitic, we will not want to feed the beast. But, I don't see it that way. I don't see a parasite. I see our tender woundedness. I see opportunity for growth. We should not be describing parts of our emotional life as though we are discussing a car part. As though there is a distinct entity called the pain-body, separate from who we are. It's not separate. It's part of us. And it's no less divine than our capacity for joy.

M: Do you have an example of how this healing-your-shit actually results in significant life change?

JB: I can give you an example from my own life. During one particularly difficult economic phase in my adult life, I became overwhelmingly triggered. I grew up in a poor family, and bear an active poverty consciousness wound. If I am doing well, I don't sense it. But if I am in a weak place, it begins to surface. At this time, money was very tight and my debt was dangerously high, and I was utterly overcome with anxiety. Once it reached the pinnacle of discomfort, I found myself dissociating in order to function. I began to spiritually bypass, telling myself that none of this mattered. After all, money was only an illusion created by a distorted world. Not the absolute truth. That sort of thing. I began to smoke pot to numb the pain. I found myself planning a move to a beach-hut in Bali, so I could start over. What I really needed to do was work more, to increase my income and clean up the debt. But I couldn't... I was utterly immobilized by the poverty consciousness material. And, naturally, the more I dissociated, the more impoverished I actually became. Not just financially, but in my dissociation I was divorcing myself from the wealth of inner resources that would enable me to confront the situation and overcome it. Floating down denial river was a self-fulfilling prophecy that magnetized precisely what I feared. Funny how that works.

Then there was a breaking point. It happened in the midst of the night... I suddenly woke up and shot directly over to my Bioenergetics breathing stool. I flung my body over the stool backwards, and stayed there considerably longer than I ever had before. Soon the early life poverty memories crept in... the too-many-to-count apartments we had moved to, my parents' endless scathing battles about money, the debt collectors banging on the door. It was all there, lingering inside my chest and lungs. And so were the feelings associated with those experiences. A whole wave of trauma-induced grief and sorrow longing to be felt. Once it reached a tipping point, I came off the stool and lay down on the bed and wept with a rare ferocity. And

I raged, allowing myself to fully express my anger at a world that kept so many of us buckled down. I continued to do it off and on all weekend—excavating my feelings over the stool, releasing them on the mattress. By the following week, something had shifted. I had the energy I needed to go back to work, and slowly begin to pull myself out of the hole I had dug for myself. And I have not been in that kind of a hole since.

Simply put, when the channels are obstructed, it is very difficult to meet your authentic self. And if you can't meet your authentic self, you can't meet reality. Because much of our energy is utilized suppressing our emotional holdings. Whether we realize it or not.

M: Jeff, again, I'm not talking about suppressing. I'm talking about rising above, while at the same time, seeing clearly. As we embody a higher level of awareness, we don't need to tamper with these things. They are child's play. No need to go delving back into the sandbox. Sometimes you just need to move on.

JB: You are right, at times it is appropriate to just move on. We naturally outgrow certain tendencies, and there's no need to fiddle with them. We really and legitimately leave them behind. I honor that. But, there still may be those dark snakes writhing in the within, that we haven't truly worked through. Unhealed traumas and stubborn patterns. Being aware of them is not adequate. Especially if they are very deep gashes. But it can happen at the same time: healing and awareness, as long as there is a working through the feelings... and not just a noting of the feelings. I think of it as the difference between watching the river flow and being the flowing river.

M: Okay, let me entertain your idea for a moment. I somewhat agree with you... there are nasty insidious sophisticated "snakes" of the ego—ready to strike. And yet, I feel the perfect panacea is through witnessing them. That way, we don't accidentally get infiltrated with their venom. Witnessing does acknowledge the knots. Yet it is safe. It doesn't *turn us into* what we see. It simply sees it clearly. Neutrally. While remaining a step above. Untouched. It doesn't work with it, fueling it with the energy of self-identification and belief. That only gives it more force and momentum. Until we can no longer tell the difference between "our stuff" and "who we truly are." Play with the knots—you get tangled up, too.

JB: I wish I could agree with you. I wish it could be that easy. But that is only skin-deep healing. It's like a good massage. You can be gently touched on the surface level of skin to evoke a warm and happy feeling. While right beneath, your muscles remain in knots. But go into the deep tissue massage, feel the knots release, and experience your body then. It will be a new body. The witnessing approach to emotional resolution is not ultimately effective. It can help us to see *some* things, to be sure, but it can also blind us to the deeper blockages—those that cannot be seen by the witnessing mind.

M: We just keep returning over and over to our fundamentally different lens on spirituality. I see spirituality as something distinct from this world and you see it within the grit and grime of this world. Come on, dude! Do you actually believe you are this bag of bones and entrails? Wake up! We are more than this: We are spiritual beings. Immaterial. Eternal. Heavenly. Divine. Wearing a human costume for a short time. Can I ask you a question? You are so good at doling out the "what if's..." Let me give you one back. What if, just WHAT IF, before you were born, your soul "signed a contract" so to speak... that you would take on a human body for a short time. But during that time, you would not forget your true essence. You would not become lost and tangled in the human experience, taking it to be real. You would live your temporary human life, while always remembering your divine nature. I have a feeling inside—a vague recollection, a gut instinct—that I made such a pact. What if you did, too? What if you are becoming over-identified with your human form? Maybe I'm actually here to remind YOU. ☺

JB: For you to be here to remind me, you'd have to actually be HERE. You're not. If you were, you would understand that your spirituality and your humanness are branches of the same tree. And you would understand that there is no distinction between waking up and growing up. The more you mature as a human-being, the more you mature spiritually. Stop pitting them against each other!

If someone were watching us go back and forth, they could easily conclude that we were completely at odds with each other, waving our hands in a heated argument, like two endearing old Italian men. But I knew better. Perhaps we had been in the beginning, but no longer. Although he was speaking his contrary views with great conviction, I could sense something else happening. Beneath the surface, he was

in the midst of an intense work-out: stretching, examining, picking up and put-
ting back down, massaging the material, to distill his truth. He was engaged in a
gritty process of discernment and reflection. In the quiet background, I could feel
a magical alchemy occurring. His customary defenses were fighting for their life,
while his deeper truths were forcing their way to the surface. He was in a process
of ready-making to surrender his mechanisms, and embrace his humanness. This
man was coming back to life.

JB: I would like to share more about one of the most significant humans in my life.

M: Let me guess. Alexander Lowen. Is he still alive by the way?

JB: How did you guess? Lowen died in 2008 at the ripe old age of 97. When I did therapy sessions with him, he was in his 80s and remarkably vibrant. At that time, he was still rigorously doing 300 mattress kicks every morning to clear his holdings and energize his body. Most alive and dynamic being I have ever encountered.

Lowen understood something very deeply. He knew that spirituality had to be embodied, if it was to mean anything at all. He developed a series of exercises that broke through those defenses, and that brought his students and clients back to life. Life-changing for me. This was accomplished not simply by exercising, but by inviting us to excavate the repressed memories, feelings, and sounds that were buried at an earlier time, in the body itself. Because if we don't open up those lines, we can't experience true internal alignment. And without that alignment, we can't be fully present.

In this way, Lowen was a true spiritual practitioner. I would even call him a Spiritual Pioneer. Same with many of the other visionary somatic psycho-therapists such as Bioenergetics Co-founder John Pierrakos, Wilhelm Reich, Peter Levine, Ilana Rubenfeld, Ron Kurtz et al., all bringing forth a new paradigm. Because they invite us to fully experience reality, warts and all. Because they had the courage to get right into the guts of the people they worked with. No soft touch approaches, no cosmic band-aids, no simplistic affirmations as substitutes for the real work. In my view, anyone who supports your efforts to come back into your "spirited" body, is a spiritual worker. Anyone who steers you away is not.

Most historical and popular modern spiritual teachers are bypassing the very material that must be deeply owned and worked through before sustainable transformation can happen. That's the great irony of their teachings. They call themselves spiritual teachers, but they turn us away from our selfhood, from our stories, from our encoded, embodied wisdom, so that we can only know reality in a limited way. They are the furthest thing from spiritual teachers. In the work of many body-centered psychotherapists, there is a deep understanding of the fact that one cannot be truly present for reality, if their physical and emotional bodies are tied up in knots. It takes the same courage and sturdiness to show up for your individual shadow as it does to show up for all elements of reality. And if you don't have the discipline to see your feelings through, you simply won't have the discipline required to be with all of what this is. In this way, I view somatic psychotherapists as our truest spiritual teachers, because they actually provide a more inclusive blueprint for awakening and integration.

As I finished speaking, Michael closed his eyes and went quiet. He appeared to be in deep contemplation. I went quiet too, waiting on him to signal when he was ready for more. After a few minutes, he spoke:

M: I was getting a visual as you spoke this. Of the prison cell you are sentencing me to, if I sink deeply into my pain-body. A chamber of perpetual suffering. And then I began to see myself floating up and away from it. Like literally. I saw myself rising up, and transcending the space altogether. It was like I was looking at my avoidance patterns straight on. And then, I saw myself doing something startlingly new. I chose to return back to the prison. I saw myself floating back down, and planting my feet on the cell floor. What happens after that... I have no idea.

JB: Very telling. You are clearly tired of confusing transcendence addiction with spiritual maturation. The real spiritual journey is not about leaving the body and entering into transcendence. It's about healing the heart and coming back to earth. I sense that you are coming to know this.

Speaking of moving the body, how about we get up and walk, Michael? I'm getting stiff, and want to work off some of that delicious banana split you bought me.

Conscious Armoring

We left the creamery, and made our way back to the beach. The chill in the air was like needles. We continued our walk along the boardwalk. The lake was roaring and wild today, churning tumultuously and mercilessly slapping the shore. Pigeons and seagulls canvassed the beach, looking for scraps of supper. Muddy grey clouds hung low. It all felt like the perfect reflection of Michael's conflicted inner world at this moment in time. He shuddered and wrapped his jacket tighter around him, shielding himself from the winds. Then he spoke strongly:

M: Jeff, the world is a harsh, cold place. You act like we are all built to feel everything, at all times. We aren't. For many, particularly the trauma survivors you often mention, that would be unbearable.

JB: I actually agree with you. In a still challenging world, emotional armor is no less valid than vulnerability. It is not easy to shed, nor should it be. It has formed for a reason: as a requirement for certain responsibilities, as a conditioned response to real circumstances, as a defense against unbearable feelings. It has served an essential purpose. It has saved lives. We need it, at times, to manage reality. Yet it can be softened over time. It can melt into the tenderest at its core. It can reveal the light at its source. The trick is to never demand it to drop its guard before its time and, at the same time, not to hold on to it for any longer than we need to.

M: Yes, but how does one determine when to drop the armor and open again?

JB: Experientially. Directly. Cultivating your intuition—that little voice of knowing inside. Reading your body's subtle cues. Learning how, and when, to shed your armor without putting yourself in harm's way. And learning when to put it back on again. I call this "conscious armoring." That is, you move away from the tendency to armor your consciousness as an automatic defense, and instead you make the process entirely conscious. You make armor a conscious function, not a knee-jerk reaction. So, for example, when you go into the marketplace to focus on your job, you put on the particular suit of armor needed to accomplish your goals. Or when you go to spend time with toxic family members, you armor up to the degree necessary. The key is that you also remember to take it back off at the end of the day, so that armor doesn't become an embedded way of being. In other words, you always remain connected to your vulnerable heart, and you armor up for a limited time and clearly defined purpose. And not a moment longer. All of this takes some experimentation, trial and error, to get it right. It's like learning a new language.

M: But we pay such a high price when we drop our armor altogether.

JB: We pay a much higher price when we don't. Think of crying... all that grief that gets repressed and locked into our bones, through various coping methods: the shallowing of breath, the physical armoring of places in the body where it is held, the stuffing down of our pain with food, with drugs, with heart-severed sex. You realized this directly in the exercise with your dad and Uncle. When you re-lived that experience, your body directly repeated those reactions, even though the stimuli were no longer present. After several decades, those reactions were still encoded in your cells. Yes, there is a time and place to release that material, but what often happens is that it gets perpetually buried, layered over with the next wave of unprocessed grief and disappointment, until we become energetically, emotionally, expressively immobilized. And, naturally, that held material—which has to show up somewhere if we aren't going to grant it the dignity of release—manifests in the forms of depression, physical illness, a diminished capacity to feel alive, and a limited ability to be fully present for reality.

M: You know that biblical quote: "Be in the world, not of it"...

JB: When did you become such a bible-thumper?

M: That quote is me. I will be physically here, but I won't truly dwell here. This world is in such a state of despair. The environment is decaying, we have infantile hotheads threatening nuclear war, violence and consumerism running rampant. If I did identify with this world, I would live my life locked up in my room with my head under the covers. That's why I choose to stay armored in my own way. And that's why I refuse to bring a child into this world. It's simply irresponsible.

JB: It's interesting you chose to bring up the subject of having a child while we are discussing armor. I am sensing an inter-connection. I have to ask: Could it be that you are over-armoring yourself, in closing off the possibility of having a child...? No pun intended, but, throwing the baby out with the bathwater.

M: No. This is a prime example of healthy conscious armoring, as you would say. The world is unraveling at the seams. It's selfish to bring a child here. There's just so much to be depressed about.

JB: No, Michael, there is not so much to be depressed about. There is much to FEEL. Depression is frozen feeling. Depression is what happens when we have blocked our emotional fluidity. You can be sad about it, but you don't need to be depressed. We have repressed so much material that we are no longer energetically mobile. The very reason you hurtle into depression, is because you have not allowed yourself to truly feel the pain of the world. Rise above, rise above, that is your approach. How about go deep down in the trenches, and FEEL it, Michael. Weep for the world. Feel the pain of your human brothers and sisters. Let it pierce you. Let it rip you open. What you find on the other side just may surprise you.

M: Ugh. I can't. I just can't. It's overwhelming.

JB: It's overwhelming at first, because there is an extreme build-up of unfelt pain. If you release it, new space will be created. A new vista will rise into view. We need to keep the river of feeling moving. Sadness and grief are a fluid and vital experience. You feel it deeply, you cry and cry, and then it lifts. And you come back to what I call a beginner's heart.

M: You mean beginner's mind?

JB: No, I mean beginner's heart... the freshness of appreciation that arises after we truly, madly, deeply feel and liberate our emotional holdings. You can only heal your heart with your heart. To do that we have to open the heart wide enough for its healing elixir to rain down on our pain. Why bury the tears that heal us? Why bury the emotions that fertilize our expansion? Emotional release is a potent way to regain a genuine experience of the moment. Tears are God's heartshield wipers. They clear the dirt from our heart so we can see the path clearly. Let our quest for spiritual expansion begin with emotional authenticity. Nothing to hide, nowhere to hide it.

After all, enlightenment is not a head trip—it's a heart trip, gusts of God blowing through the portal of the heart, the aortic love valve merging with the love that courses through the universal vein. If we want to expand our spiritual consciousness, we have to shake our heart tree often. Opening the heart unlocks the heart of the universe, and we see what is always before us. May we be committed to shedding the armor around our heart a little more with every breath.

Healthy Anger

M: That sounds like quite a weak and debilitated way to live. Nothing like the way my father conditioned me.

JB: And how did he condition you?

M: To face the world with a measure of solidity. To be strong and assured in the world. Not vulnerable and sensitive.

JB: I understand. That's the survivalistic world we come from. One where we need to bury our feelings to get by. But I am inviting you toward a different world, one that armors up only when necessary. One where you move authentically, from the heart outward. At the heart of our expansion is the capacity to be vulnerable again. Although the world rewards insensitivity with the prizes of war, it takes more guts to surrender than to numb. Better hurt than hardened. I am not talking about a weakened form of vulnerability… but one that is emblazoned with courage. I bow to those who keep their hearts open when it is most difficult, those who refuse to keep their armor on any longer than they have to, those who recognize the courage at the heart of vulnerability.

M: To be honest, highly sensitive people disturb me. Sensitive people end up being empaths, absorbing everyone else's pain… from the people sleeping on the streets, to children not properly cared for, to war-torn countries far across the oceans. I know this directly… I live with one. Fuck, I can barely manage my own pain. Yet alone opening up to the collective consciousness.

What an agonizing way to live. I'm not about to be yanked around by everyone else's emotions. That's not me—I'm not hyper-sensitive. I need to stand strong and firm, towering above the emotional cesspool.

JB: We're all sensitive, Michael. Some of us just hide it better. On my journey, I came to recognize that sensitivity isn't a sign of fragility. It's a sign of life. It's the quality that makes us most human. And this is not to say that there aren't unhealthy forms of sensitivity—there are. But it is to say that it is possible to be both deeply feeling, and solidly unyielding simultaneously. My life is one of sensitivity, but not fragility.

M: Sounds disempowered to me. I don't want to be that vulnerable, dude. I have to be able to function at my job. I have to meet all my responsibilities. The world will eat me alive.

JB: It's not disempowered, Michael. We are powerful beyond measure, and so deeply vulnerable at the same time. This may seem like a dichotomy, but it isn't. We have misunderstood real power. It has been seen as a force that is assertive, non-surrendering, pushing on through. This is not real power. This is simply willfulness. Real power is something else: receptivity, vulnerability, the courage to keep your heart open on the darkest of days, the strength to feel it all even when the odds are stacked against you. Real power is showing up with your heart on your sleeve and absolutely refusing to waste one moment of your life hidden behind edginess and armor. The art of enheartened presence. Now that's power.

M: Why bother to open the heart if it's gonna hurt so damn much?

JB: Because it is only through the open heart that we can feel truly alive to our path and in communion with life. And because we won't be able to perpetuate the species if we don't. With our hearts closed, we don't recognize our shared humanity. We don't care what we do to each other or the environment. We don't see what really matters. Everything real comes through the heart. When it is truly opened, everything secondary falls away—egoic glory, fame and fortune, substitute gratifications. The heart doesn't care about such things. It doesn't hold it against you if you don't own your own home, achieve your goals, have a perfect body. The heart doesn't care what you have earned or accumulated. No matter our seeming differences, we are all the same when the heart gate opens. Deep feeling levels the playing field. Deep feeling brings us back into connection with each other and the earth that houses us. In the end, it will be essential for our very survival. After all the malevolent warriors have destroyed each other, it's the open-hearted who will inherit the earth.

M: You sound like Hannah. So embroiled in the suffering of this world. If I allowed her, our house would be packed with orphaned children, puppies, kittens, and oh, let's throw in a few homeless people, too. It's just not practical, dude.

JB: Deep bows to Hannah. She sounds like a stunningly courageous woman. It was heartbreak that showed me the courage of the feminine. The gift of having your heart smashed open by love and its related disappointments is that you remember what it's like to feel everything again after days, years, lifetimes spent below armor. Through enheartened eyes, we see the courage it takes to stay in the feeling realm. We reward emotional armor because it allows us to 'succeed' in a survivalist world, when we should be honoring those who have the courage to remain emotionally receptive and open on the battlefields of life. It took me this long to realize that remaining heart-centered in this world is the greatest achievement of all. A lesson well worth learning.

M: Surely you don't feel this way about every form of human emotion. What about anger—the emotion that has caused untold suffering on this godforsaken planet? Anger isn't remotely spiritual. It is like a ticking time bomb waiting to unleash destruction. If I do meditate with one primary intention with respect to my emotions, it's probably to subdue my anger.

JB: How's that working out?

M: Intermittently effective.

JB: Good, then there's hope. At least you haven't been so effective at burying it that it remains entirely hidden from view, stewing and squirming its way into horrifying disease or, perhaps, the kind of outburst that does terrible harm one day. In truth, anger is no less spiritual than any other legitimate emotion. In a mad dash to react away from anger's perils, we went too far and lost a key piece of the emotional integrity and expression cycle. By discouraging and shaming its organic expression, we actually disrupt our natural emotional rhythms and encourage inauthentic ways of being. This is not to deny its perils, but we have forgotten its fiery wisdom, its contribution to positive change, its profoundly revealing and healing nature, its connection to a passionate life. Anger is a productive force that will get your ass moving to take care of business, and bring positive change into form. Here and now. And, anger is a legitimate emotion that signals that a person has been violated. Without it, we are only half alive.

M: I recall throwing the vase against the wall. That did feel relieving. Then it was followed by the sweetest lovemaking ever... Mmmm... I can just taste how Hannah's...

JB: Yes, I remember. Please enjoy that recollection privately. That occurred because anger is a river. It is no different than our tears. It wants to flow naturally. It wants to be released into the vaster ocean. When we repress it with premature forgiveness, block it with false positivity, repress it in the name of pseudo-peace, we just dam(n) our natural flow. The river then turns inward, against the self, or explodes outward, against innocents. Better we express it when it is in our awareness—not in a way that is destructive to humanity—but in a way that is authentic and that restores the integrity of our being. Anger isn't the enemy. Misplaced anger is. Let the river flow...

M: How does one express it in a way that isn't destructive? I can't break all the glassware in our home.

JB: The important thing is to honor its wisdom and meaning in ways that are appropriate and not physically threatening. This can certainly include healthy and direct communication of anger (verbal, written, legal, boundary assertion, among others), and can also include various methods of embodied release. The important thing is to be true to the emotions, without doing needless harm.

The first step is to do the work to unearth and dispel the old anger you are holding. Anger unexpressed creates a compound effect. Which then ultimately erupts in a dramatic or destructive manner. The key is to keep your anger healthily moving. Like a roaring fire, it blazes through your body, consumes all impurities, and actually leaves you cleansed and invigorated. Body-centered psychotherapies can help with this. They can show you how to open the body and bring the anger to the surface. They can also show you how to move the anger healthily. For example, many Bioenergetic and Core Energetics practitioners have a foam hitting cube, where clients can use a baseball bat, or their hands and feet to move their anger, without doing harm. I have one in my home office that I purchased when I was in the Bioenergetic training program years ago. It has served me well.

M: Ahh, yes, I recently watched your film *Karmageddon*. I know the hitting cube.

JB: That's it. My trustworthy ole cube. Best money I ever spent. It has proven to be quite an ally on my journey. It has helped me to release old stuff, which then makes any new forms of anger manageable and free-flowing. It's important to work in both dimensions—the past, and the present.

M: I always figured that if I spent that much time being angry, it would be like a tap that never turns off.

JB: It's the opposite. If you don't engage and release, it grows inside you like a virus. A toxic well that quietly seeps into your garden and destroys your roots. The negativity has gone subterranean, living itself out in a myriad of destructive forms, including passive aggressiveness, self-destructive behavior, and all manner of disorder. That's where these horrific mass shootings emerge from, it's compressed anger that has accumulated over time, finally erupting into rage, and unleashing destruction. Better to activate it, and move it sooner. Let me show you...

I stepped off the boardwalk and onto the beach. Michael followed. When I got to a clear patch of sand, I grabbed a small stick and drew a circle.

JB: Imagine yourself as this perfect circle. You are intact. Now, imagine yourself being violated by someone, or by something that happens to you. You become angry. You have a choice, you can express it, if possible, thereby preserving the integrity of your being. Your circle is still intact. With your anger expressed and resolved, you can experience the moment with genuine presence.

I marked a dent in the circle.

Or, you can bury it, and watch as it undermines the integrity of your being-ness. If there are too many dents in your beingness, it becomes very difficult to function healthily in your life. You end up hobbling through life as a dented circle. The only way to restore your integrity, is to push that dent back out. Not violently, unless self-defense is necessary, but assertively, expressively, with vigor. In other words, you own that you are angry, and you take action to release and express your rightful rage.

It's time we raised healthy anger back to the rafters of acceptability Michael, and work together to clarify a way of expressing it that both holds everyone safe AND allows us to honor its inherent wisdom. There is needless, regressive conflict, and there is healthy, necessary, forward-moving conflict. The distinction lies in our intentions. Anger is a sacred force when it is honored authentically, without needless destruction. In fact, I am certain that we will not create the world of divine possibility that many spiritual beings long for, unless we get angry about the injustices that many of us face. The world actually improves when people express legitimate anger, because it communicates a message that certain acts and occurrences are not acceptable. As we move toward a healthier collective vibration, appropriate anger shows us injustices that would not have even been noticed at earlier times. If we fully condemn healthy anger, we condemn ourselves to endure realities that don't serve us. There is a place for healthy anger in an evolving world.

M: Now I feel confused. You want me to be vulnerable, and to own my anger at the same time. That feels counter-intuitive.

JB: Not at all. You can't be in your vulnerability if you can't express your anger. Both because it clears the debris so you can open your heart again, and because we cannot touch into the deepest parts of our vulnerability without it. Until our inner child knows that we have the capacity to protect his tenderness with ferocity, he will not fully reveal it. She will only open so much, until she knows that we can hold her safe. This is one of the reasons why those who grew up unprotected as children will often keep their hearts closed. They weren't given a healthy template for self-protection. Sometimes we have to forge that template ourselves, in the fires of our own empowerment. The more sturdily we can touch into and express our rightful anger, the more comfortable we will feel embodying and expressing our vulnerability. The more powerful our roar, the more open our core.

M: Dude, you have an answer for everything. And right now, all I am feeling is tired. So very tired. Whatever is going on inside of me, is draining me big time. The world is feeling especially harsh right now. I feel like a baby who just emerged fresh from the womb, into a mad world.

JB: I understand. You have so much opening, processing, churning right now. It's an important time for you, Michael. Whether you realize it or not… you are re-entering the world of feeling. How about we stop the talking and just walk in silence?

M: Sounds like a plan.

We began to walk, this time without speaking a word. I noticed our footsteps were rhythmically in sync. We had come a long way in our recent meetings. It felt nourishing to be with Michael, a fellow path traveler. We had reached the point where we could be entirely comfortable together, in silence. When we reached the end of the boardwalk, he finally broke the silence.

M: You have another exercise for me?… Maybe something a little gentler?

JB: My instincts, exactly. Yes, I do. If you feel up to it this week, give this exercise a try. You are going through a tremendous amount of upheaval right now. Sending some love in your own direction might be the best thing you can do to support these transitions. It might feel a little hyper-sensitive, to use your word, but take my advice… and stick with it anyway. I actually recorded this exercise in audio format for one of my courses, and had a sense to bring you a copy today. Here's a CD—take a listen.

M: I'm at the end of my rope. I'll try anything.

He grabbed the CD out of my hand, and abruptly turned to leave, without even saying goodbye. And then, perhaps paying heed to his deeper feelings, he turned back around and gave me a quick man hug. And then, in the blink of an eye, he was gone.

I decided to stick around the Beaches for the rest of the day. This had been one of my hot-spots in my youth, to chase women, to attend jazz festivals, to rest on the sands. It had always been a place that brought me back to life. I felt sentimental as

I walked the boardwalk, and wandered the neighboring streets, reminiscing about days past. Just before sunset, I received a text from my wife Susan. She wanted to come down to meet me for dinner. How delightful. Moments later, an unexpected text from Michael:

> I just arrived home to a note from Hannah.
> She's had enough.
> She's gone to stay with her best friend.
> Most of her clothes are gone.
> I told you, I'm fucked.

I didn't feel surprised by the text. A pivotal time in Michael's life. No way he could hide, bypass, sidestep, or float beyond any longer. Fascinating, the intelligence of life, and how the Universe supports our return. Change was clearly afoot.

EXERCISE 5
"THANK YOU, I LOVE YOU": AN EXERCISE IN SELF-LOVE

We all have been wounded in the course of our lives: painful childhood experiences, challenging parents, an unkind environment. Sometimes our inner voice can be our harshest critic, carrying the imprint of our prior experiences. It is no easy thing to shift, but it can transform over time, particularly if we are determined in our efforts to solidify a new way of relating to ourselves. Such tender healing can happen when we change the voice of our inner self—from a critical tone to a tenor of kindness, tenderness, and love. This exercise will help you hold hands with your self again. I invite you to do it often, even if it feels uncomfortable, until it feels complete. You can do this exercise lying down, or looking at yourself in the mirror. You can be clothed or naked. You can also do it in the shower or bathtub. This exercise invites you to thoroughly touch your body, all of it. Touch yourself with as much presence as you can. Be slow and gentle with the process—don't rush. Be fully here for each part of this exercise, intimately experience your own contact, really hear and feel your words.

If you are not comfortable doing this in reality, try doing it as a meditation, getting into a relaxed state and imagining yourself going through the same steps. Or, if you don't feel prepared to imagine yourself expressing this magnitude of love to yourself just yet, imagine it being expressed to you by a loved one, or by a presence or guide. And remember that you can do this exercise as often as you want. Each time will be different. Be aware of what comes up in the experience. Be aware of any voices that attempt to undermine the message. Be aware of them, and do your best to continue.

Begin by using your right hand to touch your left hand. Touch it as lovingly as you can, with gentle strokes. Say out loud, "Thank you, I love you."

Now use your left hand to touch your right hand in the same way. Say out loud, "Thank you, I love you."

Now use one or both hands to stroke your head. Say out loud, "Thank you, I love you."

And touch your nose. Say out loud, "Thank you, I love you." Your eyes. What a marvel they are. Say out loud, "Thank you, I love you." Your ears. Say out loud, "Thank you, I love you."

Your face. Take time with your face, caressing it with great care, letting it know that its authenticity is valued. As you touch, imagine any masks melting away, revealing your vulnerable true face, beneath. Say out loud, "Thank you, I love you."

Now move your left hand over your right arm and shoulder. Say out loud, "Thank you, I love you."

Now move your right hand over your left arm and shoulder. Say out loud, "Thank you, I love you."

Now put both hands on your neck and your chest, caressing them with kindness. Place your hands over your lungs. Rest them there for a moment, feeling the breath of life rising and falling. Say out loud, "Thank you, I love you."

Now put one or both hands over your heart. Feel the pulse of life. Let yourself feel it speaking to you, let it remind you that you are here for a reason. Allow yourself to feel grateful for its gifts. Allow yourself to imagine the armor that protects it, melting. Say out loud, "Thank you, I love you." The heart loves to feel gratitude.

Now run one or both hands over your stomach and your internal organs. Again, take your time. Self-love has no time constraints. Feel into the magnificence of your human body—all the functions that happen outside of your conscious awareness, all the millions of ways the body regenerates and enlivens you, the countless ways it echoes your value. Really let yourself feel its love for you. Say out loud, "Thank you, I love you." Say it as many times as you need before you can really feel it.

Now move one or both hands down your legs. Caress your legs—they work hard and seldom get affection. Say out loud, "Thank you, I love you."

After touching your legs, let your hands gently wander into the sacred power center between them. Move one or both of your hands to gently caress your genitals. Experience the wonder of the magnificent energy center of creation. The transmitter of love. As you touch, let yourself open past any sense of shame—into pure wonder. Touch yourself with kindness, gratitude, and compassion. Say out loud, "Thank you, I love you."

Now move to your feet. Touch your toes. Rub your hands over the bottom of your feet. They so dependably carry precious cargo. Tickle them. Stroke the tops of your feet. Your ankles. Your shins. Massage the whole area. As you do, say out loud, "Thank you, I love you."

Now touch your buttocks, with affection. It's not easy to be sat on for hours per day. ☺ Give them some lovin'. Say out loud, "Thank you, I love you."

Reach up for your kidneys. Rub your hands over them. They are such hard workers. Let them feel your gratitude. Say out loud, "Thank you, I love you."

Now touch the small of your back. Massage and stroke it with gratitude and affection. Say out loud, "Thank you, I love you." Now rest your hands for a moment.

Now look in a mirror, or imagine yourself in your mind's eye. Look at your self before you: all of you, the you that God(dess) created, the you that came into being, the you that is breathed by the Universe, the you that is still here, the you that has overcome, the you that has found the faith to go on, the authentic you that lives below the world's disguises... And say aloud, "Thank you, I love you. Thank you, I love you. Thank you, I love you, Thank you..."

7 Enrealed Love Relationship

I didn't hear from Michael for two weeks. I began to feel concerned. The transition from the transcendence bypass back into the body can be a jolting fall from pseudo-grace. It can be quite a shock to suddenly come into contact with a whole web of unintegrated feelings and memories. It's similar to the re-entry trauma experienced when you come off a drug trip. We can hope that our defenses will contain and regulate the process, but it doesn't always work that way. Sometimes, it's a soulnami of epic proportions.

Very early one morning, I finally heard from Michael. We agreed to meet on Toronto Island bright and early the next day. He was waiting for me right when I got off the ferry, eager to share. We began to walk the Island.

M: Feels like two years since I saw you last. This was the most intense two weeks of my life.

JB: I had a feeling.

M: Hannah left, as I told you. And she wouldn't return my calls for days. Normally I stay pretty calm when there is a disagreement, but not this time. I went into severe panic mode. A whole ton of shit came up, including agonizing feelings of abandonment that taunted me each night. When I did finally fall asleep, I had excruciating nightmares about loss and peril. Being alone on a ship, lost at sea, smashing into waves in the pitch-black, with sharks surrounding me. It was hellish. Jeez, I didn't even know I had an abandonment wound.

JB: I suspect we all do. It runs deep in the collective psyche. What happened then?

M: The abandonment wound was only the tip of a whole gamut of feelings:

sorrow, anguish, anxiety, fight or flight reactions. I was completely defunct at my job, so I took a full week off. I don't think I left the house once. I couldn't cope. I was overcome with paranoia, possibly from the fatigue. And, I was calling my father and raging at him. Shit! Life has struck me in the bone marrow. All this stuff is churning and roaring up. I think I am having a nervous breakdown.

JB: As I mentioned before, it's a nervous break-through. Big difference. Michael, right now you are stuck between worlds. I want to reassure you that these feelings are actually cleaning you out, and carrying you to a more genuine life. But I know it doesn't feel like it when you are in the throes of it.

M: All I know is that I am completely unraveling, Jeff. My instinct is that if I don't figure out how to meet life in a real way, it will be the death of me. I can no longer just get by. I just don't know if I'm ready.

JB: The important thing, now, is that you allow the process to unfold as you can. You may be more ready than you think. If not, your psychological defenses wouldn't have allowed these doors to open. What you are going through is not uncommon. So many breakdown because they cannot carry the weight of falsity any longer. They are actually breaking through to a more authentic consciousness. It may feel crazy—but it actually is a life-saver. Sadly, this is often stigmatized as a 'breakdown,' as though they are machines that stopped working. We need to up-frame these experiences and see them for what they are: break-throughs for inner freedom. Pivotal points of our life. At some point, we just can't carry the bullshit anymore and long to be real. It becomes imperative to wake down. I believe that this is what is happening to you, Michael. This sounds like a turning point. With this new break-through—what does that mean for your relationship with Hannah?

M: She finally got back in touch with me this past week. We've been getting clearer on our issues. I have agreed to do sessions with a couples counselor Hannah has been wanting to see for a long time. Amazing what desperation can do. It's going to be a long road for us. Change is not going to happen overnight. But I'm willing to work at it more. I have no real idea how though. Wish there was a map for this stuff.

JB: Well, I actually have my own "map" per se, that I have developed over the decades. I would be happy to share it with you. It may be helpful. Can we spend some time exploring this concept of "true relationship"—and how it applies to you and Hannah.

M: Sounds like exactly what I need right now.

The Enrealed Love Relationship Map (ELRM)

Before we began, we decided to sit down across from the beach on Ward's Island. My favorite part of Toronto Island, a holistic-minded community with a fascinating collection of creativists, intellectuals and artists, all living in a unique, self-crafted patchwork of Hobbitlike cottages. It's kind of like visiting the Shire. You can expect to see Bilbo Baggins walking down the trail at any moment.

JB: Okay, in order to be of service to you, fill me in on the primary relationship issues, Michael. What feels most pressing right now?

M: There are a number of themes, Jeff—different ideas of a spiritual life, conflicting goals, certain ways of being that don't align, incompatible wounds and issues. They are all pressing, but the greatest challenge is the baby thing. It's imperative for her. She admits that she didn't take me seriously when I first told her that I didn't want to bring a child into this fucked-up world. She felt that our love would soften me over time. It hasn't. If anything, I probably became more definitive after we married.

JB: And now?

M: After this recent unraveling, I am coming to more fully admit that I have been hiding out in the so-called "higher realms" because I haven't wanted to feel the pain of the world. Witnessing an innocent child being subject to this harsh world would inevitably bring me right down here, in the grit and grime, to truly feel again. And to tell you the truth, I have been scared shitless of that. These past days when I had my breakdown—or break-through, as you call it—I had to *feel* my way through it. There was no other choice. It was feel the pain, or go over the edge. And after I began to feel again—I realized it wasn't as bad as I thought. It was horrible, and it fucking bloody hurt. Yet at the same time, it was strangely liberating.

JB: You look different, Michael. It's like—I can see more of you.

M: But I'm not through the layers of my resistance. Not even close. After I touched into that pain, another layer of steel emerged.

JB: That's good. Don't look at it as a setback. It's progress. That is often the case with growth—we work through one layer… and that invites the next layer to open up. You know, like those ever-blossoming Zen lotus flowers. So, tell me about the next layer.

M: What compels me to resist the idea now, is that I feel like having a baby is the greatest attachment of all… and I am someone who finds his peace beyond attachment. So first it seems I was afraid of feeling the pain of the world. And, now, it seems I am afraid to feel *love* within this world. Hannah has no issue with this, she finds her peace, and her purpose, inside of attachments. We have conflicted purposes, it seems.

JB: That's very insightful. Being in the dark these weeks has actually brought you more into the light. Now putting thoughts of a child aside for the moment… tell me more about Hannah, and your relationship with her… in terms of this love and attachment. Is it safe to say you are not deeply attached to Hannah?

M: I do love Hannah. But I struggle with attachment and with feeling engulfed. I am protecting something that I hold precious: my individual path and practice. I feel that her yearning for a fully merged connection will require that I lose my self altogether. Her love is like a raging fire… it will consume me. So I cling even tighter to my path, even if some part of me does long to be more relational. I don't want to lose her, but truth be told, I have no idea how one would have their cake and eat it too? How does one hold to their individual practice, and, also sustain a co-created practice?

JB: By making no distinction between them. Allowing them to co-exist and simultaneously flow into each other. You no longer see one as a place to hide from the other. They become spokes of the same wheel. The wheel of life.

M: Sounds terrifying.

JB: I am curious as to how your sexual relationship plays itself out with respect to attachment. You mentioned earlier that it had been stagnant for some time. What about before that, in the earlier years?

M: I've been happy with it, but Hannah often complained after we got married. She wasn't satisfied. I can hear her voice in my head, reciting her many demands: "I want more eye contact. Look deeply into me. Let's play and have fun, babe. Let's explore new techniques…" Blah blah blah.

JB: You lucky guy.

M: She didn't feel truly met, or seen. She often said that I made love like I did mantras—controlled, repetitive focus. She doesn't realize what it's like to be a man… and the intense focus and discipline it takes not to leak my seed.

JB: And why would that be a priority for you?

M: You know, it's the tantric way. It's as if Hannah wants me to bring my cock and my heart together and get consumed by our connection. But that's not how I do anything. My sexuality is framed by my spiritual practice. I contain my energies so I can use them for the evolution of consciousness. All of the greatest tantra teachers purport that ejaculation drains your energy and weakens your practice. I see sex as a vehicle into higher levels of awareness. Not as a tunnel into our dense humanity.

JB: That doesn't sound like a whole lot of fun.

M: Not entirely true. When I can get into the zone, I feel as though I touch the Divine. I am having a mystical, ecstatic experience.

JB: It's interesting to me that you don't say "we touch the Divine." Only you.

M: Yes, that is true. I am beginning to see it now. I have been directing the energy of sexuality, in the same way I have used meditation and chanting. Not to come deeper into connection with the world, but to leave it.

JB: Yup. Another way that you became an expert at 'mastery-bation.' Particularly appropriate term if you are essentially in your own world while making love with Hannah. Don't you find mastery-bation to be a little ungratifying? Solo and isolated, devoid of the magical alchemy of inter-relational mingling. The tendency to confine your awareness to mastering a very limited individualized path, to the exclusion of all else. Michael, has it ever occurred to you that you might have a more mystical experience in the merging than you will ever have in your isolation? Haven't you ever experienced the moist folds of the yoni as your path home?

M: Honestly, I haven't.

JB: I am fairly certain that we are not just here together to keep each other company. We are here together, to show each other God. The portal is each other. In other words, our experience of the mystical realms is often far more depthful and inclusive if we ride the energy of love connection into the great unknown.

M: Yikes. I'm terrified to dive in.

JB: To not dip into that pool, is to both deny yourself the benefits of some-thing very real and to hold your marriage back.

M: I don't see it as being held back. I feel that Hannah has unrealistic expectations. I'm a solo traveler. She knew that when she got into this. I don't want to go too far into attachment, into the complexity of human relatedness. I will lose my connection to my core. Isn't it safe to say that some people's purpose in this life is more individualistic than relational? To each their path, no?

JB: Yes, to each their path. You always have the right to choose your path, but Hannah also has the right to challenge your resistance to intimacy, particularly in the context of a marriage.

M: Yes, she does. But I do feel there is value in the relationship. I just can't seem to give her what she wants. If it was just one issue, for example, working on the shadow stuff that comes up between us—that would be manageable. But when you add in the baby conflict, it takes me over the edge and I feel like running away. It's interesting that she took off, given that I was often the one with an urge to flee.

JB: I can relate. I was often a runner in relationship. I ran for all kinds of reasons. Sometimes it was a healthy flight: I wasn't ready to love, I had other priorities, I had preparation work to do before I could deeply connect. But sometimes I ran for unhealthy reasons—I imagined every woman my difficult mother, I associated family with trauma from my early life, I assumed love meant imprisonment. Distinguishing between healthy and unhealthy motivations took me many years, but it may have been the most important clarification work I did on my life's journey. Because if our flight from connection is motivated by our unresolved life history, our defenses can convince us to run for the rest of our lives. And then we lose the opportunity to taste a different reality, one that meets our needs and heals our hearts. It's worth examining: Am I running to something better, or am I running away from something unresolved? Am I retreating to heal, or am I simply delaying my liberation?

M: Good questions. I suspect that my resistance, which is a form of running away, is delaying my liberation. But when it comes to having a child, I honestly don't believe I can handle the triggers that would arise in two primary connections in my life. I am just beginning to heal my own stuff. Hannah and I already have a lot of pain rising up between us. We have so much to work through. I don't feel I can handle another being, especially one I feel forever responsible for. One is enough.

JB: I hear you, but still, you have not left the connection. Why is that?

M: Despite the way this all sounds, there is a lot of light in the connection. When we came together—there was an unmistakable knowing… it was undeniable. There was this fierce magnetism—as if two cosmic forces propelled us together, to land in this time and space. My knowing to be with Hannah was one of the few guiding lights of my life. Should I just throw it away?

JB: Well, divorce is an option, my friend.

M: Woah, wait a minute. How did we go from discussing my relational challenges to divorce in 30 minutes? I didn't say anything about divorce. I was just laying down my perspective, I didn't say that there wasn't room to grow. I have been making progress.

JB: I'm a little surprised by how you are reacting, Michael. Your ideologies and your feelings aren't lining up. Help me to understand… where is your desire to keep the connection alive coming from? The benefits it is bringing you on your individual path, or some deeper sense that the two of you have a specific destiny or purpose together. Isn't it possible that both can be true?

M: Perhaps. It seems challenging to hold and maintain both—the individual path and the co-creative. I just don't know.

JB: In fairness to you, few do. Few of us know how to hold love safe. Few of us are trained in the art of love. The entire world has been organized around masks and defenses. Adaptation and disguise are our specialty. It's all we can do to manage our individual material. But love is a different world—an unmasked, surrendered, naked landscape that few of us have explored with any great depth. It's complex, co-creational terrain that challenges us at every turn. Even the spiritual community has neglected it. Millions of books and scriptures have been written about the individual path to God, and so very few about the relational path. As a result, it's very easy for most of us to articulate concepts, but to *hearticulate* feelings is another planet altogether. We are only at the beginning of the enheartened way. We haven't yet downloaded the ways of the heart. There is so much left to learn.

M: I feel a sense of relief when you acknowledge this. Probably because of my male ego, or in your philosophy, the unhealthy aspects of my ego, I have always felt a little triggered by Hannah's more evolved understanding of feelings and emotions. I don't like feeling so inferior.

JB: The dark side of the male mastery thing?

M: Yes, that, and also my relationship with my own father as a child… he was so impatient with me when I wasn't immediately good at something, so I developed the tendency to perfect things on my own, before sharing my interest with him.

JB: This feels connected to your reluctance to explore new pathways with Hannah until you have first mastery-bated them. ☺ Now you're getting somewhere. So how about I hearticulate a lens and perspective that paints a vision of possibility for a love relationship. I call it ELRM: Enrealed Love Relationship Map. It's the map of the journey from soulmates, to solemates, to wholemates. One that meets in all places. Let me know how it lands in you.

M: This past week kicked my ass. So maybe it's time I just sit back and listen. Go ahead, my friend. I'm all ears. I'll try to save my rebuttals for the end.

Relational Element 1: The Triad of Co-creation

JB: The map has a series of core elements. The first element I refer to as the "Triad of Co-creation." An enrealed love relationship honors the three entities at the heart of each connection: the individual world of each participant, and the world that they co-create together. So, in this dynamic, you would each honor one another's paths—your individual practices, needs, interests, and purposes. And, at the same time, you would value and prioritize your co-creative path together. So, you would not have to worry about losing yourself to an engulfing relationship, because both of you would be holding your individual paths and practices safe. Each of you would regard the other's unique and autonomous path as sacred, and treat it with great devotion. In this way, there would be very little chance for the dynamic to enter co-dependent terrain.

At the same time, you would both make a heartfelt commitment to honoring the third branch of the relational tree: the dynamic force that you become together. In other words, you don't merely love each other as separate entities, you love, honor, and cherish what you co-create. It's as if your relationship becomes a living breathing beingness all its own. You see it as a grand co-creation, a piece of shared art that you are working on together, one that morphs and changes form as your connection deepens. One that beautifully reflects the experiences and lessons you have actualized together. "Wow, I'm beautiful." "Wow, you're beautiful." "Wow, we're beautiful." Because, when it's just the love you honor, there is a way in which you are still in two different worlds. You love her, she loves you, but what stands between you? What of the bridge between your hearts? What also of the world you bring forth together? A grounded, conscious relationship is also about the third element—the alchemical combination of two souls merging, the living breathing world that you co-create in love's cosmic kiln. It's the difference between loving and *serving* love. It's the difference between the narcissistic quest for ecstasy and the joys of deep devotion. You serve the self, the other, and the wondrous universe you create and cultivate together. You serve loving. You are a devotee to the dance. The conscious-nest is a world unto itself.

And, perhaps, in the deeper recesses of the mystery, there is the possibility: Could it be this symbiosis that actually transforms the universe, itself? Perhaps the more humans push forward co-creatively, the more we mobilize Consciousness itself to expand further in scope. To weave new galaxies, each more vivid and expansive than the last. We work in tandem with the Divine. Co-creators in evolution.

M: Wow. This is high level material, dude. Entirely different from the way we have been taught to view relationship.

JB: Yes, that's not how we were conditioned. Historically, it's been about letting go of the self and loving another. This has been the great measurer of relationship: simply how much you loved each other. But, there was still a way in which we were lost in the individualized self. We were missing the most profound out-spilling of love: the new world that is birthed at the point of merger between two souls. That world is remarkably different from one that you see through your eyes alone. It is a world unto itself. A new galaxy to behold. And it must be acknowledged, honored, and cultivated if a love relationship is going to sustain itself and continue to evolve. This three-pronged perspective is an essential girder in any evolving and enrealed sacred love relationship. In my imaginings, I envision two trees side by side, separate but interwoven at the roots, always connected at the roots. Two human beings sitting side by side, hearing the raindrops beating on the temple roof, feeling the presence of the other everywhere. Grateful and gracious, jointly whispering, "I love you, I love we."

M: I need to interrupt. I have something surprising to say: what you speak is actually resonating for me. It's strange and foreign and unfamiliar. And yet, these are the words I have been longing to hear. You are saying that I CAN fully and completely be given to my own life purpose, my own path. And, *at the same time*, honor the bridge that is my connection to Hannah. One is not to the exclusion of the other.

JB: Exactly. Quite the opposite in fact. Each propels the other to new heights and depths.

M: I have had a long-time fear that me and Hannah's roots will become so entwined, I can no longer differentiate where I begin and where she ends. I've been scared shitless that if I truly open my heart wide and surrender to her, I will become imprisoned in her world. For instance, the sheer force of her obsession with having a child will swallow me whole. And I will find myself becoming a dad, not because I consciously chose it. Not because it's truly my path. But simply because I've been consumed by the relationship. I'm afraid of that. I don't feel that's my destiny. That's why I cling hard to my independence, to my individual path and practice.

JB: I hear you. I too had to learn to navigate this tricky area of interwoven-yet-independent-relationship. I have found: Real closeness is not hiding co-dependently in another's presence. Real closeness is not getting so lost in another that you no longer exist as a separate entity. Real closeness is two sovereign beings far enough back from each other to see a separate other, yet close enough to bridge their hearts. Two interconnected soulitudes. When you reconnect at the end of a long day, it's the perfect balance—a fusion of two sovereign entities, intermingling your distinct universes, to form one brilliantly new co-created universe.

Relational Element 2: Meeting of the Souls

As though divinely timed, a pair of swans soared overhead, and landed right in front of us, on the edge of the lake. They began to float harmoniously in unison. Michael seldom acknowledged occurrences around us, but this time he lit up, spontaneously uttering under his breath, "Ahh. Synchronicity." I gave him a few moments to ponder the significance.

JB: The second element of an enrealed love relationship is "Meeting of the Souls: Authentic Soulmating."

M: Like those swans over there…

JB: Yes, and as they clearly demonstrated: It's one thing for a couple to sketch their legacy in the sky, riding high on the wings of a new love—but quite another to carve their legacy on the earth, where they stand a much better chance of developing together. To accomplish this, the couple is dedicated to cultivating those practices, perspectives, and rituals that invite them to break through their blockages and blind spots, connecting them from the depth and breadth of their being. To ground their connection in their authenticity, and to open the portal to a more expansive consciousness. This can take many traditionally spiritual forms: soul-gazing, tantra, conscious sexuality, dance. What is most important is that it takes a form that is attuned to the couple, whether this means utilizing traditional templates, or co-creating some of their own. Whatever it is that takes a couple deeper, and ensures that they can shed their energetic armor, seeing through the veils and recognizing the bridge to each other's vulnerably essential nature. So, one of you might say, "Let's schedule some unmasking time this weekend. I miss your soul."

M: Hannah would eat that right up.

JB: As she should. In a world that is predicated on adaptations and disguises, conscious unmasking processes are essential so that the lovers don't lose sight of each other and the love that sources their union. And because it is damn near impossible to meaningfully grow the connection if either lover is not seen in their authenticity.

Intrinsic to this meeting is an ongoing commitment to shed any and all agendas that either person has around how the other should live, how they should love, how they should manifest or walk their path, or who they are. Because those agendas take the connection out of reality, and into a fantastical, or conditional, landscape. Real Intimacy is *in-to-me-see*. It is a meeting between two souls, an invitation to truly see with open eyes, without expectation or agenda. To hold one another in a safe space of neutrality—without judgment or personal bias. To keep out your own preferences, baggage, hopes, dreams and filters—and simply behold the other, in their raw and naked form. It doesn't demand gifts and benefits, sexual prowess, conditional offerings. It merely asks you to show up as you are, fully revealed and present. It invites you to shed any pretenses, and to drop into whatever is authentic for you in that moment. Real intimacy meets you where you live, not where anyone else wants you to live. It's the big sigh of relief that arises when you finally know that you don't have to put on a show to feel accepted. Here we are, just as we are. Hello. Welcome home.

M: Mmmm. I'm in my 42nd year. And I'm not sure I have experienced this before. It feels like time.

JB: This kind of holding is the cornerstone of a matured and grounded spiritual relationship. When we are young, it's the illusion of perfection that we fall in love with. As we age, it's the humanness that we fall in love with—the poignant stories of overcoming, the depthful vulnerability of aging, the struggles that grew us in karmic stature, the way a soul shaped itself to accommodate its circumstances. With less energy to hold up our armor, we are revealed… and in the revealing, we call out to each other's hearts. Where before wounds turned us off, they are now revealed as proof that God exists. Where we once saw imperfect scars, we now see evidence of a life fully lived.

M: I wonder if Hannah and I will sustain a lifetime of love, until we are old and wrinkled.

JB: The key is to cultivate a space where you can continue to see into each other's essence and to be replenished by each other's divinity. For myself, the one key ingredient I have found that sustains my love is a genuine fascination with my partner's inner world, with the way she organizes reality, with the unfathomable mysteries of her essence. To hear her soul cry out to me again and again, and to never lose interest in what it is trying to convey. If there is that, then there will still be love when the body falls apart, when the perfection projection is shattered, when the sexual charge dissipates. If there is that, you will swim in love's waters until the very last breath.

Relational Element 3: Solemating

JB: The third element is the grounding balance to the Meeting of the Souls: Solemating. "Solemates" is the embodied, grounded counterpart of soulmates. The other side of the coin; the yang nested within the yin. Often forgotten by couples who are riding the skyways of ecstatic love, solemating enreals the connection and ensures that the love can deepen and sustain itself in the world. It is the marriage between sky and earth, the transcendent and the immanent, the subtle and gross realms, essence and pragmatism. It's the steps that a couple take to bridge their timeless soul-deep connection to their everyday life in human form. Not just to prevent it from crashing down to earth, but also to ensure that the connection finds its way into the fertile soil of human existence. When a connection is restricted to a vertical trajectory, it can't even begin to glimpse the fertile possibilities that arise when it also moves downward, celebrating and exploring the self and its connection to earthly matters, spreading its tentacles deeper and wider into the world. Enrealed Love Relationships are a sole-to-soul proposition.

M: You keep talking about landing a soul-deep connection on earth. It all sounds nice… but following your purported principles, what does this actually mean in daily life? What does it look like? Tell me.

JB: Essential question. So, in practical terms, solemates make no distinction between their spiritual and earthly lives. They recognize that their connection doesn't just have a place in the cosmic and divine realms, but also has a perfect place down here and now, in human existence. With that in mind, they put a strong emphasis on integrating their relationship into everyday life, ensuring its rootedness and sustainability. Instead of looking for their love in the heavens, they search for it down here. They participate in society, not to the extent that they abandon their uniqueness and morph into homogeneity, but in a way that keeps their timeless relational energy grounded in the flow of time. And as they solidify as solemates, they are better able to impact this earth plane, touching and affecting humanity. They cultivate a genuine integration with the real world—staying on top of chores and obligations, remaining reliably connected to emotionally significant friends and family, leaving their love bubble and spending real time in the culture at large. They prioritize financial responsibility and societal structure building. They don't camouflage the state of the world with positive affirmations—they are both citizens of the beyond, and citizens of the here and now. They stay aware of politics and policies. They vote, they educate themselves, they tune into their media of choice. They have regard for each other's earthly skills and achievements. They celebrate the courage it takes to deal with the world. They don't hide away in the face of challenges and difficulties, but enter into the heart of the fire like love-warriors. This is not to say that the relationship does not prioritize ecstatic moments, or reaching a stage of profound grace, but both partners remain rooted, real and healthily boundaried, so that there is a sustainable foundation for those subtleties and delights.

M: Gosh, I'm not even that much in the world myself…

JB: Solemating also has a psycho-physical quality to it. Recognizing how easy it is to dissociate from life's challenges, solemates make sure to maintain a disciplined embodiment practice to keep them here on earth, planted in their bodies. Perhaps they practice yoga, Feldenkrais, dance, martial arts, or Holotropic Breathwork on a regular basis. Or perhaps they cycle, swim, kickbox, hike nature trails, or do archery. Or they co-create their own embodiment modality. Whatever they do, they remain heartfully connected to an experience of the body as sacred vessel. They don't just work the body. They live the body. Any work is done with reverence for its divine humanness, and for its role as temple of the soul-self. They engage it with feeling, cultivating it as an instrument of acute sensitivity. This emphasis on grounding one's consciousness within the body is particularly necessary for those individuals that are most at risk of floating out of their physical forms in search of bliss and ecstasy. Some connections have a strong energetic tendency to float into formlessness. It is essential that they recognize this and prioritize embodiment to ensure that they remain in wholesome balance. They must make a conscious intention to bring their formlessness into formfulness. Enrealed love connections develop a keen sense for when they are losing contact with material life, and strive to strengthen the cords. The more freely they fly, the more deeply they ground.

One of the benefits of engaging in embodiment practices together is that it tests the connection. Does it have the ingredients to become an enrealed relationship—encompassing the full range of the human experience—not just the heights? Or, perhaps it's designed to be a fleeting carrier of soul-lessons, but is not meant to take a walk through time. This is only revealed through taking it down from the heights of love, and into the nitty-gritty of daily life.

Because ecstasy and love are not the same thing. We often get them confused. There are some connections that open us so wide that we cannot help but call them love. But they may not be. They may just be a transcend-dance, an invitation to delight, the heart opening that we so desperately needed after years encased in armor. We call certain people into our lives to awaken us, to reheart us… but that doesn't mean they are the beloved. That doesn't mean we can remain together for a lifetime. Love is far more than floating to the heavens on a dreamy magic carpet. Love is sustainable. Love is inclusive. Love has feet that walk it through time.

M: Yah, but I do looooove the floaty kind of love. That was Hannah and I during the early phases. The ecstasy and bliss were delicious.

JB: Who doesn't? We all do. Only difference is, some of us want something else, too. If all you want is a loveship, shared essence will serve you well. You can meet in the mystic, in the soul-gaze, in the cosmic kiln of mutual divinity. You can ride a twin-flamed magic carpet into eternity, or until it crash lands in denial river, whichever comes first. But if you want a *real*ationship, if you want something that deepens and sustains itself over time, something else is required. *Real*ationships cannot ride on essence alone. They need earth to ground them. They need soul to soil. They need humanness to harvest. They need essence to hoe. Lasting love is not just a question of cosmic chemistry. That's the easy part. *Real*ationships are a soul to sole proposition. We land our loveships on Mama Earth, and begin bridging our purest intentions with our messy humanness.

And I have some advice for you, Michael. The eyes are a mirror of the soul… but so is the sole, reflecting one's capacity for sustainable presence. It's easy to stare into someone's eyes and fool yourself and them into believing that your love is true, but the greatest test is how we actually live and love—on earth, with our feet on the ground. If you want to gauge how sustainable your love connection to another will be, check out the way they walk on the planet. If you really want to know someone, start by looking at their feet. How do they move about? How fully do they make contact with Mother Earth? Are they light and lithe, dancing through life like a flitting fairy; or heavy-stepped, seeped in this world. How grounded is their spiritual life? Do they come crashing back to earth when the truth hits the fan? How present are they for the whole of the human experience? What is the inner-face between their earthly and Godly lives? Are they integrated, or are they positioned as two different realms, one more credible than the other? If they come crashing back to earth when reality comes a calling, you know you will have a problem when the ecstatic phase wanes and the next layer of truth arises.

M: Hmmm. I'm certain Hannah has both her feet on the ground. I love her feet, by the way, so sexy. But, me, I'm not so sure. How do I know if I'm ready for this? We both know my history of flying.

JB: Fundamental to enrealing a relationship, is the prioritization of shadow work. Which you have been slowly delving into. That is, a determined and consistent willingness to work with the relationship to acknowledge and heal the pain each partner carries, to move the feelings through to completion, to identify the issues and patterns that shape our individual and relational lives. In the survivalist world we come from, married couples were conditioned to stay away from the deeper issues that plagued their connection. In the more authentic world we are now moving toward, these mechanisms are no longer effective, and we are called to a more genuine reckoning. We are called to invite the material to the surface and to work with it deeply, both healing ourselves and, ultimately, the collective. Whether it's because the structures of society are evolving to support it, or because we have matured individually to the point of readiness, we are more open to the possibility that love connection—in both its light and its shadow—is intended as a vehicle for transformation and divine interfacing.

Solemates aren't interested in a rarefied connection. They are interested in a realified connection. They are interested in cultivating a connection that cuts a swath through all manner of authentic terrain, not only the pleasant, bliss-filled landscapes, and not only the mired, murky swampland of endless triggers. Everything, everywhere, is their terrain. They don't see their psychological issues as unreal, in contrast to their ecstatic experience—they see *all* of it as real. They are committed to finding the love everywhere they can, going deeper and higher into the regions of the heart. They don't only pray to their union when it tastes sweet. They also pray to it when it tastes bitter, because they recognize that it has the capacity to grow them to the next level of awareness. Peeling away layers, ever-deepening. Sacred compost, *Holy* shit.

M: Holy shit, indeed.

JB: In their commitment to healing and deepening their emotional body through the connection, solemates come to understand something very deeply: The brighter the love, the darker the shadow. They no longer see the triggers and reactivities as an indication that they were wrong about each other—they see them as evidence that there is work to be done to bring all of their aspects into alignment with their love. They see the shadow material as the grist for their individual and relational expansion. And, of course, it's not just previous pains and traumas that threaten to undermine the connection. We also come into contact with dysfunctional ways of being: defensive patterns, relationship-avoidant issues, reactivities and game-playing, that we have adaptively developed in response to embedded pain and trauma. And not just our own. When we open the door to great love, we also open the floodgates to collective and ancestral wounding as well.

M: Again, holy shit. This is a big responsibility.

JB: If real love reveals anything, it is that finding your solemate does not mean finding perpetual bliss. If it does, then it is love flying at half-mast. If a love is that deep, it is a portal to the everything, shredding through the adaptations and disguises that disconnect us from reality, unearthing shadow and light from their hiding places. The glory and the gory rise in unison, calling us to the earth and the sky in one fell swoop. This is in the nature of genuine intimacy—the more we open the heart, the more fervently we open the gateway to the pain we have known in this lifetime, and perhaps, in other lifetimes. The more we have to lose, the more fiercely we remember the ways we have lost before.

And then we recognize that we have a choice. We can pretend none of it is real—as ungrounded spiritualists will often do in their seemingly heightened love relationships—and watch as the connection implodes on itself, leaving a pile of charred smoking embers, or we can end the connection as soon as the truth hits the fan. Or, there is another choice: We can actually invite the material more fully into our consciousness, working with it individually and co-creatively as the fodder for bringing forth an ever-deepening relationship. Solemates invariably make the latter choice, walking on fire if necessary, to bring the connection through to the other side. They only choose to end their connection if depthful exploration reveals that it will no longer serve their individual growth, or their co-creative bond. They do not take this or any other significant step lightly, both because they are grounded enough to know that any unconfronted material will invariably need to be attended to in their next relationship, and because they recognize that what seems impossible at one moment, can become beautifully possible in the next, as the underlying layers of stubborn material heal and soften in the warming fires of their devotion.

M: This is a lot to take in… but continue on… I'm transfixed. I feel I'm a child being read a bedtime story. Dad used to love to read me stories in my early years.

JB: Very nice visual, healing… So, more about solemates. Solemates have come into the maturity to recognize that we are all part of a collective. Intrinsic to the shadow work, is a recognition of the sociological context we are embedded in. In a world that has just begun to cross over from survivalist relationships to those rooted in authenticity, solemates that take on the brave task of confronting the unhealed material, understand that they are not just confronting their own unresolveds, but that of the collective as well. Generation after generation that didn't have an opportunity to confront the baggage that they carried through life with them. That's a lot of dynamite going off at once!

I think of the alcohol and drug addicted, alone in a dark room, trying to push down their feelings because they were not provided with other effective tools to deal with their pain. I think of all the individuals, often women but not only women, who longed for a deeper level of emotional intimacy in their marriages but who had no idea how to cultivate it, nor to inspire it in their partners. I think of my grandparents, mired in their patterns of relatedness, who stuck together through thick and thin, but never had an opportunity to take the connection deeper. Those who open the door to this material, are some of the first to ever do so on this planet. They are the vanguards of a new way of being. This is a task of great magnitude, and they must be gentle with themselves, and patient as they work through the layers. There is much we can accomplish in one lifetime, and yet, we must be mature enough to understand that we cannot do it all. This is not just the work of our individual lives. This is the work of *all of our* lives. With this in mind, it's essential to step back from the fire, from time to time, both because it's essential in order to integrate the transformations, and because it is important to celebrate these extraordinary paradigm leaps forward.

M: Whoa. We're on the cutting-edge of a new consciousness. And here I am, trying to step off the wheel.

JB: A new consciousness indeed. Then, a magical alchemy occurs. After some time in the fires of co-creation, solemates become "Wholemates." No longer caught in the polarizing transcendence-immanence construct, they experience themselves as both solemates *and* soulmates. The connection is mutually sourced in essence, and grounded in the earth dimension. A love relationship that spans all realms and ways of being. Soul-to-Solemates, they have mastered the sky—the higher, deeper, soulful levels, and the earth—the healthy, grounded, balanced life, and personality levels. They have finally become a complete 'Realationship.' A restful wholesomeness and Homeness. There is still an innocence in the field between them, but it's an informed innocence, as their previously naïve understanding of love alchemizes into a maturely integrated understanding of the ways of the heart. Wholemates experience love relationship as a spiritual practice—not one that is fixated on the heavens above—but one that is grounded in the everything. On the river of essence, everything flows in the same direction—toward the ocean of wholeness. A harmonized and mutually inclusive consciousness. The path of the Wholly Holy.

M: This is quite a new vista you opened for me, brother. A lot to absorb, particularly for someone like me, who hasn't spent a lot of time exploring relational states of consciousness. Hey, the ferry is pulling up. Next one is not for another 90 minutes and I have a deep-tissue massage tonight. Definitely need it. How about we jump on the ferry and talk more on the boat? I want to bring these ideas into my current circumstances to see if, and where, they land.

JB: All aboard, partner.

Hope is a Traveler

We ran to catch the ferry. As always, Michael moved swiftly, efficiently, while I lumbered along behind, taking in the scenery. Just as I stepped foot on the boat, my friend—author Philip Shepherd stepped off with his brilliant wife, Allyson Woodrooffe, on their way home. Together 30 years, they raised two lovely and intelligent daughters, while staying committed to their own magical creative work and meaningful contributions to the world. Renaissance people. They were coming, we were going, so there wasn't time for chatting. But I quickly introduced Michael, and they exchanged pleasantries. I took it as significant that they would show up on our path, right at this juncture of our dialogue. Another meaningful sign.

Michael and I climbed the stairs to the top floor of the ferry and sat down at the front, looking ahead to the vast cityscape. The trip allotted more time to further open the relational landscape.

M: Jeff, your map is a fantastic vision to strive for, but I am not sure where it lands for Hannah and I. It's very idealistic. As I mentioned, I do feel that we have a deep soul connection that has always been there, maybe from time immemorial. Lots of chemistry, too, even if it has been derailed by our issues. And I do feel that there are many ways that we work very well together in the practical realms. We meet in the soul, and we function easefully in daily life. What has not developed—probably because of my own patterns—is the co-creative aspect you mentioned. For that to happen, I have to be more willing to do the individual and relational shadow work, and to examine my issues around participating in the world. The world of people, feelings, humanness. That's a lot of change being demanded. I'm not sure I'm up for it, and even if I am, it can't happen overnight. And she has a burning desire to become a mom soon. She is approaching 40, after all. Her clock is ticking. So there is this battle between her stage of readiness, and mine.

JB: I wouldn't call it a battle, you consciousness warrior. I would call it an opportunity. To either own that this connection is no longer your path, so you can both be free to move in the direction that now calls you. Or to accept that it's time for your relationship to move to the next level. If there is a mutual willingness, there is the hopeful possibility that you are at the precipice of a profound shift in your individual and co-creative lives. What is truly being symbolized in the story of having a child is the essence of co-creation. It's now a question of whether you can both find a point of merger that will serve the next phase of your relationship: the co-creative path. Can you?

M: You mean you can't answer that for me? That would make it soooo much easier.

JB: Nope. Besides, you wouldn't listen.

M: Shit, foiled again! I do feel that I am coming into a real willingness to do more healing work. That step I can commit to. But the baby thing, well, that feels years ahead. First I have to get comfortable in my own skin.

JB: Yes, but let's not underestimate the significance of your willingness to heal. That's monumental. Because love needs an entry point. If our emotional body is all blocked up with unresolved material, there's no way in. The more we empty the vessel, the more space there is for love to flourish. Healing our hearts gives love a place to land.

Once you go deeper into the work, you may be surprised to find that you actually want what Hannah wants. I have worked with many trauma survivors who fled the world, and returned very quickly once they set the intention to heal and re-open to the world. Those who flee connection the fastest are often the ones who long for it the most.

M: Maybe, or maybe the fact that we have wanted different things for years, means that we simply aren't meant to walk together for the rest of it. We're at a cross-roads, with cross-purposes. Perhaps it's time to accept that and move along.

JB: That's possible. I do believe that each of us has a unique life purpose. And we all have a creative life-force that demands expression in this life. For some, it includes the creation of new human life. For others, the creative impulse takes on manifold pathways and forms. Each expression is valid, as long at it matches your soul-shape. For myself, I was compelled to make books instead of babies. This is a deeply personal question that only you can answer.

M: Yes, I see that. But I am also seeing that I may have confused my trauma-induced spiritual quest with my true purpose. It's hard for me to admit, but that's probably the truth. I thought I was fully on my path of purpose all these years, when I may have just been running from my destiny.

JB: I wouldn't say that. No need to negate your path altogether, Michael. It may well be that the path you took was a stepping-stone to your purpose, at that time. Just because we move from our defenses, doesn't necessarily mean we are off path. The whole collective is making reactive decisions at this stage of human development. Perhaps this is part of the road you needed to take, to arrive at your truest purpose. Some of us need to first experience what we are not, before we can experience what we are. I took that route as well. And here you are, Michael, once a cosmonaut, now a miner, returning back to earth to do a deep dig you weren't ready for until now. Perhaps you needed to visit another planet before you could fully inhabit this one.

M: I appreciate your optimism, but it doesn't change much. Because even if that is my next step, it doesn't answer the question as to whether I should stay with Hannah. Even if I envision that I might reach the stage where I want what she wants, it is impossible to know how long that will take. It may be too late to meet her need to become a mother. And not responsible to ask her to wait, based on a hypothetical. I do love her, and I don't want to hold her back. Although it sickens me inside to say this. I feel like I'm going to hurl right now.

JB: Pay attention to those bodily cues. A key inquiry in determining a relationship's longevity is whether there is still work to be done within the relationship, or whether the work has come to an organic end. All too often, we remain locked into connections that no longer serve us. And, all too often, we let go of connections before our work together is complete. You have to discern—is this relationship a laboratory for my own expansion, or now a prison of our own making? Does it invite growth, or induce sleep? Can we find a way to grow together, or are we better off apart? This is the (he)art form of relatedness—knowing when to dive in deeper, and knowing when to step away. Once we perfect this art, we can grow forward in our relational life.

M: I have a long way to go before I can perfect that art. It's all I can do to stay in the building when she speaks from her heart.

JB: Yet you are staying in the building. She's the one that left it this time. Perhaps there is more hope here than you imagine. In my beloved wife, poet Susan Frybort's words, "Hope is a traveler." Hope is a not a stationary thing. It moves as we move. It changes form, as we change form. I would suggest you hold these questions gently for the time being, Michael. Don't seek a concrete answer yet. Let your process unfold a little more. You are at a transit point in your consciousness.

M: But I want to jump ahead to the answer!

JB: That's not how it works. True answers don't conform to our demands. They are a gentle unfurling that ripens in their own time. You committed to the step of counseling. Stay with that for awhile. It will be valuable to see how your sessions unfold together. It's quite special that you have remained married for so many years, despite your differences. Don't reach for an answer, before it's ripe. Sure, this has been a long-standing question for you. But you are now approaching a new consciousness. You are a new Michael. A new Michael needs new answers.

The boat lurched, as it slowed down to dock in Toronto. Michael grabbed on to my arm to secure himself. He was clearly feeling skittish as he rode the waves of transformation. I put my arm around him to let him know that he wasn't alone at sea.

After we disembarked, I invited him to sit down with me for a few more minutes. We perched ourselves on some large boulders surrounding the lake. I didn't want him to leave without offering him another tool to support his process. Especially now, when so much hung in the balance.

JB: Open to another exercise?

M: I suppose.

JB: Try this before we meet again. It may bring more clarity. Perhaps even do it with Hannah. It might be the just right thing for you to do together. It perfectly blends two of your passions: your love for meditation and her love for the ways of the heart. A perfect co-creation.

EXERCISE 6
BELOVED MEDITATION

This exercise is a valuable tool in discerning the relational-form of a loved one in your life. In a relationship, there can be critical junctures where we reach a crossroad: Do we split paths at this juncture, each venturing in a new direction? Or, do we continue together, on one shared trail? In either case, it can be obvious that love still runs deep. Yet significant relationships can take different forms, serving various purposes, at different times in our lives. This exercise can be used as a supportive tool at a critical cross-roads, in determining or re-assessing, the specific form the relationship must now take. You can either envision the subject (your loved one) in your mind's eye. Or, use a photo of them. (This exercise is not limited to romantic connections. It can be used to clarify the future of any relevant personal connection, as well.)

Sit on a chair, on the floor, or on a cushion, in whatever position feels most comfortable. Or lie down on a firm but comfortable surface. We want your body as rooted and relaxed as possible in this exercise. Feel your body making contact with the earth.

Either close your eyes, or keep your eyes opened and focus on the photograph of the beloved you are contemplating.

Invite your breath to move evenly throughout your body. Do not direct the intensity. Just gentle, even breaths.

Now gently touch the area around your heart. Stroke the flesh… feel the tensions… notice the energetic armor… the protective plate… the beat of your heart… your lifeblood. Feel the rise and fall of your breath as you.

Imagine the person in question. Invite them into your heart space. Feel them inside your heart. Imagine their face, their breath, their scent, their little blemishes and imperfections that only you may be aware of. Remember moments together, and then let them circulate through you. If there is anger in the way, breathe through it. Feel free to make sounds that express it. If tears arise, allow them to fall. Allow yourself to stay with the image until you can see their essence come into view, without resistance or defense. Unmasked, like in your clearest moments of seeing… before becoming burdened by difficulties or conflicts. Allow yourself to clear any fears, anxieties, emotional debris, that prevent you from seeing them and your connection clearly.

Once you can see them… see yourself, too. Breathe into a clear image of both of you, in your heart's eye. Now go deeper into your heart… allow your breath to stroke your heart with love, like a feather's touch. Connect with your deepest feelings around this relationship. Allow yourself to feel the darkness, the light, the spectrum of possibility in between. Feel beneath your armor, into what your heart is saying within and between the breaths. Feel into your intuitive knowing around the connection. See yourself on the path ahead.

When you are ready, place your hand over your heart and ask these questions:

Is this person still part of my future?
Are there still lessons we need to learn from each other, or are we now complete together?
Are there lessons I now need to learn on my own, outside of this present relational form?
Are we meant to walk together in the coming moments, or is it time to take leave of each other?

What do I feel? What do I see?
Are we walking hand-in-hand together, a shared path?
Am I now walking alone, a separate path?

Hearticulate until the truth reveals itself.

When clarity emerges, stay with the truth of your feelings. Stay there, and hold them safe. Before you rise, send love to yourself, to your person of significance, and to all of us who are trying to make sense of the path of the heart.

Michael listened closely, and then said goodbye. No hugs this time. He nodded his head somberly, treading uncharacteristically slowly toward the subway. He had something to face—heart-on. I remained seated, feeling surprisingly emotional. As I was describing the beloved meditation to Michael, I was dipping into the pool of my own remembrance. So many past loves, lost and found, summoned and dispatched, on my journey to my beloved Susan. The ones that came before were not the ultimate beloved, but they were remarkably meaningful nonetheless. Every time we dipped into love's wells we paid homage to this one great life. We tasted God, and saw proof that God exists.

I had been where Michael is. Loving another deeply, but unwilling or unable to co-create in the way they desired. Sometimes it was timing, sometimes it was just the wrong fit. One thing I learned: It doesn't matter how much two people love one another, if they are directionally incompatible or if there is not a mutual willingness to grow together. If all you have is a loveship, you are unlikely to survive troubled waters. With no ability to work together to overcome love's challenges, it will be very difficult to remain afloat. At some point on the journey, your ship is going to capsize. What is love without relatedness? If all you have is a relationship, then you may well remain afloat, but there will be a longing for something more—a love that sets your soul ablaze. What is relatedness without love? But if you have a loveship AND a relationship—there is no limit to how far your bond can travel. Love that is grounded in healthy relatedness has a compound affect. The more difficult the challenges, the stronger the bond grows. The bigger the soulnami, the sturdier the foundation that meets it.

Whatever happens, we must always remember that love is a brave path. It is like taking a long walk in a deep dark forest and never quite knowing where your soul will land. It is not for the faint of heart, nor is it ever to be taken lightly. Real love is heartcore. You have to be tenacious. You have to be innovative. You have to be willing to drop to your knees time and again before its wisdom. And you have to forge the tools you will need from your own imaginings—as very few who have walked the path before can fully describe the terrain. Most fell into quicksand soon after the romantic phase ended. Relationship is always a spiritual practice, even when we imagine it otherwise.

Speaking of which, Susan was waiting for me at home. I got up and grabbed a cab. No sense taking my time to get there tonight. After all, it was Wednesday: burdock root burrito night. My glutton-free favorite. ☺ That, and my beloved herself, in all her shining glory, the fruit of my soul's decades-long labor.

8 The New Cage Movement

Michael and I arranged a meeting the following Friday at the CN Tower. His inner journey was accelerating, and he was eager for our meetings to come quicker. Kind of like the last stage of giving birth, where contractions come close together, fast and furious. Something new was being birthed in Michael. We met at the bottom of what was once the tallest free-standing structure in the world, and took the elevator up to the revolving restaurant. Michael still preferred the bird's eye view, after all.

We sat down and ordered a late lunch. I opted for the Caesar salad. Michael opted for indulgence: a heaping plate of lasagna smothered in sauce, meatballs, and three different cheeses. I could tell his mind was churning.

M: So, there's been some breakthroughs. I did the Beloved Meditation and it became clearer than ever: Hannah is my life-long beloved. There was no escaping it. Every time I imagined the path without her, jarring pains would surge through my body. A twisting in my gut and intestines. Once I felt my neck cramp up with a pain that was almost unbearable. It was like my body was being distorted, completely out of alignment.

JB: Metaphor for your life. Glad to hear you are finally heeding the cues of your body.

M: I know it won't be easy, but I have to hang in there, and see this through. We did our initial therapy session this week, and it went pretty well. It was just the beginning, but I was able to be very present with her, and to hear her. She's been coming over the last few nights to talk. She hasn't moved back in yet, but I'm hopeful that she will.

JB: Sounds like things are moving forward.

M: Not quite. On other fronts, Jeff, I am finding myself back-tracking. I still feel like I am in a dark night of the soul. This job is grueling. It's impossible for me to perform up to par. So I've been resorting to old coping mechanisms just to get by. And it's been working. Such a relief.

JB: That's what we do as humans. Don't take it too seriously. I guess you need to put your training wheels back on. You will take them off again. In the midst of that, something is being integrated. Progress is being made.

M: Thank you for understanding. Since my meditations are no longer effective, I have switched to a crystal healing technique, followed by positive affirmations. I begin by holding the crystals in my hand, allowing their energy to cleanse my thinking and attract a more satisfying outcome. And then, I end with three positive affirmations, "This job is good for my soul." "This job is what I need to evolve." "This job will bring me abundance." I wrap it all up with the Ho'oponopono prayer: "I love you. I'm sorry. Please forgive me." Then I start my day. Gets me through to 5 o'clock.

JB: You're shitting me. My friend, that's a cute technique, but I'm fairly sure it's not going to truly help you on a deep level. More a band-aid than a real solution. Watch out... your wishful thinking will simply fall to the bottom of the fountain with the rest of the pennies. It sounds like the New Cage movement.

M: You mean New Age.

JB: No, New Cage.

M: What's the difference?

JB: Big difference, my friend. What I once respectfully honored as a new age for humanity, I now often refer to as the "New Cage Movement," as I witness seekers fleeing their humanness—and opportunities for deeper transformation—in droves. This movement does not liberate us—it actually imprisons us inside of our own unattended to issues. It has the effect of taking us so far away from reality, that we may not be able to find our way back. Here, let me pull up my definition of New Cage. It's on my website:

> A term to describe the more ungrounded, dangerous, and sim-
> plistic elements of the New Age movement, including but not

limited to: wishful thinking mantras, spiritual bypassing, premature forgiveness practices, superficial healing techniques, the perpetual denial of common sense realities, and the insistence on inflated fantastical perspectives—i.e. "Everything is an illusion," "It's all perfect," "There are no victims," "Everything that happens is meant-to-be," "All judgments are bad," "Suffering doesn't exist," "You are responsible for everything that happens to you," "Just ask the universe for what you want and you will get it...," "Everything you see and feel is a reflection of you," "Change your thinking, change your life," etc.

There you have it. Enbullshitment, at its truest.

M: But bro, as you like to say, don't throw the baby out with the bathwater. The New Age Movement has served greater purposes. It's taken us from our base chakra, our hunter-gatherer survivalist mentality, into our elevated nature. It's granted us a glimpse into the potential of a new Golden Age for humanity. It's brought us out of the dark ages, and into the light. It's taken us from being hateful and self-serving into our true nature: beings of love. It has restored hope. The New Age Movement has moved us forward. But now, here you are, taking us backwards.

JB: I'll give you credit here, Michael. These perspectives do have their place in certain circumstances, and they have served genuinely uplifting purposes. They do provide us with tools that foster our awakening. But taken too far—as they have been through the years—they actually become a prison, a 'cage,' of their own making, locking humanity in with its unprocessed pain and patterns, substituting the real work with addictive flights of fancy. Individuals who go too far into this way of thinking may alleviate their issues for a brief period of time, but invariably come crashing back to earth, even less prepared to deal with reality than before.

New Cagers pride themselves on their seeming spirituality, but are actually falling apart at the seams—unboundaried, ungrounded, and controlled by all the congealed emotional material that they have sought to avoid. In their determined efforts to float above the world, they actually perpetuate and deepen their own suffering, and miss the opportunity to do the real work to become conscious. The key to escaping New Cage prison is developing a willingness to do the required work to ground, embody, and heal in authentic terms. There are no substitutes for genuine, hard-earned transformation.

M: The killjoy strikes again.

Honoring Victimhood

Between his bites of lasagna, Michael said something indistinct under his breath. He was clearly annoyed. As we ate, an attractive middle-aged woman was involved in an emotionally-charged conversation with a friend at the next table. It was impossible not to overhear: "I hate him. He stole everything from me. That's 18 years that I can never get back. The prime years of my life. When I could have had children. He intentionally weaved me into a web of deceit, while living a dual life. Then he pulls out, and takes my best years with him. How can I recoup lost time? Bastard." Her lips quivered as she spoke, and I noticed a tiny tear rolling down. Her emotions pierced me. The enduring plight of human beings. Bad things happen to good people. Life is intrinsically unfair. My heart went out to her—a comrade on this perilous journey we call life. The conversation also piqued Michael's interest. But he clearly had another take on it.

M: Ahh, she's a perfect example of why I get bugged by your teachings. Universe must have plopped her on my path, just to confirm my point.

JB: What are you speaking of, specifically?

M: You are determined to keep people trapped in their victimhood, by making it all about endlessly feelings their feelings.

JB: Trapped, or merely acknowledging it, so that they can heal and empower themselves?

M: Trapped. Because you and I both know how easy it is to get stuck inside of a victim consciousness. Forgiveness is what releases you from that trap. The only way she can regain her lost 18 years is by forgiving the jerk. Now he still has a hold on her consciousness. She is wasting even more time, stuck in the past.

JB: Stuck, or just not sure how to find her way through it in a culture of denial?

From my perspective, the ones who actually acknowledge their trauma are far more awakened than those who deny it. They are the ones calling us to a more authentic paradigm. They are the ones who whisper our own shell-shocked hearts back to life. We are back at a similar place we often land, Michael. Although you have opened tremendously, part of you is still averse to digging deep inside and accessing those compacted and hardened emotions.

M: I disagree, I'm not afraid, or averse, as you say. I made the conscious choice to not be held hostage by my past. For example, it really helped me to stop seeing myself as a victim of my childhood mishaps. I went through this brief phase in my younger years, before my spiritual journey really took off, where I would meet people and tell them how hard it was. Poor me, poor me. I would feel angry at God for how hard I had it. Just like that woman over there, still babbling to her friend. How many times has she rehashed this same story? When I embarked on my spiritual path, my perspective changed radically. When I began to embrace the idea that I had chosen everything, I began to feel a kind of relief. I began to realize that I had selected these people in order to accelerate my evolution. They gave me the perfect example of who I wasn't meant to be in this lifetime. And the stuff they put me through, actually grew me forward.

JB: Are you sure that was a realization, and not just a mechanism or technique? Because, as you have acknowledged in these past weeks, you have not resolved your relationship with your parents and worked through all the primary issues and repressed memories. They are still seething inside you, and they still have a hold on you, Michael. You are not yet free. You are only at the beginning of that journey. So you can't really say that you weren't victimized, or that you chose all of it for some karmically beneficial purpose. You can say it in words… but it won't ring true in your whole body. It's a cover-up.

M: Ugh. You are right… it doesn't ring true throughout my whole body. I will admit that. Where do I grow from here?

JB: First, you have to acknowledge yourself as a victim, before you can recognize any choices you may have made to become one. It's one thing to go through a deep and embodied healing process, and then come through the other side with a realization that you chose those experiences and circumstances for some beneficial purpose. It's quite another to jump to the belief that there was never any victimhood, and that every experience is perfectly beneficial and pre-destined. Let's look at each situation on its own merits, rather than sweeping every circumstance under the same magic carpet.

The truth is that we have been shaming and denying victimhood for centuries. There is nothing evolved about it. The New Cage "no victims" mantra is only one more way this has been manifest. Before, we merely shoved our traumas under a rug, never looking back. The plain fact is, this planet is riddled with victims. Many. Just open your eyes. There is trauma, everywhere. And we aren't going to co-create a more humane world if we keep denying it. Diminishing it. Belittling it. Burying it. This is just victim-bashing. Instead of normalizing repression, we must co-create a world that invites every trauma survivor to share their story fully, and without shame. In so doing, they both heal themselves, and they give permission for everyone else to self-reveal as well. Honest naked vulnerability. Where real healing lies. The collective then begins to heal, and just as importantly, feels ignited to make the kinds of changes—relationally, societally, culturally, and legally—that minimize future traumas. If we keep denying the existence of victimhood, then what will inspire positive change? Nothing.

M: That's fair, but there are many situations where suffering is a gift, Jeff. I do believe that I chose certain experiences and relationships, because I needed to learn specific lessons. I have seen this in many others, as well.

JB: Sure you did, but not always. Let's keep it grounded. EVERYTHING is not a gift. There may be valuable transformation that arises from many experiences, but that doesn't mean that EVERY experience is a gift. If we lean too far in that direction, we will deny trauma and victimhood all together, something we have already been doing for centuries. Some experiences are horrors, and it is all we can do to heal from them. To suggest that someone MUST find the gift in them, is to add insult to injury. It is also to create a culture that welcomes all horrors, because, after all, "everything is a gift." Let's keep it real—sometimes, it's a gift. Sometimes it's a horror. And the only one who can decide that is the person who had the experience.

M: I understand that I did not invite these situations at a conscious level. It was not me "Michael." I am referring to a sublime soul-level, as the point from which we choose and direct our life-circumstances. On the covert subterranean level, everything happens for our highest good. In the place where our Soul is the Director, and interacts with the Universe to bring lessons through.

JB: Are you sure that is true? Have you heard that right from the soul's mouth? Is there any real value in believing something that is only a hypothetical? Missing the myriad opportunities to deal with actual human concrete realities, due to some prospective belief? Simply put, you don't ask for every bad thing that happens to you. You may learn from it in some cases, but that still doesn't mean you—or your soul—asked for it. Telling someone who has been victimized that they asked for it on some karmic level is shaming and isolating. They alone can decide if they invited it in, but they don't need to hear that from others. And, the great irony is that those who deny victimhood with the most ferocity, are usually the ones in the most pain. It's just a smokescreen.

M: But, in the great cosmic order of things—everything happens for a reason.

JB: Not so. The "everything happens for a reason" mantra emerged as a necessary counter-balance to the idea that we are ALWAYS victims in situations. Sometimes we do play a role in what has been manifest. And, as you implied, often in those circumstances, it *is* our unconscious patterns and beliefs that are doing the choosing. But, like all polarized mantras, it goes too far in one direction, and ignores situations where suffering is needless. Yes, everything happens for a reason, but it's not always a good one. There is always some degree of misguided action on this planet. Since we can't determine why something happened to someone else, it's always better to come from a place of compassion when confronted with a person's hardship. Let them decide if the reason was a good one. Let them decide if it was a gift. Blanket statements like: "You are exactly where you are supposed to be"—no matter what someone's life circumstances and challenges—have become hollow, empty platitudes. Yes, there is no question that we can often learn something of value wherever we are on the path, and yes, we may have, in some situations, attracted the exact challenge that we need to grow… BUT that does not imply that we are ALWAYS where we are supposed to be, or that we chose our every reality. Sometimes we need a kick in the ass, and sometimes we are just a victim of terrible circumstances. Sometimes our suffering is needless and the result of other people's wrongdoing. Compassion demands that we hold the space for each other's challenges with a wide-open heart. Let each person decide if they are exactly where they are supposed to be.

Let me read a piece from my wife Susan's poetry book, *Open Passages*. It speaks to precisely this issue:

> Not everything happens for a good or cosmic reason. Not everything has been orchestrated by otherworldly forces to present a life lesson. Why bad things happen to the innocent is a mystery that will never be unraveled. Thankfully there is no mystery in the wonderment of healing. And by picking up the mortar and pestle that are the emotional healing tools, we can be the alchemist that takes charge, remarkably exchanging the seemingly irreversible energy within the violations against us for the precious elements of restoration. As we place them into the crucible to be processed and exchanged for indisputable strength and with a more supportive and affirming existence, we overcome and create real meaning. We come into our wholeness as a triumphant human being.

M: Wow, that's beautiful.

JB: Yes she is.

M: I have actually experienced this myself. People who perpetually denied my own victimhood when I shared it. It was very common in a spiritual community I lived in. They had a pat answer whenever someone spoke of their suffering, "No victims, only blessings." I suppose I have adopted this mentality.

JB: To deny victimhood is to further victimize. And the more we dismiss victimhood, the more we actually perpetuate and enable victimization. I understand that many of us reach a stage where it is essential that we move beyond victimhood, and, in certain situations, recognize how we may have manifested our circumstances. But this is not true for everyone; nor is it true in every situation. For many of us, it is essential that we own our victimhood, that we are seen in our victimhood, and that we do not re-frame our suffering in positive terms, unless and until we feel it is true for us. There is no shame in owning our woundedness. In fact, it may be the only thing that saves us.

M: I hear you, but I have witnessed countless people I have known get physically ill because of their inner attitudes and beliefs. I get impatient with them sometimes, wondering why they won't see how their own think-ing created the problem.

JB: The notion that we are always responsible is one of the tragic miscon-ceptions at the heart of New Cage thinking. One place this manifests is in the condemnation of those who become physically ill. If only they had dealt with their past life issues, if only they had become more aware, if only they had processed more of their emotional pain, if only they had developed a healthier lifestyle, if only they had done the Ho'oponopono Prayer daily, if only they had done more sweat lodges, if only they had used positive affirmations, if only they had turned their thinking around. Not only are these comments presumptuous—only the person with the illness can know their truth—but New Cagers ignore the very simple fact that illness is often sourced in many factors, a number of which are not easily identifiable and certainly not always attributable to karma, or awareness, or emotional health. SOMETIMES PEOPLE JUST GET SICK. We live in an imperfect world—where DISEASE EXISTS. A prime example of where the New Cage movement abandons basic common sense.

M: True, we haven't reached the Golden Age of humanity yet, where ill-ness and strife will no longer exist. Although that's what I am striving for.

JB: We'll never get there without compassion, dear man. I have seen way too many New Cagers working someone else's illness as an egoic boost, narcissistically using it as evidence of their own superiority: "Well, I didn't get sick, because I am a more evolved person." Nonsense! If you are more evolved, you will move from compassion and humility. A microscopic cell of bacteria can wreak havoc on a nervous system. It can happen to any of us—we are all fair game. If you can't respond empathically, keep quiet. Let the recipient decipher where their illness comes from. They don't need a lecture. They need our presence.

The Law of No-Traction

M: This feels too simplistic. I practiced the Law of Attraction for a few years, and I found it effective. When I was able to get my thinking and my energy positively aligned with my desires, many good things came into my life. I would make requests of the universe, and often, they were granted.

JB: And often they weren't.

M: Hmmm, can't deny that.

JB: I see it this way: Aligning our inner worlds with our desires can have a positive impact on our capacity for manifestation. Yet, I don't believe that this is always or necessarily true. If it was, then every person who did deep inner work and became positively aligned, would summon positive outcomes. But they don't. Many become more positive in their thinking, yet their reality remains the same. In some cases, it even gets worse. And many others don't do a lick of work to overcome their negativity, and they become abundant—at least materially abundant—without even trying. In short, like does not always attract like. Our universe, and our interwoven lives, are much more intricate than that.

Having said that, the idea that there is an interface between our thoughts and a responsive universe is a vast improvement over the belief that we are alone down here, and that no one is ever listening. This was the hopeless perspective that my mother carried, and it didn't serve her. The universe is a vital living organism. There are unseen levels of interconnectedness. We humans are a brilliantly complex network of pulses and charges that transmit signals across the cosmos, no doubt. And the cosmos responds to us. But this is quite a different reality than merely "visualizing and thinking it into being." It is seldom as simple as asking the universe for what we want and we get it. Too many have followed this approach to transformation and lost their way, making major life changes without the ground to support them. Many of them lost everything while chasing a dream before they had built the necessary foundation to manifest and sustain it. I call this the "Law of No-Traction." This suggests that without the necessary groundwork—psycho-emotionally, energetically, and practically—to sustain our callings and dreams, they will never gain traction and eventually take full flight. We may get close to them, but they will seldom fully come to fruition. It's just another cage, Michael. Anything that isn't grounded in reality is a cage—a limiter of our true freedom.

M: This isn't going to be very appealing to *The Secret* crowd. That was a huge best seller. So basically, you are saying you need to work hard to manifest your dreams.

JB: Yes. Don't be intoxicated by the allure of wish-full thinking. Instead, focus your energy on genuine foundation building, doing the painstaking work to clear the inner channel and learn essential lessons, so that your quest for true-path is solid and reliable. Divine perspiration begets divine inspiration. There are no magic potions on the trailways of transformation. The universe doesn't respond to feigned positivity, flights of fancy, starry-eyed imaginings with little ground to support them. If it does respond to anything, and again, there is no guarantee that it will, it responds to authentic transformation. Deep inner work, clearing, and aligning—from the inside-out. If we want to improve our chances at manifesting our callings and dreams, we have to do much more than re-calibrate our thinking. We have to actually change from the depths of our core. We have to shape and mold ourselves in the fires of hard-earned transformation. We have to get our emotional world consistent with our requests, before they will be taken seriously by the universe. The more emotionally repressed we are, the denser and more inauthentic the message we transmit. If we are all blocked up with pain and anger, our "positive thoughts" will not be authentically sourced and organically positive. The trick is to clear ourselves out from the inside-out so that we are emanating from an unobstructed and unified channel. Then our request might carry more weight, then it might fall on open ears.

M: You are making this far too complex. I think you are a glutton for self-punishment. Always addicted to the hard road. This must be rooted in your early life traumas. I have found that simply articulating my intentions to the Universe is key to manifesting the life I desire.

JB: Cut the crap, Michael. Come on back to reality. You have already acknowledged that you hate your job, and your marriage is close to crumbling. Something isn't working in your technique. The trick with manifestation is not to think about it, but just to do it. You can tell everyone your plan, you can ask the Universe to support you, you can even hold a special fire ceremony to usher it into realization… but it won't mean anything if you don't ground it in reality. If you have a dream—do it into being.

M: Got me there. The universe is not responding favorably to my requests. I guess I'm playing devil's advocate for now. A last gasp to hold on to some philosophies that bring me comfort. Basically, you're piling a helluva lot of work on me right now. There's all the emotional work. And now you are saying I have to take grounded action steps to turn my life around. My plate is heaping, dude.

JB: Look, you've already inhaled all of your lasagna. ☺ I believe you are up to the challenge. Yes, hard work is required. Even when we do manifest that which serves us, it is an equally interesting question as to whether it was the Universe that made it happen, or simply our own efforts. Or, perhaps it's a magical alchemy of cooperation and co-creation, our consciousness and universal consciousness working in tandem. In the same way that some have a tendency to look beyond the self for their divinity in other spiritual circles, the Law of Attraction entices people to do the same. It makes the individual accountable for their vibration, but then focuses on the universe as the ultimate determiner. This is actually disempowering. It is the same self-bashing we discussed earlier in our dialogues. Many of us don't actually see and acknowledge the Divine within the self, so we attribute the ultimate blessing to something outside of us. We remove ourselves from our true seat of power. The universe that rode in and saved the day.

What about our own abilities and capacities to create and craft our path, by making wise choices one tiny stitch at a time? To weave the tapestry of our lives, by flipping our unconsciousness into our consciousness, so we aren't ruled by buried emotions. This is true power. We do the deeper work to transform our consciousness and our ways of being in the world, and the energy of our transformed humanness fully shifts our trajectory, in and of itself. It is not the universe that provides the abundance—it's our own shift toward a more abundant way of being. Not so much the grace beyond the self, but the grace within it.

M: Gosh, this is a lot of fucking responsibility. Let's order dessert—I need some comfort food.

JB: Let's. What will it be? I'm looking at the Mixed Berry Tart.

M: I need something more hardcore. The Triple Mocha Caramel Cappuccino Cheesecake.

We called our server, and he brought us two plates of decadence, heaped with mounds of whipped cream. As we dug in, we continued to dialogue. I secretly enjoyed watching a small smile form on Michael's lips as he ate his dessert. In a quiet and unassuming moment—simply enjoying his humanness. Sometimes it's those private moments when you catch someone unaware that are the most endearing.

JB: I'm not going to disagree with you. It's a colossal responsibility. This is the primary reason why so many avoid the path. As I said before, reality is not for the faint of soul. It's messy and it takes a momentous amount of work and determination. We have to harvest, plow, and till our landscape. Only this shift will attract other humans and related opportunities. It's not the universe that we attract with our healthier and improved attitude. It's our own alchemical shift. And it is that vibration which opens the portal to a more abundant way of being. Then we are working from the inside-out.

M: Hmmmf.

JB: And it is that lens, which attracts the attention of our fellow humans, more inclined to connect with us and seize opportunities because we have become a lighthouse of hope, calling out to each other on the road to abundance, supporting one another, pushing further, digging deeper. This is actually more self-empowering than fixating on a universe that may, or may not, be receptive or even remotely interesting in our doings. Why look UP for our destiny, when it's staring at us in our own mirror? That's why I am careful with the word "manifestation." I call it "humanifestation"—as it's all about manifesting our divine humanness, in this world, in this life.

It's Not ALL Good

M: I have to challenge you on something. You are gung-ho about emphasizing the value of feelings, but you seem determined to strike down positive emotions. What's with that?

JB: I don't shun positivity, Michael. I shun pseudo-positivity—the kind of feigned happiness that prevents us from dropping down and doing the real work to bring forth our authentic optimism.

M: Sometimes positivity saves our lives. Let me give you an example of what I mean. During one very trying period, I recognized that I had a choice in front of me. I could lean into the darkness and make it my home, or I could look on the bright side, and focus on the light. It wasn't a situation where I was bypassing anything. It was one of those situations, right after a series of losses and disappointments had devastated me, where I had a real choice as to whether to become super vigilant and defensive, or to remain open to what comes next. I chose the latter… and each night before going to bed, I would end my day listing five things I am grateful for. I met Hannah soon thereafter.

JB: I don't have any issue with that. It's wonderful to have gratitude in your attitude, as long as you genuinely feel it. If not, stop the lies, and get in touch with how you really feel. Not every positive choice is a bypass of reality. Not even close. I wouldn't be here today, if I hadn't taken a positive path through the heart of the darkness. This doesn't mean that I didn't have to work through the shadow material later in life, but it does mean that it served me to find any little sliver of light to hang onto to see me through the worst of it. What I am most concerned about are those who use positivity undiscerningly, rather than as a healthy means of overcoming challenges. I call this tendency "Perpetual Positivity Syndrome." Here's another one of my definitions. Let me grab it from my notes. Gosh, I should know these by heart by now!

> Perpetual Positivity Syndrome (PPS) is the addictive need to default to positivity under any and all circumstances. One of the most common obstructions to awakening on the healing path, it prevents a maturation in the deep within because sufferers refuse to be present for all that is. Symptoms include: a constant need to find the light in every situation, a tendency to forget or "rise above" the negative aspects of their partners, an inability to fully support and hold the space for another's suffering, and a turning away from the painstaking work demanded by life's challenges. Instead of forging a grounded, discerning optimism

in the grit and grime of daily life—they jump to the light, while averting the shadows that inform it. They habitually bliss-trip, when lessons are waiting in the wings to be integrated and embodied. Those who suffer with PPS are often of the illusory view that they had perfect childhoods or that they have moved beyond the shadow. In most cases, their obsessive clinging to the "positive" is rooted in their own unresolved emotional material: pain and anger that will only come back to haunt them. At the end of the day, there can be no light without shadow, and no substitute for hard-earned transformation.

M: This is yet another nail in my coffin. You are turning all my methods upside down, again. It's like when you look under a rock and uncover something gnarly. You wish you could just flip the lid back on and pretend you have never seen it. Too late.

JB: Too late is right, Michael, you are really into the nitty-gritty here. I get that we prefer it to be happy and positive, but that's just not where much of humanity is. Many of us are overwhelmed with pain, undigested sadness, unexpressed anger, unseen truths. So, we have two choices: We can continue to pretend it's not there, cover it over, shame and shun it in ourselves and others, distract and detach whenever possible. Or, we can face it heart-on, own it within ourselves, look for it in others with compassion, create a culture that is focused on authenticity and healthy emotional release. If we continue to push it all down, we are both creating illness, and delaying our collective expansion. But if we can just own the shadow, express it, release it, love each other through it—we can finally graduate from the School of Heart Knocks and begin to enjoy this magnificent life as we were intended. Pretending the pain isn't there just embeds it further. Let's illuminate it instead.

M: Well, I've got a shitload more work to do. In the past when crap would come my way, my go-to mantra was simply: "It's all Good." It's a way of approaching the challenges of life with a relaxed equanimity, and not getting hooked into the bullshit.

JB: It's easy for people to "It's all good" themselves into illusion. It all comes down to: Do you want the truth… or do you want a counterfeit version of reality, forged by your defenses and mechanisms? Sometimes all is genuinely good, yet we cannot see it because our consciousness is too burdened, or we are too lodged in our own experience of victimhood. And sometimes an experience reveals its benefits much later in time, becoming more obvious as our understanding of the relationship between challenges and growth gets more refined. If we learn to stay in the fire long enough, we will often find the needle of goodness in the heart of the karmic haystack. But to jump immediately into a casual, "It's all good," can undermine our expansion. Of course, there are exceptions to every rule of nature. This perspective can actually be helpful to those of us who have a tendency to see the glass as half empty. But it's not helpful for everyone.

For example, telling a woman who has been brutally gang-raped or telling a village where hundreds of people were murdered, that "It's all good" is not empowering—it's simply ridiculous. It's not "all perfect," just as it is. Not every act is "intended for the highest good." Because the collective consciousness is still at a stage where it's awakened by horrors, it's easy to make the assumption that every tragedy was God's will. It isn't. Sometimes people are just acting out their malevolence. Sometimes acts are merely tragic errors in judgment. The shock of a tragedy can prompt our armored hearts to open. But that doesn't mean the universe planned it for our highest good. There is necessary suffering, and there is also needless suffering. As we become more acquainted with our inner lives, we get better at making the distinction.

M: So how do I apply this in my own life? After being perpetually positive for so long, how do I find the balance again? Have you started a PPS support group?

JB: I tried, but they all said, "Life is good," and refused to come. ☺ The way that we find the balance is to simply acknowledge that there are some painful situations where good will somehow emerge—perhaps in the form of a gift or lesson… and there are many situations that are just plain tragic. End of story.

M: I guess it's safe to assume that you don't resonate with this quote, "Whatever transpires—love that." My friend keeps repeating it to me when the chips are down.

JB: Very safe to assume. It is just the latest in a long line of teachings that hand us the illusion of non-duality, before we go through all the steps painstakingly and organically. It's just another way of saying "It's all good." It is a dangerous—and potentially deadly—quote.

M: I don't interpret this quote as meaning that I have to see everything that happens as good, but, instead, that I find a way to keep my heart open and loving, no matter what transpires.

JB: No matter what! That would be inhumane. This would imply that the woman who was brutally gang-raped should keep her heart open to these perpetrators... So, along with them pillaging her body, she is also expected to open the door of her heart and welcome them in? My friend, we discussed this before. Establishing healthy boundaries is a legitimate human ability. Boundaries exist to keep us safe and intact. Human suffering has been denied, re-framed, up-framed, re-languaged, since the beginning of time. Telling people to love their every experience, and to keep loving those who violate them, is just another bypass trip. The "love everything and everyone" bypass. We won't heal until we can hold the space for the truth of each person's suffering. No bullshit bliss bypass. No artificial forgiveness. Face it all heart-on.

M: But what about unconditional love? As human beings, that's our highest aspiration.

JB: What many fail to understand is that we will not reach the stage of "unconditional love"—assuming for the moment that this is actually possible or desired—until we go through the TRUE emotional processes of owning how we REALLY feel about what has happened, and healing it. I can understand that we want to live in a world where we are safe enough to keep our hearts opened, but we aren't going to get there by denying our rightful anger and pain. We are going to get there by feeling it all, and learning how to co-create a more loving world, while living fully in the heart of reality.

Let's face it, Michael. Acceptance and love are not synonymous. Contrary to common New Cage teachings, acceptance does NOT mean pretending to love something we don't. It means accepting that it happened, and allowing for ANY of the vast spectrum of feelings to arise. *Love may not be one of them.* What is most important is that we are true to how we feel. No fake smiles, no dissociative head-trips. The world has been seeking band-aid solutions to real problems for centuries. There aren't any. We need to get real with the feel if we are going to heal.

M: "Get real with the feel if we are going to heal." Maybe I should tattoo this on my arm.

JB: Let's take that ungrounded quote you mentioned and bring it more into alignment with a grounded sensibility. "Whatever transpires, *feel that.*" That feels more honest, doesn't it?

M: Right now I am contemplating how this would apply to my present circumstances.

JB: Let's take the example of Hannah, and her burning desire to have a child. I want to know how you really feel—not what you want to feel.

M: I detest her sometimes. I feel like she's trying to rob me of my freedom. I don't want a whining brat in my space demanding something of me every few minutes…

JB: Good job, Michael. I've never heard you speak like this before. Now that's legitimate. How you really feel. Only from there can we make progress. It doesn't imply that this feeling is set in stone. Instead, it's a stepping-stone. Step by steady step… we work through our feelings, and they grow and evolve as we walk.

M: I have to admit, it felt fucking good to say that. I'm beginning to see, although I am an advanced spiritualist, I am still a novice when it comes to bridging this into my everyday life. The two worlds don't meet.

JB: The "two worlds" are meant to be bridged through step-by-step grounded and real application. The real-life application is everything. Everyday life doesn't detract from our spiritual life. It gives it feet.

M: Speaking of which, how about we get up and move? I'm done sitting still.

The Forgiveness Bypass

We took the elevator down to ground level. Once there, we headed for the streets. After a few minutes walking west on Front Street, Michael turned north on Spadina Avenue and found a park that he liked just off the main road. We sat down on a bench to continue.

M: Okay, Mr. foot fetish. ☺ Can you guide me in bridging other aspects of my life? I'm just getting a handle on the application process.

JB: Yes, let's look at your dad and Uncle Russell.

M: Funny you mention it. I have been thinking about my Uncle Russell. The violent incident and the sexual abuse. I thought I had forgiven him. But ever since our trip down memory lane, he's been nagging at my consciousness again. I've had some very disturbing dreams about him.

JB: Would you be open to the possibility that you haven't actually forgiven him? True forgiveness can only arise organically, after a genuine healing process. Only then is it authentic. Forgiveness is one of the primary mantras preached by the New Cage and "Positive Psychology" movements. They often encourage people to forgive independent of extensive emotional processes, as though forgiveness is merely a thought, or a concept, or something that can be willed. Some even go so far as to suggest that you must always heal your wounds directly with the wrongdoers, and remain connected to them. Putting our focus on forgiving a wrongdoer *before* we have actually prioritized working through our anger and our pain, is another way we imprison consciousness and overturn reasonable principles of accountability.

Yes, forgiveness can be a beautiful thing… but it is essential that it arises authentically. Forgiveness is not the first place to go after an abusive relationship or a traumatic experience. Healing is. Because forgiveness is not a mental construct. It is not something that can be forced. There is the tendency to claim forgiveness while still holding toxic emotions below the surface of awareness. You know, saying all the right things about how you have let something go.

M: You mean being S.C.?

JB: You got it. While still seething with anger beneath the surface. This is little more than inauthentic forgiveness. If forgiveness of other arises organically, so be it. If it doesn't, there is no issue. We are not responsible for those who wound us. They can take that up with God, or whatever they answer to. I call the tendency to arrive at forgiveness before going all the way through an authentic healing journey: "The Forgiveness Bypass." That is, the attempt to rise above unresolved emotions by feigning forgiveness. This is not only an ungrounded tendency—because you cannot actually will yourself into a feeling of forgiveness—it's also a dangerous one. The unhealed emotional material will come back to assert itself and haunt us in various forms: internal splitting and confusion, passive aggressive behavior, and the toxic impact of held emotions. In the process, we become another step removed from an authentic presence. Because at some level—we are not living our truth.

M: Your way of thinking appeals to part of me. I like the idea that I can be true to my feelings. But how am I ever going to truly heal, if I am holding a grievance against Uncle Russell, or anyone for that matter? It's not about exonerating him. It's about exonerating myself. For the sake of my own healing, I need to forgive him.

JB: No, you don't. Because forgiveness of other is not always the appropriate response. There are actually situations where it is more healing not to forgive. That is the genuine and true response. Forgiveness of self is essential. But I don't believe that forgiveness of other is always the healthy outcome. Some of us actually heal and choose not to forgive. Imagine that!

M: Hmmm… Never considered this before.

JB: Let me give you an example. A scenario. Like the rape victim I mentioned. Let's say she went through an authentic healing process and arrived at a place where she was no longer tormented by the memories. Perhaps it's right and honest to forever hate and despise those individuals, while still moving through her own healing process. Why can't she come to a place of peace with path, a deep letting go of the memories and suffering, without also inviting her aggressors into her heart through an act of forgiveness? Have they not taken enough? What's wrong with no-forgive and forget?

M: When you present it with such an extreme example, I can kind of understand. But what about people like you and I, in our everyday life situations.

JB: Let me give you an example from my own life. There are a few people I still have not forgiven, and probably never will. And I am healthy, and clear, and at peace. One is a family friend who repeatedly stole from all of us, despite endless apologies and second chances. Another, a relative who sexually assaulted his children for many years. In both cases, I went through a lengthy grieving process and came through it comfortable with the decision not to forgive. I don't wish ill-will upon them, I simply don't feel that forgiving them is my responsibility. It is not my genuine response—and I honor that.

So, going back to Uncle Russell. I surmise that the reason he is nagging at your psyche and appearing in your dreams since you unearthed that memory—is because you haven't truly forgiven him. Let me ask you this: If you remove all filters, all affirmations: What honestly comes up when you think of Uncle Russell?

M: Let me authentically see.

Michael closed his eyes and put his head in his hands. I could feel the micro-moments creeping by, slowly like molasses. I could almost feel a palpable vortex of energy around him, as he probed his inner recesses. It was clear—he was getting HONEST. It seemed to be a touch of eternity—before he looked up and spoke again.

M: I think, "that fucking bastard." He ruined my father's life. And he has nearly ruined my relationship with my father. My dad wasn't the same after that incident. Sexually abusing your younger brother? What kind of sick fuck would do such a thing. That destroyed Dad. No wonder he was so shut down emotionally. He couldn't handle the pain and shame of what he endured as a child. And, as I am coming to realize, that incident also played a big role in turning me away from life. The more I think about it, the more fucking rage I feel.

He suddenly became very agitated, a jumbled stream of words spilled from his mouth faster than his lips could shape them. An arsenal of repressed feelings bubbling to the surface. It was clear that this was not only his rage—but also the ancestral strands from his father's repressed emotions. When we don't heal our own wounds—they are passed down. And when we do opt to heal—the balm ripples back through the past, and forward into the future. Michael was immersed in a pivotal process right now.

M: I actually want to fucking kill him.

His words were like potent daggers, severing ties to his troubled childhood. He was cutting the cords of falsity with every honest admission.

JB: That's understandable, and nothing to be ashamed of. You can make the sensible choice to not act on such an impulse, while still feeling it fully. Let it burn through you, like a raging fire.

My instruction must have sparked something. Soon, he stopped and buried his head in his hands.

M: My poor Dad. My poor DADDY.

The tears began to fall. The expression of the rage allowed room for the grief and sadness in waiting, to rise to the surface. Tears cleansing the debris of decades—God's heartshield wipers. How wondrous it was to heal. How magnificent the intelligence of our inner process—that intrinsically knows how to re-stitch and mend our broken pieces. All we have to do is give it space.

JB: There you have it. Well, it is clear, you haven't forgiven him yet. And appropriately so. Recognize that. Admit and embrace whatever feelings are there. Forgiveness doesn't even need to be the end result. Because our healing happens through a depthful, involuntary, and authentic emotional process, one that has no clear destination. The journey will take you wherever it will—and there may be some surprising and unexpected stops along the way. Layering mandatory forgiveness onto that process only artificializes it. You cannot arrive at your true destination if you carry the belief that you must feel anything in particular when you arrive. We must journey without agenda or concern for the result.

M: I feel I am understanding the real meaning of forgiveness.

JB: Yes, forgiveness is not a concept. It's a process. And, if you choose not to forgive at the end of that process, it doesn't mean that you are unhealed. It doesn't mean that you are a lesser human. It doesn't mean you are not spiritual or evolved. It doesn't mean you will come back in the next lifetime to live it out again. That's just New Cage nonsense. It may just mean that forgiveness is not actually in your integrity. The assumption that forgiving the abuser is the benchmark of a completed emotional and karmic process is the mistake. The real benchmark of resolution is whether you have gone through your emotional process authentically and have arrived at a place where the negative charge around the experience has dissipated. Perhaps you will learn some lessons, or perhaps you will eventually be legitimately liberated from the memories. Perhaps you will work it through so completely that you have very little energetic charge around Uncle Russell. Or perhaps you will actually realize that forgiveness is not essential to your healing, and not your responsibility. The point is that focusing on our responsibility to forgive a wrongdoer, sidetracks the whole process. Your sole responsibility is to arrive at whatever destination is true to you.

M: You have a unique way of seeing the world. This stuff is not out there, in the mainstream yet.

JB: Start by over-turning one stone at a time. And don't let anyone guilt you into forgiveness. Many who preach forgiveness are merely bypassing their own unprocessed victimhood. Trauma survivors in denial, they need you to artificially forgive, so that they can turn off the tap of their own remembrance. If they can push you into premature-forgiveness, they no longer have to see the reflection of their own unprocessed pain in you. It's the most dangerous game of all—to invite forgiveness of another, before a victim has been truly seen in their woundedness, before they have honestly moved through their own organic process. If you have been wounded, you have been wounded. It's that simple. And you won't heal it, and the world won't evolve beyond its hurtful ways, if we sweep that truth under a bushel of forgiveness.

I have a question for you: Do you see the connection between your previously admitted tendency to "rise above" experiences, and your similarly pain-avoidant attitude toward forgiveness?

M: Yes, I do. I see the way that I went back and forth between seeking absolute equanimity, and seeking the light.

JB: No shadows allowed on this trip-the-light-fantastic dance floor.

M: Yep, something like that. Hey, I want to apologize. I know this has been a rough meeting. I'm aware I've been resorting to old coping mechanisms, just to get by. My disaster of a job, counseling with Hannah, a possible child. I wanted to take a shortcut to deal with all this. It's obvious now—there isn't one.

JB: I get it, my friend. It seems like everything in your life is converging into one point: your past, your present, and your future. Everything is coming up to be clarified. I give you credit for not running away. You have come a long way. Crystal healing and all.

M: Haha, I secretly knew you would get a kick out of that. That's why I shared it with you. It gave my crystal healing technique no hope of survival. You've ruined me. No more running away. Damn you.

JB: Happy to be cursed if it helps to liberate you.

The Mirror Bypass

M: Well, this has been a big day. It's already dusk. I guess I should let you go. Although I kind of feel I can talk all night. We're on a roll here.

JB: Fun for me too.

M: I'm not going to head back to my lonely abode. Hannah is still living with her best friend, Robin, for now. I think I'm going to grab a beer.

JB: Ahh, nice. I'm on my own tonight too. Susan is leading a circle for young poets.

M: Care to join me?

JB: I don't usually drink. But why the hell not. There are no absolutes in life.

We got up and headed toward King Street. The scarlet moon was just starting to rise, the chilly nights becoming shorter. We were soon drawn to a quaint brick tavern: Danny Gallagher's Irish Pub. It was dimly-lit with a Celtic Band playing jovial music, and people smiling and clanging together frosty mugs of beer. Out of the foggy window, I could see the first snowflakes of the season begin to gently tumble down. We felt protected in our cozy little bubble. I thought we would use the time to laugh and shoot the shit, but Michael seemed eager to resume the topic. He was truly getting somewhere. We ordered some Guinness on tap, and went back at it.

M: I think part of my issue with this non-forgiveness stuff is that I don't want to turn into a judgmental bastard. I still want to retain my peaceful vibration.

JB: Yup, the anti-judgment mantra is yet another way that the New Cage movement sidesteps personal responsibility for their actions. Don't judge! Yet in truth, we are judging all the time. We were granted the gift of discernment and critical thinking. Thank God for that—it keeps us from walking down the wrong paths, making unhealthy decisions, destroying our lives. Even those who criticize judgment are judging. It's fundamental to the human experience. Perhaps the real question is not IF we are judging (or discerning, if you prefer), but WHY we are judging? Is it benevolently or malevolently intended? Are we judging in a forward-moving effort to distinguish unhealthy from healthy, or are we judging as a reflection of an unresolved superiority complex? Are we judging because we have a need to call out the madness of the world, or as a direct reflection of it? Where are we coming FROM?

M: Yes, I see that, but I also see how a no-judgment consciousness helped me to stop looking down on people the way that my parents did. I remember a key moment as a little boy, when I made this shift in my thinking. We were at one of those arena churches, when the preacher began disparaging homosexuals. Where before I would agree with most everything he said, this time was different. I probed into what need I was satisfying, by being judgmental toward a person I had never actually met. I saw that it momentarily eased my fears of something different, and made me feel like I was part of a community, bonded in our judgment over that which wasn't like us. And then something shifted. I began to imagine the people he was referencing, in their actual flesh and blood. I imagined their struggles, their early life experiences, their challenges fitting in. My heart began to open to them and to the possibility that much of what we judge is rooted in our own anxieties and need to belong. I realized that this so called "other" is struggling to find their way in a confusing world, just like I am. I may not understand their context, but that doesn't mean they are a threat to me. In a flash, I saw how the judgmental tendency of humanity was rooted in a kind of primal fear.

JB: I agree. Judgment can be a divisive and destructive force, often wielded as a weapon against those deemed different. It can divide us, it can undermine our connection to one another, and it can perpetuate an adversarial framework of perception that fractures rather than heals. It is one of the primary roots of the poisonous tree. As a result, it *is* essential that we become conscious of our own unconscious judgmental tendencies, and seek a more compassionate approach where possible. At the same time, we have to be careful not to swing so far in the other direction that we lose contact with reality. Again, it's about that delicate balance. In its extreme forms, the anti-judgment mantra can actually perpetuate the madness it seeks to avoid by nullifying one's freedom of thought and expression, and deflecting personal responsibility for our own actions. It becomes yet another transcendence bypass mechanism, one where individuals repress valid and fair-minded perceptions because they fear that they are being "judgmental" toward others. When this happens, the individual becomes split between an unactualized inner knowing, and an adaptation to an externally influenced "idea" of appropriate behavior. And, that which merits true legitimate judgment gets overlooked.

M: I still think that it's better to lean away from judgments in most situations.

JB: You actually don't Michael—you hold plenty of judgments about those who live in, and of, the world. You've shared many of them with me.

M: Busted, again!

JB: Let's embrace common sense. Not every negative judgment we feel is sourced in our own stuff, or in a past life projection trail. Sometimes our judgments are actually reflections of a conscious discernment process. Sometimes we are appalled by certain behaviors because we have evolved to the point where we can distinguish good from bad, healthy from unhealthy, benevolent from malevolent. If we remove our capacity for judgment all together, we will never reach our true potential, as we are muting one of our key superpowers: discernment. Conscious judgments keep us alive, and fuel the sacred activism that improves our world. If we lose the capacity to judge, we lose the capacity to effect the kinds of change that will make the world a safer and more inclusive place.

M: But look at the bigger picture, bro. There is something to be said for the idea that we don't judge, that this human drama, or *lila*, as some traditions call it, can appear horrifying, yet is actually all part of the divine plan.

JB: Michael, we can't forego our human experience here in this life, in favor of some "bigger picture." Both need to be included. The micro and the macro. And here in this world, in this here life, it's about making the distinction between arbitrary, malicious judgment, and grounded, meaning-based discernment. The former destroys, the latter honors our intuition and supports our efforts to create a healthier reality. The important thing is to enhearten our processes of discernment, so that we are both honoring our own right to choose, and coming from a compassionate source spring. In other words, to do the least harm when we are making distinctions between what resonates and what doesn't.

M: Yes, I can hear that.

JB: You could have trusted your own judgment regarding the new job position you took. Your body provided you with a stream of highly intelligent cues. You overrode them. Now you're miserable.

M: Ouch. I wonder though. So often I feel as though my judgments are rooted in my own reflection. Like the person I am judging is a mirror back to me. I dislike elements of their personality, or actions, because I dislike similar elements in myself. Perhaps everything is a projection. Everything I think I see is an illusion. Everything is a representation of my own consciousness. The universe is holographic.

JB: Ahh, the old mirror trick. You mean, you disdain the rapist because you are a rapist?

M: No, not necessarily that I am a rapist... but that I am hiding from my own dark side, that I don't want to see and own. You are really big on the "shadow theory"... why are you denying it in this context? Another perspective is that perhaps I was a rapist in a past life...

JB: So, here we again see the over-the-top counter-balancing tendency of New Cage thinking. Instead of striking a reasonable balance—one where we recognize that our judgments *sometimes* reflect our projections, and other times reflect a healthy discernment process—they swing all the way to the extreme. *Everything* is a mirror. *Everything*, a reflection. Imagine if we had not learned a single thing about right and wrong, good and bad, healthy or unhealthy, after centuries of human development. That would be a travesty. Imagine the world you would be living in—lawless, primitive, purely survivalistic. That's not true evolution.

M: Well, I am not seeing too many signs of improvement in our species. Maybe we haven't made any meaningful moral progress. Maybe we are still stuck in the starting blocks. Maybe...

JB: Let me give you an example from my own life. I met a woman once. A brilliant, beautiful woman. Fell crazy in love with her. Transported to divine places in her presence. And then the fighting began, as it often does when a connection soars away from the earth. If I had been grounded, I would have ended the connection soon after seeing how impossible it was. But I stayed in there, and suffered terribly because I was so affixed—as you seem to be—to the idea that EVERY negative judgment I had about her was actually entirely about me. If she stole from me, I focused on the things I stole as a child. If she screamed at me, I remembered moments I had screamed at others. If she fled the connection to be with another, I focused on my own wayward history. It was only when she tried to knock me unconscious with a brick that I woke up from my New Cage slumber. You see, I had never tried to do that. So I could no longer let her off the hook with the mirror game. I ended the relationship.

M: She really tried to clout you with a brick?

JB: Yep, and I wasn't the only one. I later found out she had a very explosive history. At this stage in our human consciousness, violence and wrong-doing is a very real thing. This "mirror bypass" often invites us away from reality—the reality of wrong-doing and the truth of how we really feel about someone's characteristics or actions. Even if some of their characteristics are similar to our own, this doesn't mean that we like those characteristics or have to embrace them in another. It is also perfectly fine to dislike something in another that is dissonant with who we are or with what we value. We can respect everyone's right to be who they are, while also accepting our right to dislike, or even fear, some of their characteristics.

Quite often, the mirror trick is used as a defense against accountability by "spiritual superiors," who expertly shift the focus away from their own actions by turning the mirror back on those they have wronged, "Look! It's not me you dislike, it's actually yourself!" Trickster gurus are particularly adept at these techniques. The guru claims that his questionable actions were not actually for his own benefit, but done with the conscious intention of reflecting back to you the unresolved aspects of your own consciousness. If you felt betrayed, it was because you have issues around betrayal that you need to look at. Try making a pass at the guru's girlfriend, and see what he says then. It all comes back to good ole common sense. Sometimes we are projecting, and sometimes we are seeing things exactly as they are.

M: Fair enough, but projection or not, it still all feels like an illusion. Like what is truly real, stands outside of these petty patterns.

JB: Again, countless gurus and spiritual teachers have used, "It's all an illusion," in an effort to bypass responsibility for their misdeeds. And now it has become a mutating virus that has spread throughout the New Cage community—you see people from all walks of life trapped inside this nonsense. It's all reality when it serves them, and it's all an illusion when it doesn't. We have to be careful with this kind of languaging. Healthily applied, "It's all an illusion" supports a conscious inquiry into what is real and what isn't. Unhealthily applied, it supports the manipulation of humanity. Sometimes it's an illusion, sometimes it isn't. Again, it comes back to the sacred gift of discernment. And it's for each individual to discern the difference on their own terms.

M: Hmmm…

By now, the beer was starting to kick in. After giving up drinking years ago for health reasons, I was a bit of a lightweight. I could feel my inner comedian rising to the surface.

These past months with Michael, I had maintained a generally serious demeanor. After all, we had some serious deconstructing to do together. It was time to let loose.

JB: Think of it this way, Mike. If it's ALL a mirror, then I got me some work to do. No, wait, no need—it's ALL an illusion. ☺ Wait, how can it be both? If it's all an illusion, there isn't anything to mirror. And if it's all a mirror, then none of it is an illusion. Methinks the New Cage movement is confusing its bypass mantras! My illusory head just smashed my illusory mirror into illusory bits. Watch where you step… or not.

M: You're something else. There's no one like you. You're a pain in my ass big time. And that pain in my assness—is NOT a freaking mirror. You are not reflecting my own pain in the assness. You truly are one.

JB: Hey, I have an idea. Next time you have a terrible thing happen to you and someone says, "You choose your every experience," knock them unconscious. ☺ When they wake up again, ask them to thank you for actualizing their dream. And then, insist that they forgive you before they have even healed their head wound. Then tell them, "Pain is an illusion—just be aware of it, witness it, and you will come into the 'Power of Now.'" Then, remind them that there are no victims and that they just need to "turn around" their story of victimhood. When they try to get up, push them back down on the ground, and remind them, "Everything you see and experience is a reflection of you." Tell them: "You must have had some issues that you needed to look at around violence. I gave you a gift. Be grateful." When they begin to get angry, remind them that anger and judgments are substandard emotions, and that there is never anyone to blame. If this doesn't soften their edges, inform them that the ego is the enemy, and that the part of them that is perceiving this situation as unacceptable—is merely misidentified: "You are trapped in the matrix, and seeing the world through that limited lens." Tell them you are here to liberate them. And then, steal their wallet, and demand they give you their PIN number. So they can learn another valuable lesson about attachment and manifestation.

Don't actually do this, Michael. ☺

M: Haha. You gave away your age, dude! No one under 50 calls it a "pin number!" It's just a PIN: Personal Identification Number.

JB: Words, words, words. All an illusion anyway!

We roared with laughter for some time, before I finally recovered my serious demeanor to wrap up the night.

JB: In all seriousness Michael, we must ground our spirituality in common sense before it becomes another prison. When we begin to believe that we have a choice in EVERYTHING that happens to us, that forgiveness of other must come before self-forgiveness, that all judgments—even conscious discernments—are unhealthy, that there are NO victims, that our stories are ALWAYS untrue, that witnessing our pain IS presence, that the ego in its ENTIRETY is our enemy, that ABSOLUTELY everything we see or feel is a reflection of who we are, that ALL illness is self-created... then we have just entered another prison cell. In a nutshell: the New Cage movement. With gurus as wardens, and transcendence bypassers as inmates. Better to bust out of that unreal prison while we still can. I know a few people who signed up for life, and left us by their own hand, when reality came calling and they no longer had the tools to manage it. If it sounds too good to be true, it probably is. Again, spirituality is not all fairies and unicorns. It's reality, in all its complexity.

M: Okay, its 10 o'clock. This is officially getting too serious for this late at night. How about we close shop and stumble our way home?

JB: Sounds like a plan.

We hobbled our way onto the street and stumble-walked together for a few blocks, before realizing that we needed to hail taxis. It was a frosty night in Toronto, and we needed a chauffeur. As the cabbie drove me up Bathurst Street, I thought back on the many meetings I'd had with Michael these past few months. A lot of insights imparted, many differing points hashed out mercilessly, many approaches taken in an effort to invite him back here. If I had been asked after the first moments of meeting him if he would have hung in there this long... I would have predicted that there was no way he would keep coming back for more. He seemed much too entrenched in his spiritual philosophies and practices. I was wrong. That's the thing about humans. Just when you think you have them pegged, they show you a whole other dimension, one that reveals your own limited perceptions. I'm always happy to be wrong about human possibility. It's the furthest thing from an illusion.

PART THREE

WHY

9 Sacred Purpose

You are the mystic,
set among the unseeing,
whirling in passion first believed,
fused in patterns of deep meaning.
Breathe in and stretch out,
all your senses entranced.
Skirts swirling all about,
as your purpose becomes
the dance.

—SUSAN FRYBORT

After our night at the bar, I expected to hear from Michael soon after. We were making real headway, both in our friendship, and in Michael's commitment to the unfurling of his process. Instead, eight weeks went by. It was the peak of winter. In the outside world, the hustle-bustle of the pressure-filled holiday season permeated the atmosphere. Within, a deep hibernation spell as I burrowed into crafting my next book. I thought about contacting him during that time, but a quieter voice told me to leave him be. We would reconnect at the right time. Simply trust the unfolding and ripening of the process.

And then, a month into the new year, arrived an email.

Hey my friend,

I miss our talks.

Life has been good. Not easy, but good. I feel I have turned a corner. I've been vigilantly applying your exercises. Doing loads of inner work. I've noticed some changes. My body is moving more fluidly—feels less bogged down. I am more willing to feel into my emotions. Yet my daily life is still a mess. My relationship with Hannah is at a standstill.

Something needs to break. My job is grueling. So, in some ways life is harder than ever. And in other ways, there is progress.

Anyway, can we talk in person?

His email made me smile. I invited him over to my home office. Our rapport had developed enough where my office was no longer taboo for him. He could see that even though I appeared to have my shit together, my office desk was about the messiest on the planet. ☺ It was time to ground our conversation in my everyday world.

JB: Good to see you my friend. Those few months felt like a long time.

M: How have you been?

JB: Good. Nestling deep into drafting my new book.

M: What's it called?

JB: Grounded Spirituality.

M: Should have guessed. What else have you been up to?

JB: Doing lots of Barking Dog Yoga to keep me clear while I write. Teaching an online writing course. An amazing collection of students doing brave healing work. Susan is visiting her daughter this week. I've been learning how to cook for myself again. Thus the mess in the kitchen.

M: How's that going?

JB: Let's just say that its going.

M: Haha. It's fantastic to see you. As I said in my email, I've been applying your exercises and am embracing your version of "Enrealment"—the whole enchilada. Glimmers of real progress in the inner world. Yet, life on earth is still a mess. Both personally and collectively. So much insanity going on in our world right now. I can't remember things ever being this grim.

JB: Or maybe you just weren't paying attention.

M: Yes, could be. As you have often acknowledged, it's so bloody painful in the world at this stage of human development. I am actually being present for it now. At the same time wondering: What would propel me to endure all of this without fleeing? Why would I bother to embrace it? If Hannah and I do end up having a child, it feels as though the best thing I can teach them is how to shield their consciousness from the mad world, not how to fully experience it. Why invite a pristine new life-form into *here* when it seems more sane to just detach from the nonsense and find a state of equanimity, even pseudo-equanimity?

JB: Wow, Michael. That you can even let the possibility of "a child" roll off your tongue is significant, in itself. You are right, the inner clearings and work you are doing are affecting your whole body and being.

M: Yes, but the work isn't changing the fact that this world is a distorted and fucked-up place. If anything, I am more acutely aware of it than ever before. I feel like hiding under a rock. Or going into a monastery.

JB: Ahh, the ole escapist tendencies. Old patterns die hard. Take heart, my friend. The fact that the world is so distorted is simply because we have lost sight of our profound individual significance. We have not been encouraged to see our place in the world through a vaster and more purposeful lens. We have been squelched down and controlled, too shamed and diminished to recognize our individual magnificence. We have not been taught that we come into this life inherently purposeful, meaning-based, ripe for transformation, and sharing our gifts. We have not been offered a perspective that will empower us to stand in the fires of reality, knowing deep within our bones both why we are here, and that we are so very capable. We have been taught to look outside ourselves for our answers, and our security. The beautiful thing is—you can bring your child these gifts. You can impart these lessons. You can make a tremendous impact on one human being's existence.

M: Oh shit. But I haven't even learned this myself.

JB: You still can. That's why we are meeting here today. Let's try another way of being on for size. It's time. I call it "sacred purpose." The authentic antidote for a lifeless, generic way of being. It is through this lens of sacred purpose that we will be able to make sense of *why* we are here. That we will be inspired to come into here and to remain here, fully embodying all that we are. It is our sacred purpose that will empower us to live our lives with passion and healthy self-regard. It is our sacred purpose that will buffer us against the madness of the world, and allow us to transform it. Despite the seeming reasons to feel otherwise, I move from the core belief that each of us comes into this lifetime with an encoded purpose residing at the heart of our birth. And that an unshakeable connection to our purpose will empower us to remain steadfast and present in the heart of life's challenges. Because we will recognize that we are not merely here to survive—we are here to grow humanity forward. Each of us in our own way.

M: Yes, I always knew I had a divine purpose. Since a child, I knew my life was not meant to be ordinary, but extraordinary. And that I would glide a step above, in the world yet not of it. That's what launched me on my spiritual path. My knowing of my special purpose in this lifetime. Again, this is why I won't bring a child into this world. I have a higher path in life, Jeffrey. Not just to be married and have a child. That's ordinary. This life is meant to be extraordinary. Thank you for reminding me of that.

JB: Not so fast. You are speaking of Divine Purpose. I am speaking of Sacred Purpose, which has its deep roots, here on earth, in time.

M: Shit.

JB: Divine purpose implies that our purpose is emanating, again, from something outside of the self, almost as though we are being used as some kind of divinely channeled instrument. I use the word 'sacred' because it doesn't immediately imply that our reasons for being originate outside of ourselves, in some kind of cosmic field. Sacred Purpose empowers the self, and acknowledges its sacrosanct—and intrinsically purposeful—nature. Language matters. Let's begin here within our own flesh and bones, before considering our interface with The Divine.

M: So, tell me specifically: What is Sacred Purpose? I get it, it's not divine purpose.

JB: Sacred purpose is that unique combination of callings, archetypes, lessons, significant relationships, and key emotional issues that each of us is here to clarify, to embody, to actualize, to transform, and to grow through. We all have callings, gifts, and offerings to excavate, unpack, and humanifest. We all have essential archetypes that live at the heart of our expansion. We all have ancestral imprints, patterns and issues that provide the fuel for our transformation. These are not the antithesis of our spiritual lives but live at the heart of our human potential. Because of the gripping nature of survivalist codes that exist in our DNA and cultural conditioning, we have the tendency to define ourselves in linear, practical terms—the accountant, the spiritual person, the loving mother, the wife, the husband—but we are actually multi-dimensional. We are so much more than meets the eye. We glimpse this in our dreamscapes and in our nightmares—there is a much richer world within us than the one we encounter in our waking consciousness. That sublime world is a reflection of our sacred purpose—the profound significance of each birth, the deeper currents and rhythms that thread through us, the real *why we are here*. Far from being one-trick ponies, each of us is a "polyphrenic soul," entering this world with a sacred purpose to uncover: a multitude of treasures, pathways, potentialities and brilliant shades of possibility that both reflect our soul's growing edge, and our unique contribution to the world. We honor our purpose both because it grows us individually, and also because it grows us forward as a humanity. We are in this, together. We are *this*, together.

M: Okay, so what's mine? Is it working in a dim office in a downtown Toronto skyscraper, programming codes and selling cutting-edge software apps? Coming home at 9 o'clock at night, too wiped out to even cuddle with my wife? Is that my contribution to the world? That's dire.

JB: No, that's perfect. Now you are bringing your spiritual inquiry down to earth. A pivotal step. In the recognition of how misaligned your life is—is the doorway to your sacred purpose, lying in wait.

M: Hmmm.

Soul-Scriptures

JB: Could it be… that your relating to this "divine purpose," has kept you from looking head-on at the direness of your current situation? With divine purpose, you are kept safe, cushioned from the searing pain of your life. It can all stay pretty in a nebulous cosmic glow. Gift-wrapped in New Age positive thinking and affirmations. But, when you look at the nuts and bolts of it, it's not pretty. And yet only here can your life actually change to reflect a true earthly radiance that is infused throughout your whole body, here and now, in real time. You have stayed removed in this higher vision of your Buddhalike-presence that will someday come through. This has prohibited you from landing it here. Making it real.

M: But not everyone has some great calling to transform the world, Jeff.

JB: Every calling is great. It all comes down to how we define "callings." We may not all have a Gandhi-like calling to liberate millions, but we all have the capacity to impact the world. And that is precious. Don't underestimate the mountain of power in seemingly small acts. Describing a life fueled by callings and sacred purpose only in BIG terms is misleading. Some of us are called to a large, visible canvas, yet that path is no more valuable, or true, or profound than a more subtle path. For many of us, sacred purpose lies in the private unseen places, in the shifting patterns, in the warm breezes of transition. It is all sacred purpose, wherever there is authentic expression and expansion. It needn't be grandiose to have meaning, but it must be lived to its fullest. When we each live our sacred purpose, stitch by tiny stitch, we weave together an unseen tapestry that grows the collective. You having a profound impact as a father on one being, one child, would ripple on forever.

M: Stop! Enough about the child.

JB: Testy, testy… You were the one who brought it up! But okay, I will leave the child out for now. Let me contextualize sacred purpose further. Think of the world that your grandparents grew up in, and the one their grandparents grew up in. In that survivalistic world—where most of us come from—we were defined by what put food on the table. Your purpose was that which enabled you, and those in your care, to survive. And if you were good at it, if you succeeded pragmatically, you were considered a success through the eyes of the world. Because success was security, pragmatism, power over others, the ability to make your life "work." And your personal identifications, your ways of being, your life decisions reflected this framework of perception. You became whatever you had to become, to ensure your survival. Callings and gifts—"what are those?" Adaptation and accumulation over authenticity. These were the markers of a fulfilled life. At the time, we thought of this as our "purpose," but in truth, it was only our function. We had yet to discover our true and profound purpose. We are entering a different time now... We are ready.

M: Shit, again. This stuff scares me. It feels so real.

JB: Yes, it's the real deal Michael. This isn't the dawn of the "Golden Age" of consciousness you envisioned. One where we find purpose in the "enlightened" emptiness. This isn't the woo earth. We are at a new dawn... and it does not descend upon us—it rises up from within, as a way of being that is sourced in who we REALLY ARE, with solid roots here in form. Not our mastery face, not our survivalist face, but the real face, the real path, the no bull-shit, no hype, no pretense expression of WHO YOU REALLY ARE, and a life that fully and deeply expresses your inherent magnificence. In the world we are stepping into, we will define success wholly differently. Success becomes a function of our authenticity, not our capacity for survival alone. That is, we will continue to prioritize the meeting of our basic needs—we can't thrive if we don't survive—while simultaneously ensuring that the way we move through the world reflects who we really are, and why we are really here. We will probe deeply into the core questions of our lives: Do my life choices reflect the underlying currents and rhythms of my soul's journey? Are the faces I show the world congruent with my authentic inner face, or are they masks and disguises? Am I being true to path, or am I merely gratifying my unhealthy ego?

M: Bro, this is new territory for me. For decades, I thought of my purpose as spiritual evolution itself. Evolving my consciousness. That was my end-game. But you are presenting the possibility that my evolution is contained here in this human life, and that it expresses itself in a unique and nuanced way.

JB: So many of us have defined ourselves and made our life decisions by adapting our identities to the structures outside of us. The next step is adapting our structures to who we really are. Allowing our authenticity to shape the world in its image, rather than allowing the world to shape us in its image.

M: And what would that look like for me?

JB: That's for you to uncover, Michael. Our sacred purpose is innate within us—but it takes de-layering. That requires some work. Rigorous excavation and digging, clearing blocks and obstacles. Much of this territory we already covered in previous dialogues, and you are well on your way, my friend. Your sacred purpose is not far from view. And when you find it—it will seem like something you somehow have known all of your life.

M: Mmmm. I could imagine what that feels like...

JB: I often refer to Sacred Purpose as our "soul-scriptures"—a karmic blueprint that grounds us, expands us, and injects meaning into our lives. Each of our scriptures is like a seed planted in the inner field, awaiting detection and watering, eventually blooming into a bountiful field of possibility. They are the lessons we came here to learn, the "true-path" we are here to walk, the soulshape we are here to grow into. To the extent that we recognize and actualize our scriptures, we mature in our spirituality. To the degree that we misidentify, we walk a false-path and delay our expansion. Think of your scriptures as a library that lives inside of you, waiting to be read and lived. Each of us is a library of in-coded possibility, with purpose inscribed soul-scriptures waiting for us on every inner shelf. If the library is neglected, if the books remain untouched, your expansion is stilted. Again, our sacred purpose, composed of our unique set of soul-scriptures, lives at the heart of our actualization. We don't need to turn away from it. We need to turn toward it.

M: Hmmmf.

JB: The roots of this concept have been threaded through time immemorial. But now we are ready to take it to the next earthly level. Whatever words we use, I think of these inherent potentialities as fundamental to the soul's journey through time. I call this process "Soulshaping"—thus the name of my first book. That is, even if our birth circumstances seemed haphazard and unplanned, we enter this incarnation at a certain stage in our soulular development, with an inherent drive to expand beyond it. Getting to the next place and growing into more of who we are, requires that we both recognize the constituent elements of our sacred purpose, and that we humanifest them. Our sacred purpose may be difficult to discern, it may be covered in dirt, but it's still inside, gleaming with profound possibility. Contrary to the idea that we are all accidents, existential anomalies, dust in the wind—we are the opposite. We are each benevolently intended, purposeful and essential to this wondrous dance.

M: Jeff, you are starting to sound a little mystical and ethereal. That's not your usual style. Not everyone would agree that we come into life sprinkled with fairy dust and a 'sacred' intention.

JB: I tried to tell you early on, my Grounded Spirituality includes ALL THAT IS—from the magical to the mundane—all moving from and through our humanness. The juncture where form and formlessness mingle together in fertile alchemy. I am sharing this because I feel you have done the ground-work. You are ready for it. Grounded Spirituality strikes a sacred balance between our experience of unity consciousness and our connection to true-path: that place where we feel both connected to the Oneness and deeply connected to our personal purpose in the heart of it. As I said before… you must find that sacred point where the ocean of essence, meets the individual droplet of meaning.

M: But not everyone believes in a soul that is journeying through time.

JB: Even if you don't buy the idea that our soul travels through time, or that we chose a particular path for this incarnation, can you accept that for whatever reason, you have certain gifts that want to be expressed? Certain lessons you would benefit from learning? Certain issues and patterns that you would benefit from working through, certain people you need to grow toward or away from? In other words, wherever there is the impetus for growth, there is sacred purpose. How does that resonate?

M: It sounds compelling. But I told you… I have always found my purpose independent of the fluctuations of the human experience.

JB: Now *you* are sounding ethereal. It's not up there that we find our path through life's forests—the purpose is already encoded in our cells, in our bones, in our lifeblood.

M: First, you let go of your habitual or limiting ideas of who you are, and only then can you arrive at your purpose in the space beyond them.

JB: Floating into nothingness is not a purpose, dear man. You are again referencing the ungrounded spiritual skyscape you have flown through. The idea that you extinguish your self-hood, and then rest your consciousness out there, in the great beyond. One will not find their purpose out there. Save that for when you're dead.

M: No thank you.

JB: Sure, you can do some work to elevate your perspective and to distinguish healthy and unhealthy personal identifications, but then you have to come back down into your selfhood to develop and eventually embody your answers here. The universe can support that inquiry, but the information you seek is in your body, right at the heart of your lived experience. You find your directions in your lived experience, not from an All-Oneness field. There is an interface between your individual path and unity consciousness. But that interface relates more to the way that your individual purpose contributes to the oneness. Oneness is not to be utilized in a way that drowns or negates your unique offerings below a tsunami of unity. That is what happens all too often in the New Cage movement. Too much of the 'One,' too little of the "1." Again, the universe didn't go through all of this trouble for us to find our meaning outside of our humanness. Our path is not out-coded. It's in-coded. It's inside of us—it *is* us. We just have to learn how to honor it and plumb its depths.

M: Take a breath, dude.

JB: This is yummy stuff for me. It gets my blood pumping. Surely this extraordinary human birth, this powerful emotional body, this energized temple, all the threads and strands of consciousness, were not intended to be bypassed or sidestepped on a quest for the eternal emptiness. The issue is in fact not the self—the issue is that we have yet to find a way to embody our personhood without hurting ourselves and each other. That's our work, that's the natural movement of sacred purpose: to heal and to evolve this world. The disparity is when we attempt to accomplish this by detaching from the body. You can't grow it that way. You grow your soul by embodying it. You grow spiritually by embodying your humanness. Sacred purpose is the way in, the way out, and the way we bridge to the world. Sacred Purpose gives us a reason to keep at it, to stay here, to see ourselves as the artists that we are, sculpting our consciousness and that of the world's, with our heartfelt objectives.

M: Again, we come back to the fundamental tension between our world-views. I experience my purpose as independent of the world. You experience it in the middle of it.

JB: Yup, smack-dab in the center of the self, in the heart of the human experience. And I would take it one step further, actually. In other words, if we aren't in touch with why we are here, we aren't here. And, of course, the corollary is also true: if we aren't inclusively connected to the here, now, on a deeply human level, we cannot connect to the why of our existence. Sacred purpose is where Here meets Why. To the extent that you are living your scriptures, you are nestled into the moment. When you circumvent them, you are somewhere else entirely. Some part of your consciousness is showing up, but another part is in hiding. No spiritual practice is effective unless you are courageously walking your individual path.

The Little Voice That Knows

It was time for some tea. I got up to turn on the kettle. Michael called down from the office. Make that coffee, please. Black. He clearly needed a re-charge. I turned on the percolator, and brought him a cup of steaming black brew. Michael savored his first long sip, and we resumed.

M: You make it sound so easy. How then does one identify their "sacred purpose"? It's one thing to discuss it conceptually, but how does one find it?

JB: I'm not going to pretend it's easy—given that the world offers virtually zero training in identifying our true-path. Yet, since it's intrinsic to our make-up, there are inklings and indicators everywhere. Perhaps the most prevalent form they are wrapped in is something we often call "intuition."

Or, the little voice that knows. It can take the form of an actual voice, or of a subtle inner sense, a gut instinct, an intimation, a whisper in the wind. Whatever form it takes—it is the indicator within that tells you where to step next, and where not to step. We often hear this voice when we are about to make a significant life decision: to marry, or not; to go to school to study; to commit to a specific career; to move to another location. Our intuition arises to warn us, or to invite us in a particular direction. First it is apparent in the larger life choices, but once we begin to rely on it—it gets activated and super-charged. It then shows its face in our small daily choices as well. And through time, as we hone it, listen and abide, it is no longer a separate sense. It becomes the very heartbeat of our movement through the world. Seamlessly integrated into our very being. My inner voice used to have a name.

M: I'm afraid to ask…

JB: She was called Little Missy. I relied on her instruction heavily at first. Always sought her guidance. But eventually Little Missy faded away, as I began to live more in truth. She became an integrated part of me. It is my belief that our intuition, particularly when it is fine-tuned, is a direct reflection of our soul-scriptures. Ceaselessly inviting us in the direction that we are here to walk. And it is our safeguard as well—getting louder when we have walked, or are about to walk, in a direction that is not congruent with our true-path.

M: Again, that sounds good, but it's so very difficult to hear that voice in our overwhelmed daily lives.

JB: Agreed. Hearing the little voice that knows is a real achievement in a high-speed world. For most of us, there's lots of murky material in the way. Although many of us in the Western world meet our basic needs without worry, the collective unconscious is still easily brought back to more primitive points in time—alarmism, survivalism, and terror still reside close to our usual consciousness, and this tension prevents many of us from hearing the whispers of our authentic self.

M: There is so much inner and outer noise, man. I don't even think I can hear my little voice. Can you ask it to speak a little louder?

JB: Yes, there are many obstacles. Our inner listening is also impaired by unresolved emotional issues, and unexpressed feelings that block up the inner channel. And perhaps the biggest obstacles of all are the comforts of falsity—there is something that feels safe about living falsely. We never really risk failure, because we are not actually living our truth.

M: Even when I can hear my intuition, it often leads me in a direction that makes matters worse. It has led me to situations that were downright dangerous or stupid.

JB: Hmmm, you sure that was your inner voice that knows? You see, there is an alchemical relationship between the efficacy of one's intuition and the depthfulness of one's emotional clarity. If you haven't done the deeper work to clear and grow through your emotional debris and hone your internal voice, either because you put your focus more on the mind, as you have, Michael, or if you are like most of us, and your consciousness is more attached to survival strategies than authenticity, it is very unlikely that you will be able to attune to your most clarified intuition. What you experience as intuition, is something more akin to patterned subconscious programming. In order for your intuition to be consistently attuned to what will serve you, you must polish the rough diamond of the soul to such an extent that it gleams with your encoded sacred purpose. If you don't, you will continue to confuse intuition with intermittent murky messages that arise from your hazy inner world.

M: That makes sense. Well, I've begun that path of clearing. I hope it pays off soon. Surely, there are markers of which way to walk, even for those who have not done all the preparation work.

JB: You've got that right, buddy. Because our sacred purpose is ever-determined to find a way to reveal itself. It's an unrelenting bastard with the tenacity of a pit bull. If it can't reach you one way, it will come through another way. The most prevalent indicator of directionality, particularly for those who are not attuned to direct messaging, is something I call "truth-aches," which I define in this way:

> A truth-ache is a persistent cry from within, a symptom of our
> alienation from true-path, a sign that we are not honoring the

sacred purpose encoded in the bones of our being. It can arise in many forms, in its earnest efforts to call us home: physical and/or emotional illness, ceaseless dissatisfaction, a nagging sense that something is amiss, a voice that wakes us up at night fraught with worry. When we don't adhere, the more persistent the voice will become, and in its extreme forms, may urgently demand change. Although uncomfortable, it is a blessing in disguise, an echo of essence, a call to a deeper and more bona fide path. Better we face it while we still can.

M: Sounds miserable. I am still having a hard time imagining that something painful is working for my highest good.

JB: Truth-aches are actually a necessary and positive component of internal exploration and growth. If you listen to the Law of Attraction philosophy, it's easy to buy into the ungrounded idea that misery or discomfort means you are not on the right path. But if you listen to your inner knower, you realize that it's often precisely the shadow material that signals us home. Truth-aches may be uncomfortable, but this is often the nature of expansion. Old archetypes and patterns dig in their heels, clinging to what they know best, and new pathways of possibility push up against them, in an effort to become woven into our ever-expanding soulshape. I learned a lot through pleasure, but even more from pain.

M: Gosh, I think I have a truth-ache. Is this why my body feels like a dead-weight when I am at my job?

JB: No doubt. Because there is a strong energetic charge around that which calls us, there is an exponentially stronger counter-charge that surges through when we deny it. It refuses to die, and shows up in all kinds of different ways to remind us that we have another path to walk. Dissatisfaction with our job is a common one because our work is seldom a reflection of our truest gifts. Truth-aches are a beacon of our multifaceted possibilities, illuminating the next steps on our journey toward wholeness.

If this sounds too abstract, think of the work of Abraham Maslow around the hierarchy of needs. He posited that every organism has a natural actualizing tendency—that is, an inner force that propels it, when unfettered and alight, to strive toward becoming all that it is capable of becoming. Once we meet one need, we plateau there for some period of time, before we begin to feel the deep inner stirrings to reach for the next need in the hierarchy. The quest for sacred purpose is very similar. We have an inherent tendency to grow to the next stage of personal development. It may show up within a relationship, a calling that demands expression, an experience we gravitate toward in an effort to grow, a longing to explore a particular archetype. If we delay it, we experience an internal tension and frustration. We feel stymied because we are longing to grow forward and something—circumstance, fear, belief—is holding us back.

M: I relate to this. Lately I have been feeling encaged in frustration. It seems in some ways I am becoming more clear internally, more fluid, more alive. Yet in my daily life, I feel like I keep banging my head on a ceiling. The walls are closing in on me. Hannah is back, but we are sleeping in separate bedrooms. It's just a matter of time until one of us packs up for good. Lately she is berserk in her clarity, like a madwoman. She needs to have a child, here and now. I'm not there yet.

JB: It sounds like that is her calling, currently wrapped in a truth-ache.

M: Well it's not mine.

JB: You sure about that?

M: I plead the fifth.

JB: Remember I mentioned how callings grow louder and more demanding when they are not adhered to. Sounds like Hannah's calling is at its wit's end.

M: Sure is.

JB: I remember that phase... When I was being propelled to write *Soulshaping*. That bugger would keep me up all night long, tossing and turning, tossing and turning. Sleepless in Toronto. The only thing that would cure my insomnia was following my calling. Hannah, wherever you are, I relate to you. Michael, you are finding yourself smack-dab at a vital crossroads—I call it Sacred Purpose Junction. It's an essential threshold—a precarious point where unseen forces may even rise up to stop you. In order to make it through, you have deeper work ahead of you. You are at a natural point where your external life is no longer a match for your internal life. That is not to say that what Hannah wants will serve you—but it is to say that your work now is to get real clear on what calls you, so that you can align your outer with your inner life. Sacred Purpose is not about walking an easy path. It's about walking an honest path—the path that is truly your own. You walk it because it grows and reflects you, not because you are elated at every turn. At this point of human development, walking sacred purpose often means that you will forge a more challenging path through a minefield of truth-aches, but only there will you find peace with path. Not because it's easy, but because it's yours.

M: Sacred Purpose Junction. That's exactly where I stand.

JB: And, of course, it isn't just the voice inside of us that signals the way home. We are also called in the direction of our true-path by various synchronicities. Of course, we can easily spot synchronicities—interpreting their meaning is the great challenge. Many of us have made the mistake of assuming that every act of synchronicity is an indicator of destiny. It may be, but not always in the ways we imagine. The trick is interpreting what it is trying to tell us. It could mean to walk toward something, or it could be testing our commitment to the path we are already on.

M: I think I did have a past experience of being tested in my commitment regarding my relationship with Hannah. Years ago, I bypassed a calling, and it nearly killed me.

JB: Say more, if you would...

M: We had met, as I mentioned earlier, in New Mexico. We were drawn to each other like bees to honey, for months. It was unstoppable—I couldn't get enough of what I felt when I was with her. It was intoxicating.

JB: What did you experience in her presence?

M: There was the feeling that a great door had opened. Like a passage to another world. Very different from the experiences I have when I am alone with God. You are right about that—there is something vastly different about life when we are connected to certain significant figures on the path. Like they are destined, or necessary to our growth. In those early years, we would make love, or walk together side by side through town, and I would experience a wholeness and completeness. A seamless rightness, like all my pieces had fused together. Not meditating, not doing yoga, nothing other than walking with Hannah. In fact, for awhile I gave up on my meditations. Didn't need them. Our relationship alone was a spiritual practice that set everything right. I knew from the beginning that I had to be by her side, for some if not all of my journey, even if it hurt. That knowing has kept me there, despite the challenges.

JB: Exactly what you realized during the Beloved Meditation. Now, Michael, let this be your guiding light. Especially through these dark and trying times. Anyway, I'm sorry to interrupt, continue on with your story…

M: There was one point in the first year, where my resistance rose up so fiercely, I tried to sever the connection. She was pushing for a commitment, and I began to feel engulfed, like her love was going to consume me. Burn me alive. So, I broke up with her, by text… I know, so cowardly… but I just couldn't face her, or the implications of what I was doing. She didn't even respond. She was so distraught. She just disconnected, or so I imagined. In fact, I found out later that she went into a prayerful state, communicating with my soul and begging that I would wise up and come home to her before it was too late. For a brief time, I went back to my solitary life, and re-focused on my individual path. At first, and I mean for about a week, it felt wonderful, because I was liberated from the feelings of being trapped. I was free, again, or so I imagined. But then, I began to feel like I wasn't here anymore. I mean, I was physically here, but I wasn't truly present. The field of awareness that I had nestled into when in her presence, faded away and I was back to the same lackluster reality I had known before her. It was at that point I knew that there are certain individuals who are fundamental to our journey. Despite my obsession with the individual path, I knew Hannah was essential to my life.

JB: I have a name for those individuals. I call them our "soulpod." Included in our sacred purpose are those significant individuals that we are here to learn our lessons with and through—family of origin, intimate connections, landmark figures, people of similar resonance, mentors or way-showers, fellow path travelers—as we recognize that our challenges with them, and our joys with them, are fundamental to our individual and collective expansion. When we deny their significance, we suffer.

M: That's exactly what happened to me.

JB: Makes perfect sense. Because your soulpod is part of your truth. I'm referring to the specific truth of "Michael." The truth of your distinct path, the truth of your unique soul-scriptures, the truth of the lessons you are here to learn, the truth of the people you are here to learn through. It doesn't matter how much we achieve or how many things we master, if we are not walking our true-path. The moment we lie to ourselves, we leave the moment. This is why it is so excruciating when we deviate from our encoded path—we alienate ourselves from the source-spring, the well of wonder that each of us is born to swim in. Without the connection to truth-source, our breaths are somehow stifled, our presence eclipsed, our intimacy half-hearted—because we are not fully there for it. When we shed our cloaks of falsity and shamelessly embody our truths, the God-Gate opens and our Essence steps on through.

M: Yes, this is consistent with what I experienced when I returned to Hannah. A deep sense of relief, like a homecoming after years lost in the wilderness. My optimism returned. I felt it in my body again—I would get shivers whenever I was near her.

JB: Yes, I call those "truth-chills"—the physical and energetic sensations we experience when we are living our truth. The moment we own our truths, we get little sighs of delight from our body temple—as the veils to clarity fall away. Because the body knows why we are here, and it gets shivers all over when we have the courage, and the good sense to walk it and live it. It says 'yes,' and those shivers, or chills, or goose-bumps ("truth-bumps"), actually bolster us immunologically. This is the state of the new consciousness—woven from the inside out. Not descending upon, but being stitched from within our cells, our neurons, our neurological pathways—even re-wiring our hormones. One day, there will be studies done to confirm the relationship between our physical well-being and the honoring of our uniquely constructed sacred purpose. This will be the antidote, the panacea, the cure-all for much physical "dis-ease." Not to say that actual "dis-ease" won't exist—but living sacred purpose will be one of our primary wellness boosters. From what you have shared, it has certainly been part of your destiny to be with Hannah. She has been a fundamental figure in your soulpod. Perhaps a wholemate, if you continue to walk and grow together.

M: This is a lot to absorb. I'm going to take a breather. Be back in 15.

A Grounded New Earth

While he was gone, I made a pot of peppermint tea and heated up a spinach-feta casserole and home-made chocolate babka Susan had left me before her trip. I could at least heat them up without burning down the house. Michael returned just after I pulled them out steaming from the oven. Perfect timing. We sat down at the table to share food and sacred purpose.

M: So, I had a bit of a revelation on my walk. You had mentioned destiny. I definitely felt a sense of destiny, a directionality, throughout my life, but it was difficult to fully own it, perhaps because of the patterns of avoidance that we have been uncovering these last weeks. I made the assumption that leaving the world was my particular destiny—that the world was trying to distract me from my "true-path"… but I am left to wonder if I had it backwards.

JB: Uh-hmmm. Some wise man has been incessantly trying to tell you that.

M: By the way, this babka is to-die-for.

JB: You mean to-live-for. Susan has a magic touch. It's called love.

M: Anyway, perhaps my destiny was not to leave the world—except for fitting moments when I needed perspective—but to learn how to be *in* it in a different way. I always thought I had a special purpose for being here. That I wasn't just an average person in a sea of billions. But what if there's nothing special about me. What if I have merely been running from my actual contribution, because it seemed so menial? And utilizing my inflated "evolved consciousness path"—to evoke a sense of grandeur.

JB: This is a pivotal realization, Michael. To recognize that you do have a purpose within the world. An offering to bring to all of us. And it doesn't matter how seemingly small it is—it is the substance of it that determines its value. Just like the love sprinkled in that babka. Embracing our contribution is the only way progress can happen. If we keep leaving the world on meditative reveries, everything remains as it is. But if we can find a way to be fully present—and I believe our unique sacred purpose is the grounding bridge—we can have an impact here and love humanity forward. In other words, to let go of the idea that the 'world' is something we have to flee—which is inherently weakening—and to get inside the idea that it is something we co-create—which is inherently empowering. The world is not ours for the taking—it's ours for the making.

M: How does this view empower humanity?

JB: Because it reminds us that each and every one of us has a unique value. Each and every person has something special to offer, however humble it may be. Something that takes the world one step closer to the light. The intimate relationship between honoring our individual path and helping to move the collective Soul forward.

Let me give you an example. I have done much of my writing in a rough-and-tumble library a few blocks from here. I sit in the section where many of the addicts and the downtrodden come for a little respite. Often while writing I would stop to ask myself: how do we inspire them, and everyone, to see their sacred significance, to feel relevant, to be mobilized to bring their gifts to the world and to effect change? How do we energize their incarnation and remind them that they have something to offer, a deeply relevant contribution?

One day, a quiet, rugged-looking man sat down near me. I had seen him before, and always noticed his radiant smile. This time, I decided to engage with him. At first, he was a little reluctant, perhaps shy. But soon enough, he became more transparent, sharing details of his life. Born in Africa during a period of war and strife, in a large family of eight brothers and sisters. They came to Canada as refugees. Being a middle child in such a large family, he often felt over-looked, unseen, isolated. Not special, just another mouth to feed during difficult times. Eventually, he turned to drugs to feel alive, and to stop feeling the pain of the world. He had dreams, but no encouragement and no conditioning on how to find his own unique path—he was blended into a homogenized mix of siblings. Then, years later, after many rounds of rehab and living on and off the streets, he found a purpose. He didn't have the material means to actualize his real dream, of helping others to get off the streets. So, instead he took to something so simple: SMILING at everyone he saw. Not easy for him—since he didn't trust the world much, after his harsh early life. But he kept at it anyway. Smiling and sometimes telling the people he encountered what he always wanted to hear as a child... "You are very special. There is no one like you. Let your light shine." One day a teen girl came to him and said, "Gerald, you saved my life." She was in a state of despair a few weeks prior, standing atop a bridge, considering ending it all. Then she remembered his words: "You are very special. There is no one like you. Let your light shine." At that moment, she turned around and walked back home.

You see, no one is ordinary. No one is plain. No one is run-of-the-mill. These are diminishing terms that reflect and perpetuate a shamed collective. In fact, each one of us is unique. Each one of us is extraordinary. And each one of us has a sacred purpose to humanifest.

M: That's a beautiful story. I wonder what my sacred purpose would be.

JB: Imagine a world where each of us is taught sacred purpose from an early age. Taught that every offering we make, every calling we actualize, every wound we heal, every issue we process, every lesson we learn, carries the world forward. That each of us is here with the blueprint for our own holy book. Not reading from the same holy book, as if a single book could be true for everyone, but our own uniquely constituted holy book. Sacred purpose as the new religion.

If we can achieve this, and stop pretending that all those man-written religious books are gospel, there will be much less war and strife. There would be no need for war, based on one sect trying to dominate the other. By honoring the uniqueness of each person's holy—and wholly—path, we get away from the ridiculous idea that one group has all the answers, and that everyone else is sub-standard. This all begins and ends with the inherently misguided notion that there is a single omnipotent book for all of humanity. When you are firmly rooted on your path of sacred purpose, you will have little concern about anyone else's path. You will be too capti-vated by your own. This also dismantles an entire marketing ploy that sells product by pressuring each person to become something that they aren't, just because it's "cool." Through the eyes of sacred purpose, what is truly cool is humanifesting your uniquely authentic path. The next step world...

M: This is truly a new world. A Golden Age, indeed. Just not the one I had in mind.

JB: Yes, a grounded new earth. Not one that imagines itself smiley-faced *Shangri-la*, but that acknowledges the shadow as well. That empowers us to keep going when it's difficult. That realizes that we are *Souldiers* of a truer order, fighting for our mutual right to the light. A society that empowers us to recognize our value and that conditions us to seek our authentic voice from an early age. Not above the world, but smack-dab in the heart of it.

M: I can't argue with that vision for a new world, but I am left wondering what the rest of us do in the meantime. Those who were not exposed to this framework and who still carry our load of heavy conditioning. I mean, I have so many patterns and parts that are out-of-step with a participatory sacred purpose. Many aspects of my self are fragmented and antithetical to this vision.

JB: Again, it's not the self that's the enemy—it's the misidentified self, the self that is alienated from the purpose that gives it breath. In order to make the transition to a sacred purpose driven life, two primary things have to happen.

M: Go on...

JB: First, you have to do intensive clarification and excavation work. You are already well on your way. To bring yourself back into alignment with your true self, true-path, you have to apply exacting discernment to distinguish your false identifications from those that are true to your unique authentic nature. In the way you operated in the past, you have been ensnared by the ungrounded idea that all personal identifications are false. This is patently untrue. So much of who we are, and the stories that infuse us are actually our keys, our code-breakers, and the direct linkage to why we are here. The first step is to begin to unravel your identifications and ideas of who you are, making distinctions between the real YOU, and your intrinsic purposes—and the adaptations and masks that may have served you, but that do not reflect your authenticity.

Second, you have to painstakingly uncover, reveal, and identify your unique purpose, in all its forms. I will say more about each aspect at a later time… but suffice it to say that you have to stringently clarify the unique cacophony of callings, gifts, offerings, archetypes, significant relationships, and key emotional issues that live at the heart of your personal transformation. To pinpoint where the real meaning of living lies, the true nectar. To de-code your unique reasons for being.

M: I'm getting tired just thinking about it.

JB: Yeppers. It's hard work, particularly because you spent so many years believing that personhood is meaningless. You're starting from way out there, on a cloud. Now you have to come down here and find it in your bones. You have to suspend your previous idea that all personal identifications are an illusion, or of little value. You have to be burning with curiosity, passionately scoping out the possibility that the key to your personal unfolding lies within you. Not in the neutralizing of your individual voice, but in its resuscitation. You have to take your quest inside, adventuring deep within for glimmers and glimpses of true-path. And when you find them, you have to be willing to jump well beyond your comfort zone. You have to make a leap of fate.

M: A leap of fate? Don't you mean, a leap of faith?

JB: It is actually a leap of faith wrapped in a leap of fate. And a leap of fate, wrapped in a leap of faith. They exist in unison. That is, it requires a brave jump into the growing edge of your destiny. Boldly stepping onto true-path, leaping beyond your habitual range of e-motion in the direction that calls you. That's the leap of fate. Courage lives at the heart of this journey. We cling to the familiar and sometimes it kills us. Faith in yourself is everything. "I am soul. I am vast. I have a right to fully honor my sacred purpose. I decide how far I go on this path. I am here for a reason, and I won't stop until I find it." That's the leap of faith.

Without that level of trust in your destiny, it is difficult to break free from the shackles of societal conditioning and find your path. And I am not going to sugarcoat this for you, Michael. Often there is great cost involved. For example, with respect to leaving your job. There are inherent risks. You may lose money. You may lose security. You may feel fragile and vulnerable. You may feel your foundation quaking and shaking. You may feel like you are free-falling. Until the next step on your path comes into view. There are always great costs along the way, in walking our authentic path. It's not for the faint of soul.

M: Sounds terrifying.

JB: Yet, at the same time, it is not always extreme. Suddenly abandoning your decades-long career is a big leap. That may be what is required of you. Or it may not be. I cannot tell you the specific steps or give you a formula. Only YOU can discern. This process can be a very slow and gentle unraveling and unfurling. There must be faith, to be sure, but that doesn't always rush in at one time. Sometimes, it comes in small bites. As I said earlier, it's been my experience that wherever there is growth, there is sacred purpose. Any transformation, any act of healing, any breaking through of a long troublesome pattern, any movement from the shame-body to empowerment, any learning in relationship, any movement away from a polarized view or way of being, any humble shift in a healthier direction—is soulshaping, is true-path, is sacred purpose. So, again, if you are formulating the idea that your sacred purpose must be noisy and earth-shattering, I invite you to put that away for now. It has been my experience that even if it is destined to move in an earth-quaking direction, the more deeply you can work in the subtleties, massaging one piece, then the other then the other, moving one step at a time, making naked each layer—the more likely you are to arrive at your lift-off point, now truly ready to make that bolder leap, when the moment is right. It's all a leap, whenever we move beyond the parameters we were conditioned to and comfortable in.

M: Whether it happens in slow incremental steps, or one sweeping earth-shattering step, both seem difficult and uncomfortable at times.

JB: Yes, Michael, you will find that the whole process can be daunting at first. But it gets easier the more evidence you get that your inner knowing was right all along.

M: That's a relief.

JB: At first, trusting a hint or a whisper of true-path, and then, a slight breeze against your cheek, inviting you in a new direction. This is the trying and challenging phase, when you have yet to validate your intuition with actual experience. This is when you need to hang tight and do everything possible to keep your faith afloat. Eventually, the inner message becomes more direct, more seamless, indistinguishable from your very breath. That's when you have BECOME your intuition. That's when you find true-path everywhere you step. The bridge that gets you from faith to certainty is built with some combination of trust, courage and determination, along with a million steady steps. Although you may think that your sacred purpose is way ahead of you on the path, it's actually sleeping inside of you. It will appear now and then, like a butterfly flickering before your eyes, rehearting you to what lives inside of you. You may not see it often, but it always has you in its sights.

M: My previous version of spirituality felt a lot safer because it never demanded that I probe, examine, or change my life. To be honest, my previous version of spirituality didn't give a shit about my life. It all existed in the abstract, in the ethers, in the perfect pristine backdrop. Now I feel terror rising up. A knot in my throat. My heart is starting to palpitate wildly. I feel my body tensing, my feet wanting to flee.

JB: Do you have a sense as to why? Perhaps close your eyes, and feel into it Michael.

I could feel his fear and discomfort vibrationally in the air. Exciting stuff—fear fully felt equals fear transformed. I could almost feel a subtle quaking and rumbling beneath my feet. Something was shifting. Not cosmically, but humanly. It's like he suddenly reached the point of critical mass, amongst all his varied parts. His hundredth monkey jumped onboard this train. A pivotal point of no return. I could tell that we were at this point, now. He closed his eyes for a few minutes, before beginning to share.

M: I can identify a couple of things. I am afraid of what this will mean for my life. It's like I have no safe space. Everything in my life is up for grabs. I feel like I have no control. And I am also getting faint flashes of a childhood memory. Times when I would allow my personality to shine through as a child, and I would be called crazy. I would be dancing wildly, or singing gleefully, or challenging a belief, or simply trying to engage my mom, and one of my parents would start calling me "crazy-boy," and tell me to sit down and shut up. They wanted things placid, or, more accurately stated, clamped down and deadened. I guess this was the way they kept their pain from catching up with them. Makes sense, understanding the scope of Dad's traumas.

JB: I understand. This is why many of us stopped living and exploring who we were—we were shamed and shunned by those who couldn't handle our aliveness. Interestingly, it's been my experience that the one that families label the "crazy one" is often the sane one. This is particularly true in dysfunctional families where ideas of healthy functioning are turned upside down. These families often repress their authentic expression, and turn against any member who reminds them of their unresolved issues and patterns. As a result, the truth-speakers, the ones who refuse to contain their feelings, those who challenge the toxic status quo, are often scapegoated and vilified, made to feel crazy by those who lack the courage and insight to move beyond the family's madness. If you have been labeled the "crazy one," take heart. You are truly not alone. Most great creators and paradigm-shifters were met with fiery resistance by those afraid to grow. Whatever you do, do not allow your voice to be drowned out in the face of their judgments. Your voice, your vision, your ways of being, live at the heart of your unique soul's journey and are the key to collective transformation. No one has the right to bury them under a bushel of shame. No one! And remember, what is crazy to an unconscious person is often brilliantly sane to one who is awakening. Without people like you, the world is lost. Blessed be the crazy ones!

M: Thank you. I only wish words were enough to shift my paradigm. These ideas of who I am, and of who I can't be, and who I could never become, are deeply embedded. It's like I have been performing someone else's script for a lifetime. Imagining myself suddenly embarking on a whole different trajectory feels a little hopeless. I keep hearing negative voices raging inside me.

JB: What are they saying, Michael?

M: Things like, "You are going to fail. You will never make it. You failed at everything you have done so far. You have failed at the spiritual path. You have failed as a husband. You are not functional in this world. You might as well give up the fight now."

JB: Turn away from them, Michael. You have another voice that lives deep inside you. That script is your purpose, what you are here to express, to learn, to embody, to humanifest. No matter what others have mistakenly told you about who you are, no matter what missteps you have made in the past, you are here with a sacred purpose breathing at the core of your being. If that weren't true, you never would have made it down the birth canal. You never would have overcome all that you have overcome in this life. It's for you to decide which script to read: the fictional novel written by those who do not SEE you… or the HOLY BOOK written by your glorious spirit. Let me suggest an exercise to address those negative voices inside you.

They are old voices of self-loathing, just starting to be unveiled. They have been subconscious programs that are running your life. Now they are coming into the light. Let's uncover them. Each morning, instead of doing your meditation, I want you to do something similar to the self-love meditation we did last fall. This will be just the medicine you need.

EXERCISE 7
I TREASURE YOU

Position yourself in front of a mirror.

Look deeply into your own eyes.

Now is the time to honor the precious being before you.

Don't judge yourself.

Notice the beauty gazing back at you.

Notice your innocence. Those are the very same eyes you have had since a young child—gazing back at you.

Then say these words: "I treasure you."

And then say it again: "I treasure you."

Say it again, with even more heartfelt sincerity: "I TREASURE YOU."

In the course of your day, if you find yourself becoming embroiled in negative voices—find a mirror, and do this exercise.

Keep doing this, until you begin to believe it.

M: Fine, as awkward as it may be, I'll try it. One more question... If I brave the sacred purpose journey, what can I hope to find?

JB: When you walk through the gateway of your sacred purpose, you walk into yourself. Remember how you have always believed that you had a special purpose for being here. Well, you are right. There is a unique constellation of gifts and offerings that each of us carries. We made it through, because we are indispensable. We are here, because we matter. The challenge is to find out WHY. And when you do, you will be blessedly protected. Your purpose filters out those relationships and energies that undermine your expansion. Infused with vitality and a clarified focus, you will know genuine contentment, real peace in your skin. New pathways of possibility appear, where before there were obstacles. You will know a clarity of direction that will carry you from one profound satisfaction to another. Life will still have its challenges, but you will interface with them differently, propelled by a one-pointed vision that sees through the veils into what really matters. The rivers of essence rise up to meet you, lifting you from one wave of expansion to the next. You will no longer look for ways to escape being here, because you will be clearly connected with your reasons for being. When we excavate our soul-scriptures from their hiding places, we begin to walk in our own shoes. The path is not always easy, but we always know which way we are headed.

M: Yah, back to the meditation cushion, if I have my way. ☺

JB: Whatever your ways of distracting, postponing, delaying, armoring, avoiding, altering, feigning, artificializing, externalizing, superficializing your life… I encourage you to STOP IT NOW. This really is no game, this is the real thing. Sacred purpose coursing through your soul veins, crying out to break through your barriers of avoidance and find its place in the world. I cannot say this with enough conviction.

M: Dude, I was joking. Lighten up. I am open to giving it a try. And I have a hunch my life is going to look much different. Off to the mirror I go.

Michael shot up rather quickly, making his way for the door. Luckily, I was quick on the draw, too.

JB: Oh, and while you are looking in the mirror, I have another exercise for you. Here, take this.

I handed him another exercise printed out from my online workbook. He grabbed it from my hand and darted out the door. He was done for the day. So was I. It had been a long and winding exploration. Sacred purpose now demanded that I take a nice long nap.

EXERCISE 8
SACRED PURPOSE INQUIRY

Find a comfortable and cozy place to sit. Rest your feet firmly on the floor. Use a journal to make notes, or answer these questions internally. Ponder the following inquiries:

- *What does true-path mean for you?*
- *Do you feel aligned with your sacred purpose?*
- *What is your relationship to the little voice that knows? Is it far away, or is it close at hand?*
- *Do you hear a little voice whisper to you when you're doing something that doesn't feel true to path?*
- *Do you honor that voice, or do you postpone it, push it aside, layer it over, dull or diminish its conviction? Do you bury it beneath an endless flurry of activity, or do you listen in and take heed?*
- *What does your intuition tell you about the life you are living—is it true to path?*

- *Does your life honor your callings and gifts?*
- *Have you touched upon a calling that longs to be expressed?*
- *If so, what were you called to?*
- *Was the call honored, or does it remain unactualized?*
- *If the latter, what holds you back: Beliefs? Fears? Isolation? Laziness? Circumstances? Illness? Hopelessness? Unresolved grief or anger?*
- *What has to change before you can see it through?*
- *Are you engaged in work or life-activities that ignite and inspire you?*
- *Are your relationships a reflection of your growing edge?*
- *If there is a gap, as there is for most of us, between the life you are living and the life you are born to live, what do you feel has to shift before you can bridge that gap?*
- *What, if anything, stands in your way?*

After pondering these questions, position yourself in front of a mirror. Often when we look in the mirror, we are more interested in how we look to the world. Try it differently this time. Look at yourself with intimacy—"in to me see." Gaze deeply into your own eyes. Hold the gaze as long as you can. Heartfully inquire: *What do my eyes say about the journey of my soul?*

Now, try to imagine yourself in your most actualized form, and ponder these questions:

- *How would you walk if you were living your purpose?*
- *How would you interact? How would you relate to others?*
- *How would you connect to the moment?*
- *How would your eyes look?*
- *What would your facial expressions reveal?*
- *How would you interface with your emotional issues?*
- *What does a flowing and integrated YOU manifest to the outer world?*

When you are at the mirror, make a facial expression that reflects a spectrum of different parts of you. Find a posture or a movement that reflects some of the different parts of you. Perhaps exaggerate the part just to see it more clearly. Now stare deeply into your eyes and begin the process of consciously distinguishing your essential self from your adapted self. With each expression, ask these questions:

If the eyes are the mirror of the soul, what is my soul saying about the reflection before me? Does this part feel authentic, or does it feel masked?

Does the expression feel like a reflection of my true self, or is it something I take on in order to survive or feel comfortable? If I were to emanate directly from my soul, what would I look like? How would I walk? Stand? Breathe? Would my eyes be brighter? Would my smile be more sincere? How would I feel in my body? Who would be staring back at me?

Now ask your self: *Mirror, mirror on the wall, who is the truest ME of all?*

Imagine this authentic self—deeply and viscerally.

Feel it in your mind, and in your bones, and in your cells, and infused throughout your entire body.

See it shining forth in the mirror. The authentic You.

Stunning.

In the coming week, imagine that you are embodying your authentic self. When you need extra support—use the mirror as a guide. Imagine your authentic self walking through life, in all its shining glory. Stand back and watch yourself: how you breathe, how you hold your head, how connected you are to your feet, how you subtly move your body, how deeply and genuinely you can make eye contact with yourself and with others. Play and experiment with your sacred purpose. Imagine, if you can, how you might look, carry yourself, walk, interface with others—if you are embodying your truest path, if you are living all your gifts, if you are growing into your fullness. What do you see? How might your energy be different, how might you look different? Keep experimenting and embodying this—until it begins to become real for you.

10 Callings and Gifts

A week later, Michael and I met in Greektown on the Danforth. Once primarily Greek, it was now a colorful mix of ethnicities and their scrumptious delicacies. This part of the city held a collection of fond memories—from Bougatsa (a Greek pastry that satisfied my sweet tooth for years), to health food stores and herbalists that had supported my healing, to a cranial sacral therapist who had rocked my world, activating creative pathways that I didn't even know I had. Ahh, the wonders of Greektown.

Michael and I met at my favorite Greek coffee shop for espresso. He arrived late, and I was nearly taken aback by his presence. He stood tall and upright, towering over me. Shoulders squarely pulled back. As he sat down, his body had a rare fluidity. He must have taken to heart the embody your true self exercise. It was as though his outer appearance was morphing in tandem with his inner world. We sat square across from each other—his presence called me to sit taller. We began sipping our espressos.

JB: What was your experience of the exercises, Michael?

M: Unexpected. They evoked a lot of fear. Existential terror. Suddenly my own morbidity is in my face. Like I am looking death square in the eyes. This is something I have never confronted before.

JB: It could actually be a foreboding that you are dying to an old self, Michael. To an old way of being. Not your physical death. To me, this sounds like real progress. Share with me your real-eyes-ation. What did you see when you called forth your authentic self in the mirror?

M: My experience of the exercise was very sensual and impressionistic. I couldn't grasp it with my mind. But I can share the visuals and sensations. First, I was hit by a vast wave of subtle early life memories. Intuitive moments, when I sensed clear paths ahead of me, and then shut them down. I saw inner faces shining through the mirror that were more authentic and richer in sensitivity than my usual expressions, which are often cynical and guarded. I noticed inclinations—perhaps of an archetypal nature—toward certain ways of being, that haven't been embraced. I stood in the mirror, and played with various looks, walks, postures and movements, seeking to decipher which were truly me, and which were habitual patterns, or what you refer to as adaptations. I spent many hours looking, and on one occasion, watched my face rapidly morph into old selves, new selves, other selves, future selves. It was fantastical. The final time I caught a glimpse of a much more relaxed Michael, and saw him doing the job he long ago felt called to.

JB: What called you?

M: I don't feel ready to share it... yet.

JB: Fair enough. No pressure.

M: Actually I am embarrassed to tell you. It's so mushy.

JB: Mushy works. I specialize in schmaltz. Do tell.

M: Okay. In high school, we had to take a cooking class for a semester. At first, I hated it. I had never spent any time in the kitchen. Mom cooked all our meals, and truth be told, I liked it that way. Anyway, after a few weeks, I starting cooking up a storm—mostly vegetarian dishes. I absolutely fell in love with it, and had visions of cooking food for people as a living. I began to go above and beyond the norm—creating platters of delight, abandoning recipe books, and stretching boundaries in a palette of astonishing concoctions, jumping into crazy trial and error experimentations to find the perfect alchemy of ingredients. It was like when I poured the ingredients, I was pouring the very substance of LOVE at the same time.

JB: Sounds like Susan's babka.

M: Uh-hmmm. And then, years later, when I was living at the ashram in India, I requested to work in the kitchen. Suddenly this crazy super-power emerged. It was like I could read people—their inner essence was written all over their face and body. And so I began creating dishes that would reflect their particular nature. It was like I was a "cooking alchemist," adding the precise palette of ingredients to balance their personalities. If Rupinder down the street was too demure, I seasoned her food with a little spice. If Lucien the rickshaw driver, was too hostile, I would add some extra sweetness into his life. I called it "Cosmic Cooking." It felt like a calling. When I made the food, I was pulled into the moment in a more complete way. The rest of the world would fall away, and I was left with just me, my hands, a flurry of ingredients, and these crazy intuitive knowings. Like I was exactly where I was meant to be, doing what I was called to do.

JB: Wow, this is fascinating. Cosmic Cooking. Sounds like a term I would invent. I love it. This is a whole different side of you, Michael. So immersed in the elements of the world. Why didn't you continue with that path?

M: That's obvious. I took up the spiritual path instead. I loved to cook at the ashram, but the teachings there led me away from the world. I remember having a particularly impactful conversation with the guru at the ashram that sealed my direction. He said, and I remember this moment like it was yesterday, "You cannot find your true purpose in the world. You must find it beyond the world." He went on to tell me that too much excitement about worldly activity was a sign of "an overactive ego trying to create distractions from your higher path." He looked me straight in the eye, and with his thick Indian accent said, "The ego is like a hyperactive child. It runs around the house like a wild monkey—jumping from this to that. You need to quell it. By feeding it with your worldly desires, you make it more active. Find your true purpose beyond the world of name and form. Nothing of this world will ever truly satisfy you. Your real purpose will be found where there is little movement, and more peace."

JB: Not much for finding peace in the heart of passion, was he?

M: No. He saw them as antithetical. Years later, when I was living in San Francisco, I often went to a vegan restaurant for a quiet dinner alone. As I sat there watching the people, I would find myself envisioning the dishes I would cook for each one. Overhearing their conversations, I would imagine the specific and precise synergy of ingredients. Soon I had to stop going there. It was just too distracting. Passionate paths were dangerous. They disturbed my equanimity. I abandoned cooking at that point. Completely stopped it. In fact, Hannah hasn't ever tasted my cooking. She does all the cooking in our house. She thinks I'm a novice in the kitchen. Would she ever be surprised.

JB: Gosh, she's missing out. Maybe I could take some lessons from you. So, instead of following your calling at that time, you got embroiled in the spiritual path. It swept you away for two decades. And now the tidal wave has returned full circle.

Soul Doesn't Have a Deadline

JB: Michael, can you still locate this calling within you?

M: I haven't thought of it until the exercise, bro. I thought it would be dead and gone. But when I looked in the mirror, I felt it again. And, crazy thing is, it felt just as vital and true as it did over 20 years ago. And then, the fear kicked in. Interestingly, I didn't fear it for the same reasons I once did. I didn't fear it because it's too passionate. I'm now fearing it because I feel hopeless and demoralized. I missed my opportunity. I'm too old to make a radical career shift, and too proud to admit my mistake. Shouldn't I have figured out my callings by now? I'm in my 40s. If I make a big life-change at this point, I can imagine the uproar I will hear from Hannah. My family too. They have been calling my cousin Alex a flake and late-bloomer for years. My ears are already ringing.

JB: So-called "late-bloomers" get a bad rap. Sometimes the people with the greatest potential often take the longest time to find their path because their sensitivity is a double-edged sword—it lives at the heart of their brilliance, but it also makes them more susceptible to life's pains. They need more time to find their way. Good thing we aren't penalized for handing in our purpose late. The soul doesn't know a thing about deadlines.

M: But I feel like such a failure.

JB: Again, through a survivalist lens, you are a failure if you don't define a path and become successful within a certain period of time; but through a soulful lens, timelines are irrelevant. Our soul is not focused on timelines, only on truth-lines. In fact, the more deeply we honor authenticity above survivalism, the more quickly we replace linear, trivializing ideas of success and failure, with a life that is beautifully, magnificently growthful... arriving at one plateau of awakening, and then moving on to the next, as our longing for growth trumps unhealthily egoic, fear-based ideas of expansion.

M: Thank you for the reassurance. I still feel scared as shit.

JB: Frankly, I find this whole judgment around where individuals should be at by a certain stage of their life ridiculous. How can anyone know that for another? Nobody knows why you are here, except you. You're the only one that can find that. This idea that we have to have it all figured out by a certain age is a societally induced prison that ignores the depths and meaning of the human incarnation, which is about authenticity and growing towards wholeness—and not about meeting a deadline. Given that so many of us are shifting out of a survivalist self-definition, where our 'callings' are whatever enables our survival—into an authentic self-definition—where our 'callings' are that which we were born to do; it is understandable that it takes decades for many of us to find our path. We live in a world that is still predominantly organized around pragmatism—not passion—so we are always going against the cultural grain when we quest for true-path. Yet we are breaking into a new time now. And we are the pioneers. Pioneers of purpose.

M: Mmmm, I like that.

JB: People judge as though they have it all figured out, but their judgments are often just a smokescreen around their own confusion. It covers over their fear of taking a leap into their own sacred purpose. Are we late-bloomers, or are we on-time growers? This is a personal decision. The important thing is that we keep on walking toward a place that feels like home.

M: Yes, but... I wasted a lot of time...

JB: No buts about it. Sometimes we need to walk another path, in order to build the developmental girders to sustain our truer path. Think of it as a detour-with-a-purpose. Sometimes we need to do some seemingly mundane things in the world to build the egoic and economic foundation to support what we really came here to do. Sometimes we need to flee the world, before we can fully embrace it. Many of us need to go through a circuitous route, weaving our way from the outer ridges, working our way into the center of a concentric circle—where the juicy heart of the matter is. And even when we arrive there—the center itself is not stationary. Life is ever-morphing, expressing itself in ever-new colors, flavors, and facets. Once we walk in our sacred purpose, it is often self-generating, opening doorway after doorway of new possibility. There is always more to discover. And sometimes, like you, we have to take a long and winding journey through the house of spiritual mirrors. Only to land back down to earth again. But wiser.

M: That's reassuring.

JB: Don't worry about time wasted, Michael. Better to honor our path faithfully than imprison ourselves with a timeline. Timelessness is where it's at, one growth-full step at a time.

M: I wish I met you ten years ago.

JB: Wouldn't have mattered. You weren't ready for this process then. Perhaps you needed to explore equanimity and "living beyond this world" for just as long as you did, before you could re-connect with the energy of the world, without being swept away by it. I remember trying to rush the decision to write books… Then I overheard an old man in a bar say, "You can't harvest the wheat in February." The universe speaks to us in mysterious ways. Seems so obvious now, but at that time I really resisted the idea that I couldn't force my process. I could assert my will to clear the obstructions to it, and go through the preparatory stages. But my calling had an innate timeline all its own.

M: And sometimes we are cowards, running from our destiny. I appreciate your encouragement, but, in your words, it's not "all good." Let's keep it real.

JB: Haha, you're getting the hang of this. True, my friend. I understand. We don't want to sugarcoat it, but I also don't want to disparage you for remembering elements of your path later in life. You've come a long way, my friend. That anyone finds their sacred purpose is a great achievement in a world that doesn't give priority to authentic path. It is a miraculous and impactful step forward for all of humanity. All too often, I encounter individuals who beat themselves up because they haven't honored their callings yet—people just like you. They have caught a glimpse of what calls them, they have heard their truth-aches signaling that they are not where they belong, but they aren't quite ready to make the leap. This is not to say that we don't need a push now and then, but it is to say that we have to be realistic about the process. Foraging through the forests of artifice to find an authentic clearing is no easy feat. It takes courage, and it also takes time. One soul-step after another...

M: Patience isn't my strong suit.

JB: Even when you identify a calling—and, of course, there can be far more than just one—you can still easily lose your way in this distracted world. Not a day goes by when I don't feel challenged and distracted by an old pattern, another test, a false-path that appears promising. I think we will always be enticed away and have to remember, again and again. Remember, forget, remember. It's just that the remembering gets easier over time. Even those who are able to recognize their path are often sidetracked. As we deal with the challenges, pressures, and distractions of daily life, we can easily lose sight of our purpose, momentarily forgetting that there is an ocean of magnificence lying in wait within us.

Embracing Confusion

We finished our espressos and decided to get up and walking. Talking about sacred purpose was getting our blood flowing. Callings demanded movement. Outside, the chilly air felt crisp and clean. There was a touch of snow falling, evoking a feeling of wintry calm.

M: As you shared those last words, I was reflecting on other creative and career paths that have called me over the years, especially in my early years, before embarking on my spiritual path. None of them were given much of a chance, eclipsed by my one-pointed intention to advance my consciousness. Yet the ones I can remember felt deeply real and filled me with life-force. Now, here I am. Two decades of spiritual striving. Not much to show for it. I am not sure which direction to walk. Do I dare to escape the social matrix, and quit my current job? Hannah will freak. If I want to recognize my callings and gifts, where do I begin? How do I know which one is most important? What will happen to me? Will Hannah and

I get divorced? Will I be trapped into providing alimony? What about my retirement? My condo fees? What do I do?...

JB: Hey, slow down. You don't need to solve the world right now. Instead, befriend your confusion. Invite it. Surrender to it. Embrace it. Allow yourself to fully own it. Be with the unknowing and invite all of your different parts to speak. Don't attach to any specific voice at first. Just let them rise into awareness and move through you. The quest for sacred purpose is inherently explorative and intrinsically fluid, morphing into more and more clarity, as one layer of artifice after another falls away, in the face of that which shines with the light of truth. So often mischaracterized as lostness, there is a kind of immersion in the not-knowing that is actually quite focused and productive, in excavating and identifying our path. So much information can come up when we are gazing aimlessly in no particular direction.

M: My mind is racing right now. I'm hearing a lot of negative voices. My heart is palpitating.

JB: It's understandable. You weren't taught how to be with confusion while immersed in a culture obsessed with fleeing it. You've yet to embrace your confusion.

M: Easier said than done. How does one actually *do* that?

JB: It can happen in many different ways. Lie on your bed and feel into your body and your bones. Invite your confusion forward... be a safe space for it. Or move your body in whatever way calls you. Set the clear intention to bring forth the voices that call you into awareness. Invite your callings to show themselves. Let them know they are welcome in your world. Allow yourself to re-connect with prior glimpses of path that have been repressed or delayed. See what comes up, without grasping at it, without attaching to it. At this stage, just let it rise to the surface without judgment.

M: I am not sure why this idea is so unnerving.

JB: I can give you some hints. For one thing, you were conditioned by the patriarchy to be rewarded for your one-pointed focus, and chastised for your lostness.

M: You are correct. My father didn't care what career path I chose, as long as I committed to something. He funded my college education, and once I started studying Computer Programming here in Canada, I was scared shitless to make a change. It felt like a sufficient practical path. It would pay the bills, and ensure a comfortable lifestyle. And, of course, all these years focused on mastering the spiritual realms hasn't helped me to become more curious and explorative. Even though my path had an exploratory quality to it, it was also very regimented. It was a contained wandering. I was questing into unknown territories, with a very clear agenda: enlightenment. I guess I don't know how to surrender to the great mystery, particularly if that requires a deeper foray into my own embodied personhood. That's very uncomfortable terrain for me.

JB: Yes, it's like moving to a new country.

M: How long does it take to learn the new language?

JB: Sometimes, a long time. But, not always.

M: I don't have a lot of free time, dude. My life is on overwhelm. I'm currently working 55 hours a week, until the new software is launched. My sales quotas are ridiculous. I have to squeeze myself into a tight suave salesman persona—it all takes up an enormous amount of energy. With all that's on my plate, how do I embark on this kind of subtle exploration?

JB: You have to prioritize it, Michael. This is your LIFE we are talking about. As well as your health: physical, spiritual, emotional. The more aligned you are with truth, the healthier you will be. Make room for this process, even a little at a time. When you did the mirror work, what other callings came up, beyond the memory of loving to cook?

M: Many. Not all of them were career related though. I also had glimpses into other ways of being, for example, the calling to harmonize more with nature. The archetypal calling to become less of a peace-maker and more of a fierce warrior. That one freaked me out. And, I also began moving my body in unusual ways. Ever see the film "Karate Kid"? That was me.

JB: Maybe you should try out the martial arts.

M: I just might. I have a question: Does a calling always have to involve our work in the world?

JB: Absolutely not. A calling is any path of doing or being—that is sourced in your unique soul-scriptures. You can be called to a career path, a way of being, a relationship, an act of service, stillness, a lifestyle, a creative project, any pathway of possibility at all. A call can come through in any way, shape or form—a hint, dream, vision, sensation, knowing, longing, feeling, a little tug, an inner war, a melody in the distance. Any whisper that calls you home. Callings are often seen in very dramatic terms, but they can be, and most often are, simple and quiet. Some are called to become better listeners, to slow down and feel, to feed the birds. Callings are anything that we are strongly and magnetically pulled to, anything that has the energy of essential expression and expansion at the heart of it. Any path that you sense is deeply connected to your sacred purpose—your reasons for being—in this lifetime.

M: I'm reluctant to share this next impression with you. Can you promise you won't jump to conclusions?

JB: I promise. This is about exploring and embracing confusion. You're familiar with brain-storming sessions—we are now "soul-storming." It's not about making definitive conclusions or declaring your ultimate calling.

M: In one of the 'visions,' I clearly felt a child sitting in my lap. A toddler… I couldn't tell if it was a boy or a girl. I felt a palpable warmth. I even caught a momentary glimpse of the little one. And I felt this delicate scratching sensation on my face stubble. Little fingers rubbing my bristly cheeks. It was oddly comforting, actually.

JB: That's beautiful.

As he said that, Michael's pace picked up. I had to run just to keep up with him. As we crossed Withrow Park, suddenly a little girl about 3 years old ran clear across his path. He nearly bumped into her.

JB: Sometimes our calling lands smack-dab in our lap.

M: Hey, I warned you not to jump to conclusions.

JB: I'm sorry—that was just so obvious.

M: I wanted to be honest about the exercise, and not hold back. So, how would I differentiate a call that is rooted in sacred purpose from an interest, or a general passion?

JB: A calling that is rooted in sacred purpose has a life-force to it. It is inviolable, invincible, and it withstands the test of time. It will feel alive in you—a force all its own—like there is a fire in your soul, and you will simultaneously experience an alignment of your whole body with your whole being. When you imagine yourself doing it, or being it, it will be as if you are entering the moment in an entirely different way, coming into the "zone," coming home to your self after years of wandering. This doesn't mean that it will feel exhilarating. It may well be quiet and tender. But always alive.

As with all of the elements of sacred purpose, our callings are like gifts waiting to be unwrapped. When we unwrap them, when we actualize them, we feel more peace with path and we step into a more expanded version of our self. We become some aspect of who we were meant to become in this lifetime. When we ignore them, we are overcome with truth-aches, and a nagging sense of discomfort, because we are not following the tether to our own true path.

M: When I think about quitting my job, I experience a broad range of emotions—regrets, anger, a sense of loss. And, most strongly, a fear of being a forlorn wanderer, directionless and alone. I hadn't realized how attached I am to my career.

JB: Is it possible it's not the job itself, but more the self-definition and identity it has provided for you?

M: Yes, that rings true. Ironic, isn't it? Just when I thought I had transcended worldly identity, I see how afraid I am to let mine go.

JB: That's the way it often works. When we exist on the abstract spiritual path, we don't have the opportunity to confront our own fears—because we are bypassing all the worldly grit. When we really land our spirituality here in this world—we get to experience the growth opportunities the world provides. So much opportunity in the nitty-gritty friction of form. So tell me, what do you feel afraid of?

M: Afraid of the wide open spaces.

JB: You? The man who sought after wide open spaces for the past two decades.

M: Gosh, this is such a revealing. I feel embarrassed admitting that I have been wasting years on the wrong path. Afraid of admitting I am lost. I don't do lost very well. Never have. Truth be told, it terrifies me.

JB: I understand, but how can we live a complete life if we limit our movements to clearly marked trails? How can we find our path if we can't surrender to the experience of lostness? Lost is intrinsic to found.

M: Surrendering to my lostness feels decidedly disempowering. The whole process can't be about surrender. What about willfulness? What about taking action to clarify our path?

JB: In this context, surrender is anything but defeatist. It is courageous and empowered to surrender to the truths held within. But you are also right. It's not the whole story—one way of being never is. The sacred purpose journey is a balance between surrender and willfulness.

M: I feel so naked and exposed right now. I'm not accustomed to this.

JB: There are two forms of courage in this world. One demands that we strip ourselves bare-naked and surrender. The other demands that we jump into action with our armor on. At some point, surrendering to our confusion is not enough. We have to also adventure outward into life, in an effort to authenticate that which calls us.

M: Sounds like a grand adventure, indeed.

JB: It's the adventure of a lifetime. Once you excavate something that calls you—whether its an offering, a creative pathway, or a way of being—you then take the adventure to the next level. I call this stage, "Authenticating." Authentications are willful efforts to scope out and assess those pathways that have called us. When the soulular phone rings, we answer the call by giving it a try. So, in your case, you might take a part time job as a sous-chef, to see how real your cooking vision actually is. As you explore it, you compare the experience to your soul-scriptures, to determine whether there is alignment or whether it is not true to path. You authenticate the call to confirm if it is, or is not, the direction for you.

Depth Charges

M: How does one find their callings in a world that is, as you have rightly pointed out, survivalistic? So much of our energy goes into wearing masks to get through the day and grinding it out in the workforce. Are there any steps I can take to first activate all of my callings?

JB: Yes. I call them "depth charges." In the context of sacred purpose, depth charges are deliberate efforts to excavate our soul-scriptures from beneath our emotional and energetic armor. They are efforts to bring us into contact with that which calls us and longs to be lived. When you are ready to bring more glimmers of true-path into your awareness—it's time to drop a depth charge.

M: How does one do that?

JB: Many ways. You may choose to explore something that you feel actively curious about. You might study something entirely unlike anything you have studied before. Or something you feel afraid of: a certain relationship, an activity such as public speaking, a form of physical exertion that crosses bodily thresholds, or a particular way of being. Something completely out of the ordinary. You might go on a vision quest to see what directions or insights come through. You might go to a rolfing session, or explore other forms of bodywork to unpeel the callings that are camouflaged by your physical armor. Perhaps you would make friends with people radically different from yourself. Or, perhaps you would delve straight into something you have a knee-jerk aversion to, to uncover what lies behind it. You may be surprised. In order to access the many aspects and calls of the polyphrenic soul, we must approach the quest and discovery on many different levels. The idea is that you walk boldly into life in a brand new way, looking for the golden threads of true-path. What all these experiments have in common is a quest for information as to who we are, and why we are here. And you always ask the questions in the heart of the quest: What does my body say about this path? Does it vibrate with the sensations of truth, or does it ache with a longing for something more?

M: Now you have my wheels turning.

JB: Thinking of anything specific?

M: Many things. One of them is that dude over there.

JB: You mean *that* dude? Sleeping under the bench, covered in newspaper.

M: Yup. Intense aversion. I can barely even look at "them."

JB: I've picked up on that, during several of our jaunts around the city.

M: It's always freaked me out. Such a carnal way of living. So base. So primal and survivalist. Just trying to subsist day by day. And, now, as I think about abandoning my career, I have a primal fear that I could end up in the very same boat.

JB: Maybe you need to volunteer at a homeless shelter, or a missionary. Confront this. Look deeper. Perhaps there's something more, here.

M: Fuck. You may be right. But I feel an aversion to exploring my aversions. I see how this challenges me. I like everything neat and tidy, as you know. If I imagine myself venturing out and experimenting, it feels way too messy for my liking.

JB: We can't find our path without getting messy. Messy comes with the territory. We came into this world messy. We learn messy. We love messy. We leave messy. I never found my way to clarity without first befriending confusion, in all its chaotic forms. I never found a path that felt like home before falling into quicksand. I never established a new way of being without trying the wrong way of being on for size. I never found the light without stumbling around in the dark. I never tasted God before getting a little dirt in my mouth. In the heart of the chaos is the clay that shapes us home. Chaotic Magnificence!

M: I do feel compelled by these ideas. Having been around the spiritual community for decades, I've met very few who were willing to seek their path at the heart of the self. We just kept looking out there for our "self-realization."

JB: Yes, in that tricky way where "self-realization" is actually focused on nullifying the self.

M: I see how all these years, I didn't actually want to be a FINDER. I wanted to be a SEEKER. That was my identity, my comfort zone. Perhaps that is also part of my 'spiritual bypass.' Gosh, *finding* is a whole different animal. It sure gets your blood pumping.

JB: It sure does. Many of us seek that which we will flee if we find it. I have seen this time and again, both in myself and in others. We seek, we search, and then finally we find a calling or a relationship that is a perfect reflection of our yearning… and then we turn away and go back to seeking, almost as though the light of our true-path was too bright for us, too vulnerable for us, too real for us.

M: I get it. I feel the urge to flee. What is that called—fight or flight?

JB: It bears the technical term "adrenaline"—but it's actually energy. It's life-force. Embrace it. Let it surge. Use it. It will carry you forward. Seeking is seemingly safer than finding. This is a pattern that we have to recognize and heal, or else we will never stop looking for what is already there. True-path is not always around the next corner. Sometimes it's right under our feet.

Simply put, there is a time to seek, and a time to find. Seeking, exploring, excavating our true-path is essential to the journey… but we need to be careful not to miss the signs that we have discovered a treasure that is ready to be lived. Sometimes we know more than we are admitting to ourselves about our path, because we are afraid to live our truth fully. Perhaps in the past, we were not met with acceptance and support when we revealed who we were; perhaps we are afraid of the consequences of owning our path. Whatever stands in the way, let us courageously live what we find—so that we can expand into wholeness. The universe delights in our actualization.

At All Costs

M: It all sounds very good, but there is a financial component to all of this that can't be ignored. My mind is buzzing right now. Contemplating quitting my job. Our top floor lake view condo costs a fortune.

JB: It may be time to return to ground-level. That's all part of grounding our spirituality. Money is part of that, but not to an excessive degree.

M: But seriously, there's my Lexus Convertible. There's my retirement plans. There's my…

JB: For someone with such an aversion to the world, you certainly live the good life.

M: Yes, I do. My job in the software field provided that kind of security.

JB: Security? Sounds more like luxury.

M: Well, okay, luxury. I told you… I don't want to live like that dude over there. It terrifies me. I don't like to be uncomfortable. I prefer my little palace on top of the world. Up in the clouds. How will I take care of Hannah? How will I take care of myself, my expenses, my future?

JB: You will have to either adjust the way that you live, or accept that your calling is not necessarily your primary income stream. Many aren't. Those who can't make an adequate living at their callings, do them as part-time jobs, or as labors of love. All that matters is that you are doing it.

It all comes down to: What price do you pay to honor a clearly demarcated calling? If you don't honor it, you suffer. If you do honor it, your life takes on an entirely different trajectory. I paid hefty prices to follow my callings. It hasn't been an easy road. I can share some crazy stories with you.

M: Please do. I love these little glimmers into your past life. Before you awakened and got all your shit together.

JB: I'm not awakened, Michael. I'm awakening. And I don't have all my shit together. No one does. We are human, and there is always more to expand into. It is always a messy business… it just gets less messy over time. But, true, I used to be worse off.

M: C'mon, I'm waiting. How did you reach the stage where you were able to fully live your calling to write?

JB: Where do I begin? Graduated from law school, after a very intense year articling with Canada's most famous criminal lawyer, Eddie Greenspan. Did a major murder trial with him that year and was primed to go on and do extraordinary work as a lawyer-activist. But then I heard a little voice inside calling me away from what I imagined a successful and secure path. It was not telling me where to walk. It was telling me where not to walk: "This path is now complete."

Soon enough, the inner battle reached a radical crescendo—something that Stanislav Grof refers to as a "spiritual emergency"… and that I refer to as a "spiritual emerging-sea," that critical point where one pathway of possibility pushes up against another. I felt torn between two worlds: one clearly defined, one not. Over the course of many months, a ferocious battle was waged inside of me. It was the hyper-vigilant warrior vs. the tender-hearted gentle-man; the sharp savvy impeccable lawyer vs. the discombobulated falling apart-at-the-seams humanist-on-a-mission. I stumbled about, attaching to the familiar path for a moment's reprieve, before being catapulted into a holding cell of torment, sleepless and disturbed. The call to the next step would not release me. I was caught in its mighty talons. It was as though my very soul was at stake. Perhaps it was. By the time the battle ended, I was… beaten and bruised, jumbled up, unraveling, cracked open—yet ready to take my next steps. And I never truly went back. I left law. It was a pivotal moment. I shared this story in great detail in *Soulshaping*.

M: How did you get from there, to here?

JB: I took a tumble, Michael. From sleek, suave, clever, calculating lawyer, to a door-knocking window salesman, working ridiculous hours each day, in frigid Ontario winters, and somehow writing five books in the process. A grace-fall that was, in truth, grace-full. I couldn't stop the fierce momentum of forward movement, despite the endless challenges.

M: It sounds extreme.

JB: Yes, and it got worse after *Soulshaping* was released. Because I was then doing countless radio shows, writing articles for Good Morning America and other e-zines, and constantly building in social media. I would go door-knocking, sell a window order, jump onto radio, check Facebook messages at the library (I refused to use a smartphone), call window customers to make future sales appointments, grab some dinner, and then race home to write late into the night. It went on like this for years.

M: Perhaps if you were born into wealth, you could have ditched the window business. I wish that was my destiny.

JB: I don't think so. There was a time in my life when I wished I had grown up rich, so I would be able to focus on my ultimate goals without wasting precious time fighting to stay alive. You know, the trust fund fantasy. But, I now see how naïve and incomplete this perspective was. Because I developed the resilience required to see my callings through on the battlefields of overcoming. Knocking on door after door, meeting person after person, in Ontario sub-divisions—provided me the relational skills to expand on social media, one comment at a time. I came into the wisdom I write from, at the School of Heart Knocks. Working through my issues. Working endless hours. Pushing on through. No accidents, here. Blessed opportunities.

We have to be careful what easy path we wish for. We might just get it, and simultaneously extinguish the fire of overcoming that both ignites our quest and helps grow our fortitude. Difficulty grows us forward. Resilience begets actualization. I know many brilliant people with clearly defined callings—who don't have the resilience, the see-it-through-it-ness, to actualize their dreams. Selling windows and knocking on doors 10 hours a day in often frigid temperatures, was almost always grueling work, and yet it was somehow the perfect preparation and counterbalance for my creative spiritual path. I closed the business a few years ago, and what I miss most is delivering flyers and knocking on doors. It grounded me and got me into my body. So many of my most potent writings were inspired while trudging through the snowy streets of Canadian subdivisions. I needed to be firmly planted in the world in order to share a message the world could relate to. My calling is designed to course right through the world.

M: Sounds intensely overwhelming and intensely messy.

JB: Oh, goodness, it was. So messy. The house was a mess. My clothes were a mess. My car was a mess. I was always behind on my bills. I often wore hats because it took too long to wash my unruly hair in the shower, and I couldn't go into people's houses for sales appointments with my hair standing up. One night I woke up at 3 in the morning and realized I had forgot to make an essential bank deposit. I quickly walked to the corner bank machine… and only once I arrived did I notice that I still had my night guard in. And I was wearing my pajamas! I was that overwhelmed.

M: Now that's a rude awakening!

JB: Then another morning, I went out to a sales appointment in Oakville, and the customer asked to see a sample window before buying it. He came outside, and I pulled one out of the back of my Jeep. I then noticed that he and his elderly wife were staring at something. I had dressed so quickly that morning—I forgot to remove the underwear I wore the day before, from my pants. The extra pair of underwear was hanging out of the back of my pants! Luckily, I had the capacity to think on my feet, and used it to wipe down the dusty window sample. God bless them—they still placed the order. Not sure if it was because they felt pity for me, or because they really believed that the underwear was my cleaning rag of choice.

M: Oh, dude! You're killing me. I'll never see you the same. This is great stuff.

JB: And, it gets worse. One winter I was working long grueling days, and writing books far into the night. I didn't have the energy to wake up early and take out the trash. So I got into the habit of storing my bags full of garbage in the back shed. Months passed, and I accumulated about 30 bags of trash back there. Finally spring arrived and the trash began to thaw, creating quite a stink in the neighborhood. You see, this is not the picture of a man who has his shit together.

M: That must have been your garbage we smelled one spring morning on the other side of town!

JB: Haha!

M: Oh God, I can't see myself living like that. Not me. Our condo is immaculate. I'm a neat-freak.

JB: Hopefully, your calling won't demand it! But if it does, you won't care all that much. Because you will be happy as a pig-in-shit that you found it. You'll be too busy carrying out all its detailed and precise orders, to worry about such trivialities. And the cool thing is that once you find it, the momentum continues to build and peak, build and peak.

M: You've worked your ass off in your life. When are you going to retire?

JB: Never. One does not retire from a calling. One retires from a job. I will never retire. I have too much left waiting to be expressed. I feel as though I am just getting warmed up. I opened a publishing house and an online school years ago, and I want to expand them, and engage in heart-core spiritual activism in the coming years. There are too many souls that need support for me to stop. I am propelled to make my contribution to the well-being of humanity. A vista has opened wide, and I can now see many steps ahead. That's what happens as the calling matures in us—we gain vision into the bigger picture. My calling is my lifeblood. I am dead without it. As long as I'm alive, I will be humanifesting my calling.

M: Yes, but we do need to secure ourselves in this crazy world. What happens when I grow old… who will take care of me? What happens if I get sick? What happens if… And God forbid, bringing a child into this world. No way I can do that now! Not with leaving my job. I'll be a mess of a dad!

JB: If it's something that truly calls you, then it doesn't matter. You would be an authentically messy dad, with a beautifully authentic life. And you would impart to your youngling—the codes for living a life of sacred purpose.

M: Hmmm.

JB: Regarding finances, I believe it is important to meet our basic needs. Be practical, be reasonable, use your common sense. For instance, you may opt to hold on to this job until you are ready to take the action steps into your calling. It may not be productive for you to be riddled with worry about money, or trapped inside a poverty consciousness. That could be paralyzing—and paralysis won't serve your callings. But, after basic needs are met, what then motivates your action? If you don't make it about sacred purpose, you end up trapped in a misguided greed cycle, where persistent shopping becomes a substitute gratification for meaning and purpose. While never satisfying your true hunger. The thrill of the new car smell soon wears off and you need to make yet another meaningless purchase.

M: Hey, I like my new car. It's hot.

JB: I'm not referring to you specifically. This is the North American way. If this approach was so gratifying, then why do people keep purchasing? We see who this benefits—the marketers and corporations—but it leaves tremendous suffering in its wake: high rates of violence, dissatisfaction, emotional illness, depression. A world addicted to psychotropic medications to keep people numb to the fact that they are trapped in a self-defeating system, that is not designed to make them happier or healthier. If we prioritize sacred purpose in this world, we will create a healthy balanced system, one where our basic needs are always met, and where we find ourselves under far less pressure to earn money for empty gratifications. Gratification will come from knowing and living WHY we are here.

M: I'm down with it. As long as I don't lose my car and condo. I need security.

JB: There's no guarantee, Michael. To be authentic, you can't hang on tight, or try to control the process. Security is a funny thing. We long for it—but it is all too often an illusion, one that covers over our authentic path… and we end up paying the ultimate price. Security is merely a sick-cure for what ails us on the deepest levels. What we really long for is a life that is infused with meaning and purpose. I know many people who promised themselves that they would live their "real-life" after retiring from the quest for security. When they arrived "there," they were either entirely exhausted from decades of falsity, or they had forgotten the "real-life" that called them. The tragedy that happens when we bury our precious life below mountains of obligation and distraction. We can't get out from under them.

Our security blanket is often what suffocates us. It's one thing if what secures us is congruent with our sacred purpose, but if it isn't, then what have we gained? The illusion of security at the expense of our authenticity. Better we prioritize our truest path above all else. Better we trust our soul's callings. Then we can sleep without a security blanket, warmed by the fires of our authenticity. Better to live true.

M: Even if I find a calling, how to stay focused on manifesting it in such a distracting world?

JB: Once you uncover any element of your sacred purpose—you must immediately get focused on living it. Ignore everything that doesn't serve the honoring of your purpose. Not ignore as in deny reality—ignore as in find a way to keep your eyes fixated on the purpose at the end of the tunnel, no matter what is pressing up against you. When we can hold a vision of purpose safe no matter what... it deepens within us and ensures that we can see it through when the moment is right. Sacred purpose requires tunnel vision. We lose our way when we get distracted from our path. And, beware, the distractions are aplenty. So many seen and unseen forces that attempt to draw us away. We have to be the safe-keepers of our sacred purpose. We must protect it with all that we are. Because it IS all that we are.

M: Well, I could always go back to my job if I don't like the way the calling is working out.

JB: Don't count on it. You can't get away from a calling once it has revealed itself. Once you see it, you can't 'un-see' it. Unless you want to live in misery. If it remains fully buried, that's one thing... but once it surges into awareness, your resistance is futile. It only makes matters worse.

M: Shit.

JB: Simply put, essential lessons cannot be avoided. Callings don't go away. When we turn away from our lessons, when we ignore our truth-aches, the universe jumps into action, orchestrating our return—a symphony of self-creation dedicated to our unique expansion. This is the nature of karmic gravity—we are brought back to our path until we fully walk it. Return to sender, address now known…

M: I will wait to walk forward—until my next steps are clearly in view.

JB: Doesn't always work that way, either. Sometimes one lets go of one path—as I did when I left law—without having any clear idea where they will land, or what comes next. You don't always get the comfort and luxury of knowing the next step on your journey. Often it requires we follow our inner guidance one faithful step at a time—before the next clear direction reveals itself. A wise friend once told me, "Step first, and then the ground appears." Sometimes we need to remove from our path what isn't authentic—before the next true vision will arise into view. Sometimes we have to clear some of the gnarled trees that are blocking our path—before we can see the pristine and towering Mountain of Truth, standing tall in view. This is both a leap of faith… and a leap of fate. Once we take the first leap of faith, it enables our leap of FATE—to shine into view. They work together simultaneously.

M: Let's forget that for now. My security issues are too neurotic to handle that much uncertainty, at this stage. I need to slow down and be more in step with my own psyche, if I am going to live a life of sacred purpose.

JB: Do you realize what you just said, Michael? That's about the most grounded admission I have heard you make. I'm proud of you.

M: Thank you, but it's true. If I'm going to seriously consider sacred purpose as a path, I have to do it in a way that keeps me sane.

JB: Let's work where you are then. No giant leaps. Since you are not yet sure of your next steps, I invite you to do some clarifying. I have another exercise for you. I want you to go home and try this every single day for a full week. Yes, that's intense. But, as we have said—there is no more time to waste. Your true-path is waiting for you. You are ready.

EXERCISE 9
IS THIS TRUE?

In this exercise, you will work deeply within your body to clarify and confirm a calling. You can also utilize this to explore the authenticity of any component of your sacred purpose: a relationship, an archetype, an emotional pattern, any issue waiting to be worked through and healed. The purpose of the exercise is to determine if a particular direction is truly right for you at this time.

Begin by focusing on the emptying of the physical and emotional bodies. It's important to release anything that may block your clarity.

Focus on the physical body first. Begin by stretching and opening your body. Then, do any activity that helps you to energize your body and to clear tensions or holdings: dancing, swimming, yoga, rolling around on the earth, a strong walk or run, etc. Stay with it until you feel energetically vital.

When you feel ready, engage in an emotionally expressive activity, such as, hitting the bed, crying, screaming, sounding, moaning, writhing, shaking frenetically. Anything that taps into and discharges your unexpressed feelings. Give them permission to be expressed. Enliven them. Move them. Clear yourself out.

Once you feel energized, fluid and open, invite the calling into awareness. Name it, and ask yourself this question aloud: Is this true? Ask it repeatedly, if necessary. If it serves you, do a sitting meditation, a walking meditation, a sacred ceremony, a more vigorous activity. Anything that helps you to become clear. Bring all of your consciousness to bear on the inquiry. Keep asking, inquiring, investigating, and probing until you find that tiny trail of truth. Follow it. There will be clues that you have found it: it could be a relaxedness in your body, a sense of relief, a quieted knowing, or any other indication that you have come upon something innately real and true within you.

After imparting the exercise, we took out our calendars, and booked an appointment for ten days later. I had a sense he would have a lot to report—after such a spell of rigorous exercises, coupled with all that was brewing in his deep inner cauldrons.

As I walked home, I felt jolts of electricity surge through my veins. Talking about sacred purpose got my juices flowing. On par with exquisite lovemaking. I was elated for Michael, and the new horizon he was stepping into. It felt like we were now working in tandem, cooperatively, as co-journeyers on this path. There was a way in which his willingness was fueling my fires. Through him, I was re-living and remembering my own discovery of sacred purpose: the delirious excitement of stepping into the vast unknown. I felt a renewed vigor for all the expressions of my purpose that I had yet to discover, and bring into being. Sacred Purpose never gets old. Suddenly, I felt less solitary on my journey. I felt myself smiling brightly. It was now late February. Time was passing quickly, and before we knew it, the starkness of winter would abate. The days would become longer, and little tiny buds would appear on the trees. Life is full of endless new beginnings.

11 Cell Your Soul

Each of us possess a gripping life story. A continu-
ance of vital passages. An entire account of our
earthly evolution. Each story is a relevant thread in
this infinite weave of multi-colored hue. Not every
story will be spoken aloud. But every story is sacred.
Every story worth recounting. Every story true. We
must recognize the short-lived and silent threads, for
they are part of the magnificent cosmic shawl. We
must pause to give them a voice, to allow their spirit
to take space to confess their existence. We must give
them the honor that is due.

—SUSAN FRYBORT

The day before I was scheduled to meet with Michael again, I received a jarring text.

Do you know where my husband is? He's been missing for
three days.

I immediately knew it was Hannah.

I have no idea. He didn't mention anything to me.

I'm worried. He said he was driving to a cabin to
contemplate his life, but his car is still in the garage. And
he left behind his phone, his wallet, everything. I'm here at
our condo, looking through his cell for clues. Found your
interactions. He has spoken highly of you.

And of you too. We are scheduled to meet in Chinatown
Thursday morning. I will let you know if he shows up for the
appointment.

Hmmm. That was unexpected. Yet somehow I had a quieted sense not to worry. I had an inkling: Michael was up to something.

The next day I arrived at the tearoom a little early to pore over a few chapters of my manuscript. A half hour later, out of the corner of my eye I caught a glimpse of an unkempt, heavy-footed man barreling over to my table. Thinking it was a panhandler on his daily routine, I raised my eyes to give him a nod of acknowledgment. It was Michael. He now looked almost unrecognizable. His usual hipster stylish way of dressing was replaced by a bulky worn out sweatshirt and sweatpants, running sneakers with holes, disheveled hair. And yet, an unmistakable gleam in his eyes. My inclination was right—Michael was up to something.

JB: Michael? Where were you? I got a message from your wife.

M: Dude, I had a helluva weekend. It was radical.

JB: I can see that. Do tell.

M: In our last meeting, you talked about experimentation. Doing something out of the ordinary… facing fears… questing for clues about my path…

JB: Uh-hmmm…

M: I took it to heart. I realized it was time for some radical action. A jolt back to reality. So, I took off for a few days.

JB: I picked up on that. Where did you go?

M: If I tell you, you won't believe me.

JB: Try me.

M: Remember when you said to confront something you had an intense aversion to. I did it. I took to the streets.

JB: You what?

M: Yup, I went homeless for a few days. Sleeping in a shelter one night, on the streets the other two nights. Had to fight off one guy in the shelter, and a raccoon in the alley. The tenacious little varmint fought me all night for my orange. It was one of the most eye-opening and radically transformative experiences of my life. There's so much I can tell you.

JB: Wow. Please share more…

M: These people. I connected with many of them. They are so different than I expected. The stories they told me. Dreadful things many of them have endured. Childhood horrors. Yet, incredibly, many of them still have an open heart, and faith in life. I realized—there is real wisdom that gets cultivated through life's difficulties. This one guy I met. Long dreads. He went by the name "Eminence." He had this mysterious magic to him. This knowing glint in his eye. He was a treasure chest of wisdoms, that he doled out generously. Another guy I met was once a trial lawyer, like you were. Maxwell Sampson, ever heard of him? And then, one day, he began to hear voices. He was diagnosed with schizophrenia and lost his practice, his home, his wife and child. Yet he was fucking brilliant. Privy to all kinds of cosmic codes that my mind couldn't even grasp. Yet with all he went through, there he was counseling me on life direction. And this morning I met a city-planner, a woman named Sheryl Phillips, who had actually run for Toronto mayor years ago. Between tears and heart-aches, she shared profusely about her desire to make a difference. A passion burning inside. Even though she lost everything, and doesn't have a place to call home, she is still committed to making a contribution to the world.

JB: I've always said this. Most of the greatest achievements on the planet are unknown to others—private overcomings, silent attempts at belief, re-opening a shattered heart. These are the real heroes. The real path of champions truly lies within: the transforming of suffering into expansion, the clearing of horrifying debris, the building of a healthy self-concept without tools. The greatest achievers have found a way to believe in something good, despite being traumatized and fractured on life's battlefields. No matter what else they accomplish in their lives, they are already champions. One day the world will realize that it is much harder to heal a shattered heart than to excel at worldly matters. Gold medals all around…

M: Exactly. I feel transformed. I faced a long-standing fear. And you were right—what I found on the other side surprised me. Shocked me, actually.

JB: You are on fire, Michael. It's the fire of sacred purpose.

M: I suddenly care very little about my car, my condo. I want to live for the true gems of life. That pristine timeless wisdom. Oh, I probably lost my job, too. After they couldn't get a hold of me for a few days, I'm not sure what will happen now. And, yet, it doesn't really matter. I got more tiny glimpses into my calling. Serving edible creations, infused with love. That's part of it. But there is more… I want to serve magic to these people—the champions of the human heart—who have endured so much. I want to support them, as they tried to support me. I want to somehow give them hope to keep believing. And there is something more I am meant to contribute. I can't put it into words yet. It is like a nebulous cloud in my vague imaginings that has yet to materialize. I feel a passion rolling through my veins.

JB: Powerful medicine.

M: And this morning, while my head was laying on bunched up newspaper, I had the most potent dream. I was in my final moments—in the deepest, purest experience of death consciousness—and I was watching my life like an old film. Flashes of meaningful moments and memories appeared on the inner screen, some that I have always known were significant, and myriad others that I failed to recognize as meaningful at the time. But in retrospect, every single damn moment was shrouded in meaning. From doing the dishes, to taking a walk, to simply getting dressed in the morning. All the trivial moments I dismissed as the pure drudgery and density of the human experience, suddenly gleamed with poignant, soul-serving beauty. Wild. One thing that came clear was the time that was wasted on trivial worries—the perpetual distractions, the opinions of others, the pursuit of excessive money. But, it was also shockingly clear that I was wasting my time, trying to find the Divine outside of my life. It was actually right in the heart of it, all along.

JB: You had the power all along, my good man. Wait, that's from the Wizard of Oz. Keep going…

M: I lay there in a clarified, vulnerable state and longed for more time to just be here. It was like there was this giant vat of joy that always existed just outside of my habitual awareness, longing to be imbibed. A life waiting to be lived. All too often, I bounced from one activity to another, imagining the joy I would find at the end of it all. The dream was crystal clear in its message: Drink it now, man. For bloody REAL. Drink it now. I woke up parched and thirsting.

JB: That is profound, Michael. You sure did have a helluva week. You went to your growing edge and held hands with yourself. Kudos to you. That is truly awesome.

M: I can't yet articulate my purpose. Or even see the next steps. But I can FEEL it. Like in my bones.

JB: That's where it lies. Makes perfect sense. The clarity that we get as to whether a path is a calling, invariably arises from our feeling-body. What calls is not a concept—it's a visceral, palpable force embedded deep inside our bones. The more work we do to attune to our feelings, the clearer our callings become. And, naturally, they can also be blocked by the unresolved emotional body. If we're all bunked up by prior material, we can't see our path. We have to move the material that is in the way first.

M: Yes, exactly. The first two nights were a wholly different experience. I tossed and turned throughout the night, gnashing my teeth in anguish. Hit by torrents of rancid emotional material. More memories of childhood, and new ones—anger at a woman I dated when I was only 17, my first love, who broke my heart in a zillion pieces. I pushed that deep away into the ethers of my subconscious. I tapped into shocking subconscious material: primal wails of anguish, demons and goblins, and grotesque sexual lustful dreams. Stuff too weird to share. It all became so intense that I began to feel like I was suffering from mental illness. I wondered if sleeping beside Maxwell at the shelter had rubbed off on me.

JB: I don't really like the term mental illness. I prefer the term "emotional illness." Yes, I understand that our material is often manifested in our thinking, but I also believe that the mind is not the primary source-spring for many conditions. The focus on the mental keeps us looking in the mind for the core issues, when so often the real issue lies within the emotional body, and requires more embodied, therapeutic approaches. Once some-one is labeled "mentally ill," they often end up with an analytically based psychiatrist who medicates them, rather than with a psychotherapist who can support their deeper healing. It feels very similar to the spiritual and patriarchal emphasis on the 'monkey mind' as opposed to the 'monkey heart.' By focusing on the mind alone, we get trapped in a head-tripping loop and it is very difficult to liberate our consciousness. We are also much easier to control. If we focus, instead, on healing the emotional material that sources the condition, there is hope for real change.

M: I'm beginning to really get this. Every time I follow your guidance, I uncover more and more loose ends in my body—anger, grief, fucked-up patterns and issues. It's very humbling. I am also more inclined in the direction of your assertion that these unresolved emotions and issues, live at the heart of our transformation. I used to imagine divine purpose as shadowless, but I can no longer abide by that view. The shadow is too pervasive to pretend it's not relevant. At the same time, I find it hard to believe that all of these wounds, scars, and issues are mine, birthed in this lifetime. I'm a triggerfest.

JB: Good observation. You did not accumulate all this in your lifetime. Our emotional material is also a reflection of the state of the collective: shame and unresolved pain and issues are everywhere. The ancestral patterns are encoded in your DNA. The material is yours, and it is ours, and to the extent that you can heal and work it through, you transform yourself and the entire species.

I can't say this often enough: Repressed emotions are unactualized spiritual lessons. Unresolved issues and toxic patterns are brilliant opportunities for transformation. When we flee the shadow, we flee ourselves. If we ignore the material, we block our own expansion. When we deny our fucked-up-ness, we actually delay our own evolution. We remain right where we are. And the shadow that we fled with all our might, doesn't go away. It waits around the next bend to trip us up and to remind us that it needs to be seen. Not because it wants us to suffer, but because it wants us to heal. Because it wants us to grow. Our shadows aren't the enemy. Our resistance to them is. Only by bringing the shadow into the light of day and working it through, can we can evolve this humanity. Only by 'celling our soul' can we transform ourselves and bring the world forward.

M: Sell our soul? To what, the devil?

JB: Hell no. "Cell" as in living vital organism. The body is far more than a vessel for the soul. It is the karmic field where the soul's lessons are harvested. It is the alchemical chamber for our soulular transformation. To "cell your soul" is to make your essence alive and real—at a cellular level—by embodying it fully, here in this life. When we do the work of healing the emotional body, our other bodies transform simultaneously. The soul and the emotional and physical bodies align as they were intended—as intertwined threads of the same sacred weave. Again, emotional maturation and spiritual maturation are synonymous. We clear our emotional debris both because it creates space inside for our sacred purpose to reveal itself, and because inherent in those feelings and memories are the lessons we need to grow spiritually. The more work we do within the emotional body itself, the more depthful our spiritual journey becomes. It is as though the soul is shaped with toxic waste that transforms into gold as it moves through the soulshaping birth canal— from experience to lesson, from unresolved emotion to clarified realization.

M: How, then, does one 'cell the soul,' in practical terms?

JB: You turn toward your suffering, your issues, your unresolved memories. You go deeply into the material held within your body. You own all that you have been through. You feel all your feelings. You work them through to completion. Once you have gone far enough through, the transformation takes root.

You've had a profound initiation into The School of Heart Knocks, Michael. Welcome.

M: Hey, question: I know you disparage witnessing… but could it be a useful technique for wound-watching?

JB: Actually yes. Witnessing will never represent the full picture. But it can serve as a tool in the process. I did a lot of inside work with my watcher. The key is to use it for a limited purpose. Not to dissociate you from your pain, but to help you to recognize issues and feelings that are ready to be addressed. And, once you make those observations, detach from the witness and drop down into your feelings-body and work the material somatically. If you are someone who prefers to look before you leap, then imagine yourself a surgeon. You first look at the wound very closely in order to determine its origin and how it connects to the complete system—and then you get to work repairing it. You get to know the trauma before you suture it.

M: I wonder, though, if all traumas can lead to transformation.

JB: Most traumas are treasure-chests of transformation. Working them through, can radically develop consciousness.

M: You are sounding like a New Cager. It's all a gift?

JB: I said, most traumas. Others are not ripe with transformative potential, but can still be healed to varying degrees. Not every wound is a gift, but every wound holds the possibility of healing. When there has been too much pain, we often forget that we have the built-in capacity to move it through to another state. We are natural shape-shifters. The Divine gave us tears to be cried; God gave us the capacity to express our anger; Goddess gave us a vast range of emotional devices that, when healthily unleashed and expressed, can clear the toxicity out of us. In our authentic vulnerability lies our greatest power—the power to re-open our hearts after loss and disappointment. Feeling the pain is an act of self-empowerment, and the only way to make a break from the prison of repressed emotions. Reach inside and unlock the door...

M: The last few days on the street, I felt their pain-bodies. Yet I also felt an intrinsic wisdom, right beneath it.

JB: Let's stop calling it a "pain-body" for God's and our own sake. It's a gain body. No pain, no gain. While I am a great advocate for acknowledging our shadow, I also recognize the value of doing all we can to find the light where possible. Not the pseudo-light, but the light of true-path, the light of hope, the light of love.

M: So, I don't need to continue sleeping on the streets to excavate my shadow, right?

JB: Only if that's your authentic clarity. No, you don't need to deliberately get lost in the shadow. Our shadow is designed to arise, be assimilated, and move through us. When we are open and conscious—that process happens more seamlessly. I have known a great many individuals who clung to the darkness like a security blanket, cloaking their fear of the light beneath various mechanisms. The darkness bypass. It became their comfort zone. It is one thing to open the shadow chest in an effort to heal and become more authentic. It is quite another to hide in the shadows and make it our home. That won't get us anywhere. Once we have done enough work around the shadow, we have a choice. We can either open the door to more darkness, or we can open it to light. It is through making the darkness conscious—that it actually transmutes into the light.

M: I gotta tell this to my buddies on the street. Wise words. Can you write this down for me?

JB: Sure can. Having said all of that, I am under no illusion that this is easy to achieve in this world. Many people continue to dwell on their past traumas because they have never been shown how to heal. And because they are embedded in a repressive culture—one that shames and shuns us if we acknowledge our pain. The way our economic systems are structured also makes it difficult for victims to find the support to heal. Those who have been the most traumatized are often the ones who have the hardest time making ends meet. I'm sure you discovered that the past few days. People that would genuinely benefit from healing, but don't have the means to get the proper support. It's the healing of their wounds that would enable them to re-assimilate as functioning members of our economic society. Yet they are stuck. It's a catch-22.

M: I met a lot of people that are caught in that vicious cycle. Perhaps I can help them. I have a vague inclination that I'm going to play my part in shifting this. Me! What a fucking surprise.

JB: Sacred purpose. The conscious path is full of surprises. I can't wait to see what you do next, Michael. Until we have the good sense to make psychotherapies free for all, many people cannot possibly get the support they need to heal their wounds. So yes, don't linger in the shadows any longer than you have to, but don't make the mistake of thinking that all those who continue to reference their victimhood are hiding there. Some may be, but many of those individuals simply do not have the support they need to come back to light.

Michael, I was incredibly moved by what you said about street-dwellers and the disenfranchised. They are often discarded, and yet they are the treasure chests of wisdom. Moving through the fires of hell, back into this world, and still finding the faith to go on—refines their inner gold. I always take the time to truly look at each panhandler or street-dweller. Once, an old rugged looking gentleman looked me straight in the eyes and said, "We are the ones who show you your wounds." It was like a message from the Universe itself. Praises for the trauma speakers, in all the forms they arrive. They do speak for many of us. Rather than ignoring and shaming them, perhaps we should gather before them and let them whisper our hearts back to life. One thing I am certain of—those who can't embrace their shadow can't embrace their light. It's all, or it's nothing at all.

M: Amen to that. I can see it now.

JB: The inner monsters we distract from are not nearly as dangerous as the monsters we create to avoid them. As painful as early life traumas can be to confront, they are seldom as destructive and difficult to transform—as the behaviors and addictions that we develop to bypass them. As children, our defenses and distraction techniques saved us, but, as adults, they become a self-fulfilling prophecy, concretizing and locking us in with our early pain, blinding us to the fact that we are now better equipped to work through our memories than we were as children. It may have seemed insurmountable back then, but it no longer is. If we can turn around and face them now, if we can resist the tendency to cover them over with layer upon layer of distortion, we can re-claim our trauma and work it through to resolution. There is no way to escape wound-body memory. It is always there, awaiting its moment of integration. Better to turn around and embrace it. Once a monster, now an opportunity for genuine transformation.

M: Gosh, I was confronting some bad-ass monsters and demons those nights at the shelter. I hope they chillax.

JB: By the way, did you let Hannah know you re-surfaced on the planet? She texted me. She was very worried about you.

M: No, I came straight here. Didn't want to miss our appointment. She's gonna think I fell off the deep end.

JB: Let's take a stroll. The weather is finally breaking. I'll buy you a street coffee, my homeless friend. ☺

You Are Your Story (and then some)

We left the teahouse and started walking through Chinatown. I was immediately struck by Michael's gait. His steps reverberated with a striking solidity. Astounding I hadn't even recognized him when he approached me in the café. Not just his physical appearance—but his whole presence was transformed. It's like he was in a process of materializing from the ethers into solid mass form. Michael was truly changing. Giving him a sidelong glance, I smiled knowingly to myself. A work of (he)art to behold.

M: I heard so many life-stories the past few days. I was captivated, riveted. This is so unusual for me, and the path I have been on. Usually I reject and ignore stories. So I have to ask: What do you think of stories? Is it better to be free from the weight of the past? How do we distinguish stuff that is worth working through, from the silly stories that hold us back? After all, we are far more than our human lives. Surely you agree that our stories are but one small, and often delusional, fragment of who we are.

JB: No, we are not more than our human lives, Michael. We ARE our human lives. We just have to define humanness in a way that encompasses the everything. Somewhere at the heart of our stories and characterizations lie our deepest truths and our path home. That is, there are 'stories' we carry about ourselves that may be patently false, and, yet at the same time, they still contain the granules of glory that transform us.

Below the surface of the 'story,' is the real story of our lives. Because we are made of story—there's no shame in that. The illusion is illusion, itself. So, don't discard your entire story. Look below the story to the real story. There is something there waiting to be healed and converted. There is no true identity independent of the story of our lives. We just haven't learned how to read our own storybooks yet. And, once we can read their unique language, we see how they include the soul's codes for our evolution and development. Our wholeness doesn't begin beyond story. It begins within it. Either we work through our story… or our story will work through us.

M: One guru used to tell me to stop chasing my tail when I would get lost in my stories. He would utter, "Don't look back, look beyond." I get that you believe in the value of working our stuff through. And I am seeing the wisdom of that in certain situations. But it sounds like you just want us to chase our tails 24/7. Is that really productive?

JB: Sometimes what is behind us, is actually still right here, as alive—or more alive—than it was back then. Because it hasn't been attended to, yet. Pretending it's not there, won't serve us. No, Michael, it's not about chasing your tail. It's about chasing your tale—the one that accurately depicts your lived experience. It's one thing to wallow in story—it's quite another to dishonor your personhood altogether.

M: But Michael is a story, Jeff is a story. It's a fiction.

JB: Oh God, not this again!

M: Haha, got ya. I'm just being the devil's advocate for a moment. Chill out.

JB: Okay, I'm always up for a good debate. For the sake of argument: the meaning of our story may be misunderstood, but none of it is a fiction. It's as real as real gets. We just haven't been taught the ways to see our story through until the fruit is harvested. So we jump to emotionally convenient re-frames in an effort to extinguish the fires of discomfort. We turn away from them—when what we most need to do is turn toward them.

Our story contains clues as to who we really are, and our unique expression in reality. For example, in my early 20s, I self-identified as a fierce warrior. Eventually, it was evident that this story no longer served me. It was time to embody a more surrendered and tender-hearted way of being. But my warrior-self did reflect a very real part of my archetypal journey, and it was an aspect that lived at the heart of my sacred purpose in this life. Years later, after I came to embody my tender heart, the fierce warrior showed up—ready to be actualized, now in a more wholesome balanced way.

Here is another example… I always felt that my mother hated me throughout my early life. This was the story I would tell to the world. Years later, I recognized that this was not, in fact, true. She was hard on me, but not because she hated me. She had other motivations—it was more about her relationship to her own inner world. Realizing this was deeply healing. In fact, I couldn't have moved on to the next stages of my soulshaping journey if I hadn't recognized this. What got me there, was a willingness to turn toward the story and find its roots in my emotional life, revisiting the experiences that sourced the belief. If I had followed your guru's advice and refused to "look back," I would never have gotten to the core material that needed addressing: the story at the heart of the story. It was going deeper into my story that led to a significant reduction in my suffering, and a concomitant increase in my delight. It also helped me to ultimately recognize more of my calling to deepen into grounded spirituality—as both a way of being and a message for humanity. Doing the emotional work deep within our stories are like breadcrumbs on the trail, leading us to the next stages of sacred purpose.

I deeply believe that our truest path is encoded in the bones of our being, and lives in the heart of our stories. I believe in an encoded path, Michael, and that our personal stories—the details of our lives, the ways that we frame them—are hallowed ground. This doesn't mean that the way that we characterize our experiences is always accurate, but it does mean that below—and not beyond—those characterizations is the real story waiting to be seen. At the heart of our stories is the fuel that is fundamental to our expansion. Think of your misidentified stories as welcome mats, waiting outside the door of your true home. The trick is to get beyond the misidentifications to the real story.

M: I can hear my past gurus turning over in their graves—most of them disparaged the value of stories. I see it now… I wanted to flee my past, so I conveniently bought into that.

JB: It's something I wish I could emblazon on the forehead of every seeker before they step foot on the path: Beware the transcendence bypassers who deny the significance of our stories. They are often deeply unwell. It's one thing to say that we should not get trapped inside of our stories, but to suggest that all of our stories are without value and merit, is to desacralize your personhood. It's to swing too far in the other direction. I understand that they believe there is something greater awaiting us beyond the self— but they are wrong. Whatever greatness awaits us must thread through the heart of the self, so that our experience of the "beyond," is rooted in something real: our precious humanness. The only path home.

M: My comrades on the spiritual path would be aghast at what you are saying right now.

JB: No doubt. The story bypassing troupe has forgotten that their non-story schtick is a story, too. It's always story. The question is what we are going to do with it? Are we going to dive into the heart of it and expand in karmic stature through the learning of the lesson, or are we going to drown in our unresolveds, floating numb and detached down denial river. Michael, why are you laughing?

M: Oh, the irony. Just remembering the time Hannah and I went to this Intro workshop my friend was hosting, where we spent two days proving that all of our stories—about ourselves and each other—were illusory. I loved it. Hannah had a very different experience. By the end of the day, she felt like she wanted to shoot herself. She felt a void of meaninglessness, like life wasn't worth living anymore. She began to question every thought that came into her head. And suddenly life felt so dismal and depressing—like NOTHING was true anymore. Nothing had any meaning. Nothing mattered. For her, that was devastating. For me, it was liberating.

JB: I understand her hopelessness. Many of the story-bashing models have roots in cognitive psychology and the New Cage movement—the fixation with 'thoughts' as the primary problem humans face. They are bypassing models. They deny the veracity of our suffering and distract us from the deeper issue: that which sources our thoughts. Yes, our beliefs may be misguided, but there is often a deeper truth below them—unhealed wounds and unexamined stories that will simply re-surface in another way, if they are not met whole-heartedly. Turn toward your stories, and find your true-path right at their heart.

M: But you agree with the underlying philosophy, that we are so much more than our thoughts?

JB: Yes, but the difference is: this philosophy seeks to find the rest of who we are beyond the self—and I seek to find it right at the heart of the self. And there is a fundamental difference between their vision of a whole human—emotionally bereft and equanimous—and what I know to be an authentic human-being: emotionally integrated, richly nuanced, and full-bodied vital and robust. These models are presented as healing tools, but they are actually a trick. Their intention is to take us further away from the world of feeling. Many of the story-bashing models want to keep us on the surface—not because the answers are there—but because they are trying to keep us away from the roots of our stories—our wounds, memories, experiences. Let's explore the contrast. Can we engage in a process right now around a story that is up for you?

M: Let's just run with the same old song and dance. Hannah's obsession with having a child. We've been going to counseling for some time now. But I'm still at an impasse. She needs a baby. I can't surrender. I'm stuck. We're fucked.

JB: Let's start with your core belief. Your belief is… "I do not want to have a child." Is that true, or false?

M: Yes, true.

JB: Which part of you says that this belief is true? All of you? Some of you? Not really you?

M: My mind. It keeps repeating it over and over.

JB: Do you sense that this can be shifted from within the mind, itself?

M: I used to think it could. I would try to shift it by changing my thinking. Repeating a more positive affirmation over and over. And sometimes, it actually would shift. For a moment. I would hear a different voice telling me I want to be a father. But fairly soon thereafter, the naysayer would just take hold again. I couldn't shift my position from within the mind, itself.

JB: Figures. Now, let's stop in front of this store window and try a different approach. You ready?

M: Sure.

JB: If you don't feel comfortable doing this in public, we can find another place.

M: No problem at all. After living homeless for a few days, I seem to have lost a major level of inhibition. Life is too short to worry what strangers think.

JB: Great. Let's try the grounding exercise we did in one of our initial meetings. Bend down fully and let your weight fall forward. Connect with your feet, your breath, the vibration coursing through you. Allow any feelings and sounds to arise as your body opens and energizes. Invite yourself to come alive. Raise your hand when you feel like you are deeply and solidly in your body.

After only a few minutes, Michael raised his hand. Although he didn't need to. His stability was palpable. A vivid contrast from the first time he did the exercise. His breath was strong and deep, the vibration in his legs solidly rooted. It was heartening to see how he dropped deeply into his body, like it was second nature. I had to pull my attention away from simply admiring him—and back into facilitating the exercise.

JB: Now rise up slowly, and look in the window at yourself. Take the question deeper into your body and ask it again. Is it correct that becoming a dad is not right and true for you in this lifetime?

Michael stood there for some time, gazing into his own precious being. At some point, his eyes began to tear, and his face began to morph. Almost as though a mask was shedding, and another layer of authenticity was coming into view. It was like watching a human transfigure and transform before my very eyes.

JB: Go deeper into your body. Feel into your blood. Feel into your cells. FEEL. Michael, just FEEL.

He closed his eyes and inhaled deeper. He raised his neck high, and he did a few long slow neck rolls. He spread his legs further apart, to ensure a stronger stance, like a broadly-rooted oak tree. The deeper he went into the body, the more visible and fuller he became.

M: It isn't true, Jeff. This belief I've held for so long. It's false. It's a belief— it's my story—but it isn't the actual grounded truth.

JB: Speak more…

M: Before, I identified this as core truth... but now that I have gone deeper into my feelings and my body, I see that it isn't. When I keep my breath shallow, in my chest, I feel that this belief is true. But when I breathe deeper and fuller—into my belly and pelvic bowl—I feel a more prescient truth rising. It's hazy, and it is frightening, but it says that my usual story is false. It says that, below all my fire and fury, I am open to becoming a father.

I could feel the weight and gravity in his words. As he continued to speak, his voice broke and trembled. He was embracing a reality—a possibility—he had long barricaded. Michael was teetering out in the vast unknown right now—right on his sharpest cutting edge.

M: Holy shit. It's fucking terrifying. But it's true.

JB: What does your intuition say is the best way to hold safe this precious knowing... To explore it more fully... To make it real?

M: I need to continue unpeeling the layers of feeling. To get to the bottom of my resistance. In my body. Changing my thinking doesn't change much of anything. You are right about this. I can only fasten to the truth when I get below the mind, and into my feelings-body. The war may be up high—but the resolution is down below.

JB: Exactly. It's true that we can sometimes recognize the falsity of our beliefs simply by questioning our thoughts... but the deeper questions of our lives don't get resolved that way. Because the source material is still there, dictating our thinking. We have to drop down into our hearts and make our inquiries there. It's the heart that knows the path. The mind is just there to organize the steps. The real work lies far beneath the surface.

Habitual Range of E-motion

M: So, how do I identify those wounds and issues most pertinent to work on? How do I delve into the kingpin wound that is holding me back from surrendering to Hannah, and welcoming a child into my life? I get the concept of celling your soul, but where do I first put my focus?

JB: Start by putting your focus on those wounds and issues that are energetically charged. Go where the core material is. Some of this will be readily obvious in your day to day life: the anger that keeps coming up when you least expect it, the hints of irritation when dealing with practical details, the issues and patterns that continue to plague your relationships. Follow the charge. Your relationship with Hannah is the perfect ground for all of this to surface. It's a natural wound revealer. Works like magic, as long as you go into the body to reveal the source material that is fueling the issues.

In essence, you need to utilize the same depth-charging intention that we discussed with respect to your callings, this time, to get to the bottom of your unacknowledged issues and to bring your submerged emotions into awareness. You can't heal what you can't see. Continue to engage in heartfulness practices that energize and expose murky material. Some we have already worked with: somatic psychotherapy exercises, excavation meditations, Barking Dog Yoga, and there are many others. Consciously note your reactions, feel them deeply, and trace them back to the originating material. Then, work the material through to transformation. It might help you to do sessions with a somatic psychotherapist as well. It can be difficult to hold the space for our own process in the way that another can.

M: What you propose is inherently uncomfortable, kind of like you are constantly asking me to stretch myself far beyond my comfort zone. Perhaps this is what you mean by 'soulshaping'—we keep stretching our soul in new directions? Having a child would be the pinnacle of that for me.

JB: Yes, but it's not stretching for the sake of creating challenges or suffering. Remember, we stretch the soul in the direction of its own sacred encoded potential.

With respect to celling our soul, think of it as an effort to expand your habitual range of e-motion. Our habitual range of e-motion can be defined as our emotional comfort zone. It is the range of feeling that we return to time and time again because it feels familiar. Comfortable. Safe. Unfortunately, for many of us, it is a very narrow range—one that doesn't reflect our potential, a life fully lived. It doesn't reflect the true-paths we are here to walk. It's a step back from our growing edge. And why shouldn't it be? Our range has been determined and prescribed by our trauma history. Most people come in deeply vulnerable and open, and life experiences compel a tightening of the range. The narrower the range, the less vulnerable they are to disappointment and pain. At the same time, the tighter the range, the less capable they are of feeling joy and liberation. And the less likely they are to step out into the purposeful life that awaits them.

M: I am willing to go deeper into this shield of contraction I feel around the child. It's freakin' uncomfortable. But I'm used to uncomfortable now. I was thinking the other day about some of the ways that I kept myself in range as an adolescent. As I say that, I feel my solar plexus becoming hot with energy. It's no accident. That stuff that came up in today's exercise is still with me. And I do know what its connected to.

JB: What is the real root of your armor regarding this particular issue?

M: I am feeling it is linked to the engulfment wound I discussed with you before. I associate family life with suffering. When I imagine it, I feel my body tense up. Like I am going to suffer just as I did as a child, with my unattuned parents, my toxic uncle, the dark history of my dad's sexual abuse. I don't have a template for family life as peaceful and satisfying. Not in my mind, nor inside my body. I assume the worst.

JB: That's such a courageous admission, Michael. It is often difficult to recognize the connection between early-life feelings of imprisonment, and our subsequent need for space and distance in our adult lives. Many can never see that pattern in themselves. And so they run, in the illusion that the issue is the job, or the city, or the relationship; when, in fact, it's their unhealed issues that are stoking their flight. For a time, these coping strategies can actually serve a counter-balancing purpose, as our spirits breathe a healthy sigh of relief after years spent entrapped. If all you've known is engulfment, it is essential that you have a taste of safety and spaciousness. But, taken too far, these escape hatches can actually become a prison of their own making, one that deepens our isolation and prevents us from forming positive associations with the world. Any imbalanced reality will ultimately have an imprisoning quality. Just because our early-life environment felt like a prison, doesn't mean that we can't create a different reality—one that is rooted in healthy boundaries and heartfelt connectiveness. The first step is owning our fear of engulfment before it swallows us whole.

M: Thank you for the validation. I am open to doing the work to get to the bottom of my fears. I worry, though, that it will be too late for me and Hannah. She's ready to start a family now, and even if I do the work to expand my habitual range of emotion, I may be years away from making that step.

JB: I hear you. Changing the migratory direction of the soul is an incremental journey. As essential as it for us to shoot for the moon on this path, it is equally important to be realistic about the pace of the growth process. We can have all the peak experiences we want, but the real work happens between the peaks, while laying down and integrating on the valley floor. That takes time. Growers are inchworms. Lasting transformation is an incremental process, one soul-step at a time. This may frustrate us, but it's the only way to craft an awareness that is authentic and sustainable. Because sustainable transformation requires something more than intensity and process—it requires regeneration, integration, and... celebration. Celebration of the courage it took to get this far. Celebration of your steps forward. Don't wait until the 'end' to celebrate your achievement. Celebrate it now. You have come a long way, Michael. Don't forget that... whatever happens with you and Hannah.

M: If it took years to accumulate our emotional armor, it makes sense that it won't evaporate overnight, doesn't it?

JB: Correct. The healing process has a heart of its own, unfurling at its own delicate pace. Our survival adaptations may be tough, but our wounds are so delicate. As I said before, emotional armor is not easy to shed, nor should it be. We have to take our time and approach it with tenderness. It has formed for a reason: as a requirement for certain responsibilities, as a conditioned response to real circumstances, as a defense against unbearable feelings. It has served an essential purpose. To heal, we have to lift the armor carefully—it saved our lives, after all. It's like moving your best friend off to the side of the path. You don't trample on her. You honor her presence like a warm blanket that has kept you safe and sound during wintry times. Never rush it, never push up against it, never demand it to drop its guard before its time. Because it knows something you don't. In a still frightening world, armor is no less valid than vulnerability. Let it shed at its own unique pace. Only when the moment is right, do you get inside and stitch your wounds with the thread of love, slowly and surely, not rushing to completion, nurturing as you weave, tender and true. We are such wondrous weavers...

M: But I still have such a long way to go...

JB: My friend, I have faith in you. Look how far you have come. Sometimes we forget how far we have traveled while we are looking ahead to the next steps. Good to lie down and remember what it took to get this far, all those challenging hoops we had to jump through, all those courageous overcomings. Good to stroke our face with love and to remind ourselves how much courage it took to arrive here. Good to say "thank you" to the inner spirit that walks within and beside us, whispering sweet somethings in our inner ear, reminding us that we are simply and utterly worth fighting for. We ARE simply and utterly worth fighting for.

M: I do believe in my heart: this relationship is worth fighting for. And now that I caught a deeper glimpse of myself on an entirely new path, I can't turn back.

JB: With that in heart, how about I leave you with one of my favorite meditations to work with before we meet next?

M: You're giving me another meditation. Just when you got me off of them. Ha! I'm actually going to take a pass. I have enough to work with already. You have me well-equipped to take things to the next level, Mr. Brown.

Michael gave me a quick hug, and lumbered off for home. No doubt, Hannah would be waiting for him, longing for an explanation. I had to admit, I was completely gripped by this man's story. I felt like I was watching a great film—not an action-packed Hollywood melodrama, but even more enthralling: the wild, uproarious adventures of the human spirit. Climbing the mountain of healing and revealing. Summoning the bold courage to re-shape and authenticate the inner world. The best genre of entertainment. The kind that actually changes both the experiencer... and the viewer. Michael was the star of the adventure of his life—forging his own script as he walked. The film didn't have a predetermined end-point: it was shapeable, malleable, ever-morphing—as we all are. As I walked through the University of Toronto campus on the way home, I teared up... bowing deep within to him, to my self, and to all those that brave this path.

This life truly is a hero's journey. Anyone who sticks it out and gives it their best shot is heroic. What we call normal is so often extraordinary. Just overcoming the weight of the world, and making a sincere effort to identify and walk our true-path—is a profound accomplishment. The very fact that we are trying to heal our hearts in a world where so many have had to bury their hurt, is already extraordinary. It may not seem like such a big feat, but when the energy has been moving in another direction for so many generations, it is quite a challenge to turn the tide. We are breaking new inner ground, after all. It's a long path back to the receptive heart, one opening at a time. Kudos to anyone who is making a genuine effort to get through this life with originality, awareness, and authenticity.

12 Soulpods

I didn't see Michael again for another month. We had a number of scheduled appointments, but he canceled them all. When he was finally ready to meet, I chose my favorite all-day Indian buffet on Gerrard Street. Little India. Somewhere we could sit and talk all afternoon, over curry and chai. I had a feeling he would have a lot to share.

We almost bumped into each other as we entered the restaurant. Michael had gained a little weight, and it looked good on him. More fleshy and hefty, less slender and spry. He was continuing to transform. We grabbed a table and filled our plates with butter chicken and heaps of saffron rice, before beginning what would prove to be our last formal counseling session. Our teacher-student dynamic was truly coming to an end.

JB: You look good, Michael. Bring me up to speed while I scarf down my first plate.

M: Oh man, so much to share. Where to begin? Maybe with the job thing.

JB: After your homeless stint, did you go back to work?

M: It was intense. At first, I wasn't sure if they wanted to fire me for going missing in action for a few days, or seduce me with a raise. I came in to a note on my office door—see the president at once. I felt myself wanting to flee, but instead, I did something different. I rubbed my feet into the carpet and did the grounding exercise you taught me. Right there on my office floor. I grounded and discharged some feelings and fears. And when I was solidly occupying my body, I went up to see him. When I got there, he was unusually subdued. Not the austere posture he usually takes when he's ready to fire someone. He asked me what was happening with me. And, instead of doing my usual song and dance just to keep my job security, I actually told him the truth—head-on.

JB: What did that look like?

M: I told him that I didn't want to be a salesman. That it wasn't my truth. That I wanted my old coding job back. And that I wanted to do it three days per week, so I could explore other pathways. I also admitted that I didn't see myself being a computer programmer for the rest of my days. I was refreshingly honest. And as I spoke, my words felt clear and potent. My voice sounded different—as if I was speaking from my whole body. My body felt rooted and sturdy. Standing there before him, meeting him full-on, in his top-floor office. Funny thing was, he looked mesmerized as I spoke. As if it was resonating just as much in him—as it was in me.

JB: I believe it. Once we step into our own sacred purpose, we give others the permission to do the same. We light each other's flames. Sacred purpose is contagious.

M: That's not the whole story. He agreed to give my old job back part-time, as long as I agreed to fully train another sales rep. And, on top of that, he asked that I teach him meditation. Shock of all shocks... this guy is about as worldly as they come.

JB: Wonders never cease. This is fantastic news, Michael. What do you think made you so willing to take this chance?

M: A combination of many things, I suppose. Our conversations these past six months have made a real impact. All my inner explorations and excavations are finally starting to show their face in my life, in this world. And my own fierce hunger to create something more than the life I have been living. It's like a ferocious lion has awakened inside. Our tendency is to sleep—or bypass—our life away... I realized I have no time to waste 'checking-out' of here. It was just time to fucking speak some truth.

JB: Another beautiful step on your path of sacred purpose.

M: There's more. Something radical happened between me and Hannah.

JB: This is getting juicy.

M: After my last exercise with you, looking in the window, I was playing it safe for a few weeks in our couples therapy. I wanted to fully integrate the revelation I had, before speaking it to Hannah, or to anyone. That's why I canceled our meetings these past weeks—I needed to quietly see this process through to completion. And then the right moment struck me—and I pounced. I got core-splittingly truthful one session. I told her about the revelation I had. That beneath my congealed and compacted armor—there was a tiny sliver of openness to become a parent. A tiny door was ajar.

Then I made a powerful confession. That I had made a mistake when I refused to work on my issues all these years. Because it prevented me from getting on the same page as her and preparing the ground to become parents together. By evading my own healing, I inhibited Hannah from actualizing her deepest purpose. As I spoke this, a well of grief rose to the surface. I cried and sobbed from the deepest parts of my soul. Then I told her that I was prepared to release her, to actualize her calling to be a mother. And I meant it. I told her that there was more work I needed to do before bringing a child here. And if she couldn't wait for me, I was willing to set her free—to live her truth. It was the most heart-wrenching 50 minutes of my life.

JB: Ouch. I feel like I am grieving right along with you. Have you and Hannah decided to divorce?

M: No, quite the opposite. We're closer than ever before.

JB: Huh? I don't understand.

M: When I told her that, something shifted in her, too. After that session, she took a week off from work and rented a cabin up north in Muskoka. I thought for sure it was over. Instead, she came back home to me with a startling shift in her tone. She had spent the week in solitude, dancing, stretching, crying... And by week's end, she had decided to authentically release the need of having a child. She said she was done pressuring me. Done putting conditions on our love. She wanted to be with me—simply because she knew it was true. I was her home. Faced with the choice between losing me and having a child with someone else, or being with me without child, she chose the latter.

JB: She'd always had that choice, but chosen otherwise. Why do you feel that she made a different choice this time?

M: In our next session, the therapist asked her that precise question. Hannah said that it was ultimately quite simple. Beneath everything, she knew that her life was, first and foremost, with me. But she couldn't quite see that, until I fully acknowledged the value of her call to motherhood. She needed to know that my resistance was not a hidden reflection of my feelings for her—putting limits and boundaries on the depth of my love. When I demonstrated my reverence for her true-path, thus demonstrating my love for her soul, her essence, ALL OF HER… it freed her up to come into her deeper truth. She no longer had to demand I prove my love, by agreeing to have a child. She saw my genuine love shining through for her, and the vulnerable revealing of my limitations. So the war ended. She just wants to love me.

JB: Inter-relational dynamics are so fascinating, the way we can both open and close one another. What a radical breakthrough for the two of you—after all these years, to land on the same page. This is what I was sharing some time ago. The soulpod. The way that some of us are meant to walk together for a lifetime.

M: Yup, we are two peas in a soulpod—Hannah and I.

JB: And it's more evidence of the relational nature of sacred purpose. You do some healing work, which then opens the door to more healing of Hannah's path, which results in a core-deep transformation between the both of you. Everyone benefits when we live in our truth.

M: And, it gets even more fascinating, dude. Ever since she arrived at that, I have found myself feeling more ready than ever to be a dad. It's like for years, my resistance triggered her resistance, which then triggered more of my resistance. A decade-long tug-of-war between two adults, with an unconceived baby as the rope between. Poof… gone! The moment I heard her say that she chose me, my heart opened to the idea of creating life with this wonderful woman. I no longer felt engulfed. I felt accepted, and loved for something other than my sperm. Now I want to fuck her whenever we get a chance. We've stopped birth control, and are simply letting the universe take its course. We never made such connected love before. It's crazy.

JB: That's the best kind of crazy.

M: It's definitely more fun. I'm not saying life is "all good." But I am saying that some critical walls have come tumbling down... And, there's even more!

JB: More? Wow, what an incredible few weeks.

M: We sold one of the cars and got a quirky wrinkly bulldog puppy. We named her Poutine, after our favorite Canadian food. Hey, animals can be part of your soulpod, can't they? Because there were dozens at the pound, but we both knew in an instant that this was our dog.

JB: Absolutely, animals are intrinsic to many people's soulpod. On some level, you may be prepping the nest to become parents. It can start with fur-babies.

M: I've been doing some soul-storming about how to bring my sacred purpose into "humanifestation," as you would say. I'm a little embarrassed to tell you, but I have an idea that excites me. I'm looking at starting a charitable foundation. Hannah is totally on-board with the idea. Our first project would be something we call, "The Love-it Forward Café." It's a vision for a hub that will serve my 'cosmic cooking' to people from all walks of life—from the homeless, to high-end corporate executives. A place where everyone is welcomed, nourished, provided the tools to heal... and seen in their inherent magnificence. People wouldn't pay a set price for their meals—instead, the model would be called "Pay-what-you-LOVE." People pay what they feel inspired to pay, based on what it means to them. If they can't afford anything, they eat for free. If they have ample resources, they are welcome to give generously. And upstairs, we envision having a wide array of "Pay-what-you-LOVE" class offerings—from your Excavation Meditation to Holotropic Breathwork to Barking Dog Yoga to Bioenergetics Exercise Classes to traditional meditations. A broad spectrum of ways to heal, awaken, and celebrate the moment.

And, I have a question for you. If we can make this happen, would you consider being on my Board of Directors?

JB: I would be honored. But, one thing, if we move in that direction, we will have to stop our formal sessions. Professional boundaries, that sort of thing.

M: No problem. I've been feeling that this part of our connection is coming to a close. Hey, do you think we are part of the same soulpod?

JB: For the last six months, absolutely. And perhaps for far longer. Time will certainly tell.

Family of Origin vs. Soul Family

M: So, as I start to prepare a nest for becoming a dad… it's prompting me to look deeper into my family of origin. My relationship with my father. With Uncle Russell, with their mom—my Grandmother Audrey—who cloaked and enabled these dark family secrets. If a child is going to come through our soul-channel, I want to remove the static. So I've been sorting through these familial relationships.

JB: Brilliant idea. It's essential that we make conscious the question of who is our real family, at each stage of our journey.

M: Overall, I'm feeling on a completely different page than my family. They have already made it clear that they vehemently oppose my decision to work less at my lucrative computer job. My father screamed into the phone and hung up on me twice. But that's just the tip of the iceberg. There are so many ways that we don't see eye-to-eye. Truth be told, I don't genuinely like them, if I am going to be truly honest about it. I have never really liked them much, and now I feel like I am moving from an entirely different value system, sourced in a completely different purpose. If I cut them off, how to deal with the guilt and shame and keep moving forward?

JB: I understand. I went through this. One of the great consequences of finding your sacred purpose is that it shines a light into those areas of your life that are not alight with the same vibration. When the soul is on fire, it burns through everything that doesn't truly resonate with it, leaving only karmic ash in its wake. This is the up-framing nature of a growthful path—that which distracts us from the path, that which doesn't share our new resonance, asks to be shed so that we can continue to evolve. It's not always easy to say farewell to relationships, but it comes with the territory.

M: I get that, but the question is when to cut the cords, and when not to?

JB: There are many factors, but no single formula. It's deeply personal and highly specific. Do you feel that one's relationship with their family of origin is a permanent part of one's soulpod, or only for a limited time? What's your intuition? Can our soulpod change over time to reflect our own changes, even when it comes to familial relations?

M: I suppose it depends on the particular dynamics.

JB: It sure does. Blood is thicker than water. Yet it's also more likely to clot and destroy its hosts. There are two ways to understand family. One is through the survivalist lens: family are the ones you were born to. You bond together through thick and thin. You endure each other. You have each other's backs. You don't fall too far from the tree. If necessary, you hold yourself back so as not to leave anyone behind. The other idea of family is rooted in a more authentic perspective: family are those that reflect where you are at on your journey. People of *soulnificance*, you bond together on the basis of shared resonance. You enjoy each other. You support each other in becoming all that you are meant to become. You have no agenda for each other, beyond celebrating one another's uniquely unfolding sacred purpose. Two different ideas of family, two different worlds of possibility. Survive, or thrive. Cling together for dear life, or invite each other to truly LIVE...

M: Can't it be both? Can't we root in a survivalistic view—recognizing those whose shoulders we stand on, while simultaneously rooting ourselves in a more authentic way of relating?

JB: Absolutely. It's wonderful when that occurs. But it doesn't occur very often, yet. Because those that make a break for an authentic consciousness are often the only ones in their family to make that step. It's so foreign to most family structures—that when someone makes that leap, they often end up at odds with where they came from. It creates a fracture in the age-old genetic family system. This appears to be what is happening to you. You are transforming and moving forward. They are remaining locked within their fixed belief system. The simple truth is that some of us cannot preserve our dignity and well-being if we remain connected to certain members of our family of origin. The gap between our perspectives and priorities is too wide. This is not to say that we don't do our best to heal and preserve those relationships, but often it is simply not possible and it is not healthy to continue. Perhaps this is what is happening to you—with Uncle Russell, Grandma Audrey, and that segment of your extended family.

M: I hear you, but I often wonder if they can actually heal, too. Can Dad heal his wounds? Can he reveal those dark secrets seething beneath the surface? It could liberate our entire family. Hey, if I can do it, anyone can, right?

JB: It depends on them. I have seen it go both ways. It certainly feels good to imagine that the entire dysfunctional family will heal and mend. It feels good to imagine that everyone will overcome their traumas and find their way to an awakening life. I held out for that vision of possibility for many years, largely because of the unhealthily enmeshed nature of my trauma. If we suffered together, then we would rise together. But it seldom happens this way, both because of the complex nature of ancestral trauma, and because it takes so much energy and imagination to craft a healthier way of being. Most people who have been trapped beneath the rubble of family madness, don't have the energy, or the faith to get out from under it. It has become who they are. They are not able to break those chains, and often, they aren't genuinely compelled to. And that's their choice, their right. Just like it's your right to stitch together your broken places. Bottom line—if you are one who got out, you have to stay out. You have to keep going. Traversing your path. You have to give yourself permission to shed the paradigm, even if it's lonely, even if you feel the temptation to go back and wait on the others. Family dynamics can be like quicksand—they may end up dragging you down with them. We need you to stay firmly planted on your path. Because the world changes when one gets out. Because you are our best hope for a healthier tomorrow. I know it's difficult to get out alone, but you are never truly alone. You are raising the bar for all of us.

M: Just imagining the consequences of standing in my truth with Uncle Russell, and saying farewell once and for all. Being radically honest about the reason why. That would be like dropping bombs on our whole family. I don't handle conflict and hostility very well.

JB: The fact is that hostility and conflict often come with the territory. Many who have made the brave, necessary decision to disengage are met with a shaming, shunning response from others. It is one of the most destructive and imprisoning guilt trips of all time, "But she's your mother," "But he's family," "They did their best," "You owe them your life." Pay no mind to this. It's been my experience that if someone is considering disconnecting from members of their family of origin, there are usually very legitimate reasons for doing so. Even if they did their best, that doesn't mean we have to stay in contact with them. Some wounds cut too deep. Some bridges have been permanently burnt. Some people do not change. You are not a bad person if you choose to say good-bye to abusive family members. You have every right to preserve your emotional integrity.

M: Easier said than done, my friend. Way easier. I feel that because I have some understanding of where they come from, that I shouldn't hold it against them. I feel empathy towards Uncle Russell, even though he has been a poison to the family.

JB: Empathy is an interesting word, often mistaken for something quite different—unhealthy boundaries, not knowing where we end and the other begins. I think of how often I remained connected to hurtful people (and others to me, when I was hurtful), because I imagined myself empathic. And maybe I was—but that didn't mean I had to endure their madness. Our empathic capacity can be as misdirected as any other ability. Just because you can feel where someone is coming from, doesn't mean that you have to put yourself at risk. When we allow 'empathy' to keep us invested in that which brings us suffering, when we confuse it with a boundaryless way of being, it morphs into misplaced faith and self-sabotage. It becomes empathy run amok. It turns a gift freely given, into a gift freely abused. Better to not turn your compassionate nature against yourself. Empathize with humanity, but shield yourself from harm.

M: But everyone has innate potential, don't you think? Everyone can wake up and actualize their sacred purpose, can't they? Hey, I've made progress. And you know I was a tough nut to crack. Maybe I'm meant to lift my family forward.

JB: Theoretically, sure. But actually, no. Not at this stage of human development. What you are describing is something I call "The Humanism Bypass." I did it for years. I saw glimpses of someone's potential, their beautiful soul, their loving heart, and told myself that this was who they truly were, ignoring all the rest. But that menial "the rest" was actually the force that destroyed. The "rest" is where they lived most of the time. The rest was no illusion—it was real, too. In my case, this self-destructive pattern was birthed in two places. First, my deep desire to see the best in my difficult parents. Not for them, but for me. I needed to believe that there was something kind and caring living inside of them, because I didn't want to be alone. After all they brought me into this world. Without them, I wouldn't exist.

There was also another dynamic at work, a misplaced projection from my own self-concept development. I held the unyielding belief in my own potential, as a way of overcoming the shame I carried. But I made the mistake of assuming that everyone else was just as committed to finding their light. Of course, we all have glowing potential. At the core, we are all magnificent beings with profound capacities. But how many of us endeavor to fully actualize it? At this stage of human development, not so many. The key is to hold the space for two things at once: a deep belief in everyone's possibilities, and a deep regard for your own well-being. It's okay to pray for everyone's liberation without joining them in prison. Pray for them from outside the prison walls, while taking exquisite care of yourself. You can't do the work for them anyway. Remember my old adage: Boundaries, boundaries, boundaries... don't leave home without them.

M: Boundaries... That's something I have to consider if we bring a child into this world. Do I boundary them off from my parents and family? Or, give them the chance to forge a new type of relationship. Different from the one I had. Hmmm...

JB: Well, it worked magic with my Grandparents. They were not particularly good as parents. Over-burdened, feisty, unattuned. But they changed when I came along. Their first grandchild, I melted their armor, and found their soft spots. They became gentler, more patient and heart-centered. They met my parents in their shared love for the little one. Sometimes the baby becomes the generational bridge. Something positive in common. Babies can work wonders.

M: There you go again! Pressuring me into becoming a dad before my time.

JB: Shit, I forgot your resistance patterns. ☺ What I meant to say was, "If you HAD chosen to become a Dad, you might have found a point of connection with your folks. But since you didn't, there is no hope."

M: Well done, sir. Now, I'm open to baby-making again!

Lite-dimmers and Lantern Holders

We finished up another bowl of dahl. Then relaxed into a steaming cup of perfectly spiced chai. Family of origin matters were intricate and complex. I had spent years working through my familial dynamics. We come into the world riddled with so much conditioning, and deeply entrenched assumptions about what family means. It was refreshing to sit with a fellow path traveler—and bring the challenging nature of this inquiry into the light. Of course, the inquiry goes far beyond our birth families. The question of who belongs, and who doesn't, applies to all of our unfolding relationships.

M: I get that family relations are complicated, but I am also exploring the bonds and relationships with friends. I'm having difficulty discerning the place that some friends have in my life. Not just those from my 'spiritual' sangha, but also those that Hannah and I connected with as part of our Toronto life. I can see that you are right about the changing nature of the soulpod. Some friends reflected my path for a time, and clearly don't fit any longer. But there are others that I am unsure of. I mean, people go through changes and metamorphoses in the course of their lives. We don't always have to leave our friends behind, each time we transform.

JB: Agreed. There is no definitive rule. It depends on where they sit within your heart, and the nature of the path you are walking. One of the simple rules I live by relates to the distinction between what I reference as "lite-dimmers"— that is, those who dim our light—and those I call "lantern holders." Those who enhance our lives, helping us to carry our light along the path. They even light the way for us when we drift astray, or when our light grows dim, always beckoning us back to true-path. They are our lighthouses, our beacons, on this winding trail of life. As I get older, I recognize just how important it is to be surrounded by people who deeply believe in our value and goodness even when we lose our footing. No space invaders, boundary crossers, confusing messengers. It took me years to rid myself of the lite-dimmers, and it has been much clearer sailing since. My general basic philosophy: If they don't see you in your truest light, wish them well and cut the cord.

M: Sounds good in theory, but I have the hardest time letting go of certain friends. Especially those I have been connected to for decades. Actually, the most complex, high-maintenance, demanding relationships, are the most difficult to release. I seem to get ensnared in some distorted cody dance with them.

JB: Cody?

M: Sorry, it's a term Hannah uses to describe co-dependent people. I get over-attached to challenging relationships, and under-attached to healthy ones. With the lite-dimmers, I begin to do that humanism bypass thing you mentioned. I just can't seem to face the fact that they are never going to change. I suppose this means that they are still part of my soulpod, because I still have work to do around this issue. You did say that wherever there's growth, there's purpose.

JB: Yes, for sure. We do need to learn from challenging connections. But the key is to do the work, rather than to stay in those perpetually grueling dynamics because it feels familiar. Relationships aren't meant to be endurance tests. And difficulty just for the sake of difficulty doesn't actually grow us forward. Much of my greatest learning has occurred in the heart of my "Uh-Oh! Moments"—the stepping on paths that caused me pain. There have been so many of those: falling down an existential rabbit hole, drowning in the quicksand of an overwhelming life challenge, standing at the center of a firestorm I had created. I have learned far more from my "Uh-Oh! Moments" than from my "A-ha! Moments." After all, not every rite of passage is a pleasant one. Some are more like 'frights of passage'—scary moments of transition from an unhealthy pattern to a healthier way of being. But it's okay, as long as we see the "Uh-Oh! Moment" for what it is: an opportunity for transformation. So you stay in the destructive friendship for only as long as it takes to learn the painful lesson. And then you move on. Where before you would have continued to walk into suffering, now you have the good sense to step back and protect yourself. You have finally learned from your mistakes and can heed the warning. Lesson learned.

M: But, again, what about unconditional love? One of my gurus said that it would heal the planet. I believe that if I just unconditionally love them, it will be a healing balm that will transform them.

JB: Unconditional love is a beautiful thing, as long as we don't use it against ourselves. I can love all of humanity, but that doesn't mean that I will put up with all of humanity. The boundary, for me, is set at healthy self-regard. When my unconditional love for another undermines my self-respect, the fence goes up. Not because I don't believe in their possibilities, but because I have come to realize that there is no value in sacrificing my actuality for their potentiality. I make a distinction between human potential—which may well be infinite; and human actuality—which is often quite finite, particularly in those who choose, over decades, to remain asleep. Yes, they may well awaken, but we should never postpone any part of our own life waiting for that to happen. We should never hold back our own potential. Unconditional love begins at home, with the protecting and honoring of our own unique journey.

M: I feel that somewhere inside myself, I have the capacity, skills and abilities to fix other people's dynamics and patterns.

JB: I understand you want to hang in there during difficult times, but you need to recognize that there are people that you will never win with, no matter what you do. I call them "The Impossibles." The ones that always leave you feeling somewhat diminished. I have known many. Often they are members of our own family, but not always. These are the ones that we must avoid, and yet are often are the ones who are the most difficult to avoid. If we continue to make an effort to connect, we are left feeling weighted, like our light has been slightly dimmed. If we disconnect altogether, we are left feeling guilty, selfish, perhaps responsible for their isolation. Often we blame ourselves for the state of the connection, even though we rationally know that we would have remained heartfully connected to them if they had been respectful. We would have found a way, if there was a way. What gets lost in the shame shuffle is the fact that some people are truly impossible. Not just difficult, not just requiring boundaries, but impossible to maintain a healthy connection with. And their impossibility is not lodged in our actions, or choices, or behaviors. It is not a consequence of our imperfections, decisions, or missteps. It is lodged in their own issues and limitations. It is lodged in where they are at. They are simply IMPOSSIBLE. And the sooner we face that, the sooner we can live a life of unlimited possibility.

M: So, while we are on the topic, let me ask you something else. One of the things that perplexes me is the spiritual adage, "Your vibe attracts your tribe." I interpret that to mean that if they're in my life, they must be part of my soulpod. After all, I drew them in.

JB: Not always, Michael. Let's come back to earth. Sometimes your vibe attracts your tribe, and sometimes your vibe also attracts sociopaths, lite-dimmers, and border-crossers that come to steal your thunder. If you needed a specific lesson, then I suppose it's okay to call them part of your tribe for a time… but if you didn't, then it's fair to say that your vibe also attracted an abuser. I have known many who bought into this ill-conceived New Cage quote and let the wrong people through their door. Perhaps a grounded re-frame would serve us: "Sometimes, your vibe attracts your tribe. Sometimes, your vibe attracts that which doesn't serve you. And sometimes your vibe has nothing to do with any of it. Sometimes a sociopath walks through the door, one who can fool anyone."

M: I hear you, but I don't want to become an armored person again, especially after doing all this work to open my heart… Bridges, not walls, right? This is something very relevant for me to consider, in the path of sacred purpose I am about to step into, which I suspect will be far more relational.

JB: Healthy boundaries aren't walls or barbed wire fences. They are gates, portals that we selectively open when it is safe and life-enhancing to do so. Sometimes we do have to wall others off—to heal, to get a taste of what it feels like to be protected after an abundance of suffering—but eventually we come into a sacred balance. Here, we make conscious decisions as to when to open, when to close. I think of it as the art of selective attachment. Rather than responding from a patterned place, that is too open or too closed, we assess each situation on its own merits. We keep the gate closed, when it is unsafe to open it. We unlatch the gate, if there is a healthy basis for connection. Healthy boundaries are situation specific, evolving and clarifying as we grow. We sift connections through an intelligently discerning filter, only opening the gate to those experiences and individuals that enhance our sacred true-path.

M: I need to selectively attach to some Gulab Jamun for dessert. Join me?

JB: Yes. It's time for a bowl of sweetness on the path!

Woundmates

M: The process I have had to go through to clarify the truth of my relationship with Hannah, got me thinking about prior love connections. Reflecting on my history of attachment vs. non-attachment. People I had brief encounters with, others I dated for longer periods of time. I've been doing some excavating—determining how some of these relationships developed. Wondering which connections were part of my sacred purpose, which ones were mistakes. Some of them had powerful synergy and chemistry. How does one make the distinction?

JB: Some connections are only meant to exist on a limited timeline. We have a natural tendency to assume that a remarkable chemistry between two souls is confirmation that they are meant to be together for life. In the heat of profound feelings, it seems counterintuitive to imagine ourselves separate from a beloved. But chemistry and longevity are not necessarily bedfellows. Just because we feel earth-shatteringly alive with someone doesn't mean they are supposed to be our life partner. They may have come for a very different reason—to awaken us, to expand us, to shatter us so wide open that we can never close again. Perhaps they were sent from afar to polish the rough diamond of our soul before vanishing into eternity. Perhaps they just came to give us new eyes. Better we surrender our expectations when a beloved comes. (S)he may just be dropping in for a visit.

With respect to those relationships that last longer, there is no simple answer. It's the same process we discussed earlier with respect to friends and family. It comes down to: Does the connection reflect your truest paths, or serve as a vital stepping-stone in this stage of your development—or does it merely sidetrack you from the next steps? Again, it's for you to determine, when the challenging connections are serving your sacred purpose—and that includes the difficult experiences we need to awaken—and when they are deterring you from your path.

M: What do you think of "twin flames"? Let me share an example from my past, that I still wonder about to this day. A woman named Rhonda—she went by the spiritual name "Shakti." And shakti-force she was. She was a spitfire. I met her when I was living in the Bay Area. She was part of the TM community I was in. We never had a commitment, but we connected often.

Lots of deep eye-gazing, sitting together in silence, tantric explorations. Our lovemaking was explosive. We didn't have much emotional dialogue. We were both at a stage where we found that distracting. It was better to just 'be here now' together. But, at some point, I began—well, *we* began—to get into all manner of conflict. Mostly petty bickering, like whose meditation cushion should be closest to the window, and whether we should leave some clothes at each other's place, and my feeling encroached upon when she wanted to stay over after sex. Our wounds began to flare up—but we were not willing, and I suppose not yet able, to confront them. Then we broke-up in a volatile shouting match on Highway One, near Bodega. I ended up storming out of her VW van and hitching back to San Fran. Anyway, I often think of her, and wondered if we were twin flames. There was this powerful charge between us. And if we were twin flames—were we right to end it, or should we have done the work together? I sometimes wonder what my life would be like if I took that path.

JB: First of all, "twin flames" is one of the most dangerous, delusional terms in the spiritual world. It has little solid ground, and often attracts New Cagers with very poor boundaries, who desperately want to believe that their unhealthy relationship is soul-sponsored. Maybe it is, but that doesn't mean it is healthy or sustainable. The moment someone says they are in a "twin flame" relationship, I suggest that they buy a fire extinguisher and a burn kit. Because they are going to need them. What we need now are terms that reflect soul connections that are centered, grounded, sustainable, mature, balanced. I have provided some of those terms in my ELRM: soulmates, solemates, wholemates. We need many more.

With respect to you and Rhonda, err, I mean Shakti, you've made it clear that you weren't ready to do the work. That means you were there to get other needs met, but not to go all the way into conscious relating. And even if you do have that intention, and feel open to a lasting partnership with another, it still remains to be seen whether you are truly meant to be together for the long haul. Just because a couple has a strong energetic charge, and issues are provoked, doesn't mean that the connection will actually serve the bigger picture. I think of this as the distinction between the purpose-filled relationships that are meant to remain together over time—and the less healthy or toxic version: woundmates.

M: What's the diff? Isn't it part of the conscious path—to transform our woundmates into soulmates. Isn't that the work we are here to do?

JB: Not necessarily. True, it can be difficult to distinguish a soul-mate from a wound-mate because powerful connections excavate the unresolved emotional material that each of us holds. The stronger the connection, the stronger the light shining on those dark places. Some woundmates truly do contain the seeds of our soulular expansion. And yes, in some cases, woundmates do become soulmates, particularly if there is a real willing-ness in each person to do the work to convert the wounds and issues into the seeds of transformation. But not all woundmates carry the potential of becoming soulmates. Sometimes they are toxic connections masquerading as something more heightened. Sometimes they are destructive battle-grounds with very little possibility for expansion. Sometimes they are just trouble. It's an important distinction. As for you and Shakti, it's hard to say because neither of you were at a place where you wanted to explore your triggers and heal in unison. We want to go where we grow. If they don't help you glow, then let them go.

M: I'm still confused by these distinctions. Are you saying that any con-nection holds the possibility of soulmating, if there is mutual willingness to work through the stuff? Is that enough?

JB: No, it's not always enough. One of the issues I have with the burgeoning conscious relationship movement is that it often implies that if we provoke each other's triggers, that it is an indication to stay together. This is not always true. Again, I appreciate the value of not turning away from paths and people just because it becomes uncomfortable. We cannot only remain in situations when they feel good, because there may be essential lessons to learn in the heart of the discomfort. At the same time, the idea that all trigger-laden connections carry a seed of transformation is unhealthy and is not always true—even when there is willingness to do the work. There is a meaningful difference between difficult situations that are fodder for expansion, and those where the discomfort is a signal to walk away. This is as true for love relationships as friendships. Sometimes the shadow emerges because we have something to work through. Sometimes it emerges because we are simply not where we belong.

For example, we often pick partners that reflect our unresolved issues with our parents. At times, this is fuel for expansion, particularly when both partners choose to consciously work through the material and grow together. But other times, it's an absolutely impossible dream, because the same characteristics that made the parent-child dynamic impossible are still present. The idea that we can shift ourselves or the other to finally make those dynamics function healthily—is simply untrue. Sometimes, our best chance for a healthy love relationship is to pick someone unlike the impossible parent. The therapeutic movement has to be careful to not make the assumption that every trigger-filled relationship is worthy of our time. Just because stuff comes up to work with, doesn't mean that it's worth our while. Stuff will arise in healthier connections too, but that material carries a seed of hope. It burgeons with possibility.

M: So there has to be a certain element that suggests there is enough hope there, or a sense that they are truly fundamental to our life's journey, to justify going on?

JB: Absolutely. And let's never under-value the significance of willingness to do the work. Perhaps the most important question you can ask a potential love partner relates to their relationship with the shadow—their own, and the shadow that emerges in the relationship itself. That is: "How much work are you willing to do on yourself and the relationship when the shit hits the fan? Are you willing to go as deep as we have to go to work it through, or are you only interested in a breezy, low-maintenance relationship?" Few people ever talk about this during the romantic phase, because they are not envisioning the challenges to come. But it is an essential inquiry. I have known many people who were shocked to watch their 'great love' walk out the door when the connection required personal accountability and therapeutic work-through. Some of us will brave the journey; others will flee the fire. Some of us will do the work to transform our stories into the light at their source; others will run away with their 'tales' between their legs, only to find out later that their tales go with them everywhere they go. If you can determine someone's willingness at the beginning, you can save yourself a lot of trouble later.

M: That's a tough one. People often hide their shadows, or they don't even realize them, until they are tested. Like me and Hannah. We have been tested in ways I would have never predicted.

JB: It appears that you have passed. Congratulations. You get an "A" in relational willingness this lifetime. ☺

M: Yes, but it was close. I almost failed. Many don't walk the fires together. The divorce rate is severely high. I often wonder why that is.

JB: Lots of reasons. One is that we are shifting away from a survivalist basis for connection—duty, practicalities, roles—into a more authentic basis for connection. Oftentimes one partner begins to awaken, and the other doesn't join them; or one or both partners realize that they aren't an authentic fit. The relationship served a purpose for a certain time, but it no longer does. Their sacred purpose demands that they walk in another direction. And, in this fast-paced substitute gratification culture, many divorce because one or both partners simply don't want to do the deeper work required. There is a significant difference between superficiality as a basis for endings, and conscious choice-making. It would serve us all to consider our choices carefully—going in, *and* going out. Every moment of connection or severance has profound consequences on our spiritual life.

M: Yep. Like parting with this Gulab Jamun. Serious consequences. I think I've formed a bond.

JB: Me, too. Let's have some more.

Door Openers

M: This has been another eye-opening meeting. I feel like we are covering all the bases. The relational forms spanning from soulmates, to wholemates, to family of origin, to soulpod. And then there's you. You've really made an impact in my life, Jeff. I've had a lot of Gurus throughout my life… But you are something else altogether. A true wisdom-keeper. Someone who took the road less traveled and forged his own path. More effective than any of my Gurus.

JB: Thank you for that. Often gurus are blank screens that simply reflect our own unresolveds. They don't actually point you to your own inner compass. We are such a shamed collective, with no experience with, or training in seeking the Godself in the mirror. So we look for him and her everywhere. Those who had unloving parents or difficult childhoods often fall into this trap.

M: True dat. I definitely projected father issues onto my Gurus. I wanted someone to give me direction. And I wanted someone to support my efforts to avoid pain. I wanted a safe paternal fortress. There was no better place to look than the gurus who were advocating for the dissolution of the personal self and the illusory nature of feelings and emotions. They were exactly what I needed to enable my self-avoidance.

JB: In the Hindu tradition, a distinction is made between two types of guru. There's the "Sat-Guru"—a realized master. And there's the "Upa-guru"—a door opener. I believe that the Sat-Guru is disempowering for humanity. Because I believe that the idea of absolute realization is a full-on delusion— and because I have seen how the illusion of spiritual mastery has attracted, manipulated, and damaged many vulnerable souls. It's all just a big ploy that feeds on our need to believe that someone is ultimately enlightened. Mommy and Daddy surely weren't. God is elusive—existing in an unseen form. And most of us have been too shamed and disempowered to find our own inner compass and treasure trove of wisdom. So, we look to a bunch of pretenders to play "enlightened master." But they aren't. It's just another way that the patriarchy has controlled and imprisoned our consciousness.

We need to let go of the idea that there is someone out there who has it all figured out. They don't. They may have a worthwhile offering, but they are not masters of all realms of existence. This cosmos is like a giant tapestry— we each play our part in weaving a tiny thread of its majesty. There are no perfectly *realeyesed* beings, no matter what great spiritual abilities they may exhibit. Because there is no such thing as a fixed state of enlightenment. There is no stationary absolute endpoint of consciousness. Again, awaken- ing is a deeply personal and relative process, one doorway opening after another, in this fascinating fun-house of life. There is no point of completion applicable to all. It is for each of us to decide what transforms and awakens us, and to determine the state of being that most genuinely reflects our growing edge. We need to take all the so-called 'sat-guru' pictures off our altars, and replace them with a picture of ourselves. Godjectifying others isn't the path to the self-love we seek.

M: I do acknowledge that I have encountered many frauds who called themselves enlightened masters. A great many.

JB: Me too. There are many grifters in guru garb—camouflaging their unhealed inner worlds behind claims of enlightenment. Lot of sham-mans, flaky masters, and mastery-baters out there, exploiting humanity. Using New Cage spiritual principles to justify their illicit actions.

If you look at the madness that occurs in the 'spiritual' community, much of it emerges from this fundamental split between our humanness and our spiritual life. In that dichotomy, anything goes… because the guru can always fall back on the argument that their actions do not reflect their true essence. You can sleep with your devotees and call that spiritual expression. You can abuse your followers and claim that the abuser is not truly you. In other words, you can be a 'realized master' no matter what terrible things you do. And yet, if anything reflects your stage of development spiritually, it's your behavior. If you act with zero integrity, you are underdeveloped as a spiritual being. It's that simple. You can't call yourself enlightened, if you're a self-serving ass. You are either aligned on every level—from the sublime to the practical—or you're not. Enrealment, or enbullshitment—pick your path.

M: Enbullshitment is right. I've met a few Bullshit-Artist Extraordinaires on the guru-path. Seen some pretty shocking stuff, now that I think about it. I pushed it out of view at the time, rationalized and covered it over because I wanted to believe in their magic.

JB: Don't follow any one else, Michael. A true master follows her own foot-prints, encoded within her before she arrived in this incarnation. Someone else may remind you, someone else may in-power you, but no one else can possibly know the unique contours of your own true-path. The next step is right there inside of you, divinely imprinted on the souls of your feet.

M: I resonate with that. And yet, there are some gurus I truly did benefit from. Some have given me meaningful advice, and modeled healthier ways of relating to me. They're not all bullshit-artists or scammers.

JB: I agree, and I have no issue with that. We are meant to learn from one another. As long as we don't pretend they are fully enlightened humans. There is no such thing. That's just a hustle. We all have work to do. That's why we're here—to get a little closer. If one claims to be a "realized master," then they are, by definition, not. Anyone who grows in awareness realizes that there is so much more left unseen, so many wisdoms yet unknown, so many doors yet to open, a million more learnings to come. And we get more compassionate as we evolve. More humble. More subtle. We don't get superior. We don't form cults of personality. We don't think we have it all worked out. If we imagine ourselves "all that," then we have actually devolved. In my experience, claims of enlightenment are an over-compensatory, unhealthily egoic assertion that masks a profound insecurity. They are not to be taken seriously. Better we sit with those who both recognize their offerings and honor their limitations. I trust the ones who realize how far they have yet to travel. We have so much more to learn. All of us. Let's walk together, side by side.

Right as I finished, Michael closed his eyes. I knew not to continue until his eyes opened. When they did, he began to share his reflection.

M: I do remember how I would love going to satsangs, and looking up at the guru on the stage. The higher the stage, the more relaxed I became. It calmed me right down. I have to admit, when I look back now, I see my desperation. I was desperate to believe that someone up there was realized. And that someday I would be too. It was the only thing that brought me peace.

JB: It didn't truly calm you down, Michael—it calmed you 'up.' Your down was still in a state of disarray. We want to believe there is something up there, watching over us and sharing wisdom. The sat-guru trip preys on that. It represents the 'heights' of ungrounded spirituality. Grounded Spirituality is not hierarchical. We all meet on the ground level, and learn and evolve together.

M: Guess my Guru-trip is long gone. Damn, some of them were really fun to hang with.

JB: It's a different story when you stop seeing them as 'Guru,' and start seeing them as an equal. A comrade on the path. This is why I prefer the term: Door-Opener. It's more accurate. Any being can be a door-opener for our healing and awakening. Everywhere we look, we see relational opportunities for transformation. The key is to not Godjectify any of the door-openers we encounter. They aren't God—they're human. We can certainly respect and learn from them, but the moment we begin to project perfection or spiritual mastery onto them, we have undermined our own empowerment. Nothing will disable you more on the path than perpetually projecting God's wisdom onto others. Not only because they may disappoint you, but because it's all too easy to get locked into the safety of a 'seeker role' this way. Finders don't spend their lives looking for their answers in others. They cherry-pick from a patchwork of different door-openers, and come to realize that they can only find it within. Yes, others know a little something—but when it comes to your own path, only you can know what specific soul-steps to take. Others can provide us with tools that help us to remove the blockages to clear seeing, but they cannot tell us which path to walk. The real journey is not one of adapting yourself to someone else's vision, but instead, shaping who you are with your own inner resources. Your karmic clay lives deep inside your soul bones, waiting to be detected, shaped and molded, by your own two hands. You are the only person who can know the true-path you are here to walk. You are the sculptor of your own reality—don't hand your tools to anyone else.

Our reasons for being are privately held; they are encoded within us, embodied and embedded, a karmic blueprint that can only be read by the one who carries it. That's why not a single soul on earth can tell us why we are here. They can't decipher a language that is original to another soul, no matter what claims they make. It's one of the most beautiful things about this human trip: the Divine blessed each of us with our own secret lexicon, a unique sacred code that will never be replicated again. We are the book of our life. Now all we have to do is hone our inner-reading skills.

M: What about the Buddha, Jesus, the Saints, the great mystics?

JB: Each offers threads of invaluable wisdom, but each looked at the world through a particular lens, one shaped by their particular context. What one man calls the "Four Noble Truths," another calls pessimistic nonsense. What one man calls "The Ten Commandments," another calls simple common sense. I don't recommend accepting anyone's wisdom as definitive truth, unless it resonates with your own deeply lived experience. The moment you blindly accept another's truth as your own, you no longer have access to the moment, because you are no longer moving from your personally encoded truth. You are no longer *here*. Again, the degree to which you can know truth is a direct reflection of how truthful you are about the entirety of your experience. If you have bypassed intrinsic aspects of your selfhood, you cannot see the whole picture, because you are missing integral parts. I have faith that if we continue to evolve as a species, we will have access to a more inclusive, expansive, and encompassing version of truth than those who came before. Yes, it is helpful to look back in time for insight, but, again, only if it points us in our own direction. I have no reason to believe that The Buddha, Jesus, Bhagavan Sri Ramana Maharshi, have any more access to truth than you or I do. Do you?

M: No, I suppose I don't. I agree that it would be devaluing to give my power away if it doesn't reflect my own direct experience.

JB: I also have no reason to believe that those who originate from the East have greater access to wisdom, than those from the West. I mean, what if the Buddha was living in the kind of horrifying society where the only way to survive was to develop non-attachment practices? Does that mean that his first Noble Truth—that of suffering, is true for all of humankind, at all times? Or was he speaking from a particular context, one that denied him access to a more positive, or hope-filled perspective? Because if it's the latter, then it is quite dangerous to base your life on those convictions. They are circumstantial—not absolute truth. We run the risk of making non-attachment—a healthy tool under trying circumstances—into an entrenched way of being. This denies us access to a more life-affirming and relationally engaging way of being after the darkness has passed. This is not to diss all of the Buddha's offerings, it is to elucidate that he spoke from a particular context, and that his perspective and recommended practices are not the answer for every man, woman, and child on this planet. We each have our own Noble Truths to be discovered.

M: Do you consider yourself a spiritual teacher?

JB: Oh God no. Life itself is the only real spiritual teacher—and we all have access to its manifold teachings. Because I define spirituality in the most inclusive sense—as Reality—I do not believe anyone is specially qualified to rightfully call themselves a spiritual teacher. Because no single person can teach any one all of reality. Some can effectively explore aspects of reality and provide tools to others, but none of us, at this stage of human development, can access the full grand picture. All one can access and teach are limited strands. Better to reference yourself by what you specialize in: a meditation teacher, a reiki practitioner, an embodiment facilitator, rather than a spiritual teacher. That's the old delusional paradigm, one that feeds into our sense of smallness and gives the 'teacher' an artificial sense of elevated value. And it's ironic—many of them bash the ego and then seek to strengthen their unhealthy ego by labeling themselves spiritual teachers. Most teachers have not transcended their egos. In fact, their need to be held in high regard as the awakened knower—preserves it. They call themselves "spiritual teachers," and yet, many of them are merely larger-than-life trauma survivors.

I know that every time I dare to imagine myself a spiritual teacher, the universe immediately hands me my karmuppance. It's the great delusion—that some of us can teach reality. So soul-limiting an imagining.

M: I remember you saying that you have actually found that certain body-centered psychotherapists were the most effective and authentic spiritual teachers you have encountered.

JB: Yes, I said that to make a point. I wouldn't actually call them spiritual teachers. They can't teach all of reality, but they can effectively impart some of what we need to align with the intrinsic flow of life. From there, we can discover reality, on our own terms. If you are looking for a broader experience of reality, I do believe you are far more likely to find it in the somatic psychotherapist's office, than before a self-proclaimed spiritual teacher. The spiritual teacher—in many cases—will lead you away from the self; while the body-centered therapist—in many cases—will help you to both clear the emotional debris that obstructs your full-bodied presence, and will support the construction of the healthy balanced ego—required before anyone can fully honor their path. As you have experienced, many gurus will take you further from an embodied experience of reality by inviting you toward a heightened state that lacks individuation and celebrates emptiness. This may feel peaceful for a time, but it's not the place to find your life purpose.

Because your life purpose is stored in your emotional and physical body. It's in the bones of your being, at the heart of your story, in the hints and whispers of truth that course through your veins. You want to find your reasons for being here? Then you need to come into more of reality—not just a specialized pocket. Don't look up. Look down. Don't look to teachers for meaning. Look to life. It will show you the way home.

M: Speaking of which, it's time for me to go home. Hannah and I are making progress. I don't want to stay away too long.

JB: Tell Hannah I said hi. When will I see you again?

M: Let's let life decide. Since I am more grounded now, I can speak honestly. I suspect that this will be our last session, Jeff. Don't get me wrong, I am eternally and internally grateful, but I feel like I am ready now to give this life a go. Ready to meet it head-on, or in your words—heart-on. My heart is finally ON again, no small thanks to you.

JB: You did most of the work, big guy.

M: You helped save my marriage, and you helped bring me back to life, here. You arrived just in the nick of time. You know the old adage: When the student is ready, the teacher appears.

JB: Let's re-frame that. When the student is ready, the student appears. We are all students, bowing together before the great mystery. It's a pleasure to share this journey of life with you, my friend. Truly a pleasure.

With that, we got up and paid the bill and spilled out onto Gerrard Street. After some brief small talk, Michael leaned in and gave me a solid man hug. Not tentative, not avoidant—body-to-body, heart-to- heart. This man was officially HERE. Before I could say another word, he spotted the streetcar pulling up and opening its doors. He looked at me, as though to ask if I would join him. I shook my head. I had something I needed to do before heading home. He crossed the street and stepped on in. On to the next adventure in self-creation. On to the next surprise. I quietly wished him well as the doors closed behind him.

I began the long jaunt to the subway. I loved to walk Toronto streets. They kept me grounded and connected to where I came from. My roots, my history, my story. When I reached Sherbourne Street, I headed over toward a meditation store that I had frequented long ago. Months earlier, Michael had sincerely inquired if my perspective on spirituality was rooted in something unresolved in me, or even an unhealthy attachment to the world of form, the path of difficulty and suffering. I was taken aback at the time, but I promised that I would consider it. And so, I did. And while I do not feel that my perspectives emanate from unhealed material, I do feel that it is possible that I have drifted a little too far in the direction of worldliness alone. It's all about that delicate point of sacred balance. I saw so much disparity in the transcendence bypass movement, that I may well have forgotten the merits of the "bigger picture," the vast unseen, the backdrop that restores our hope and fuels our steps. I got so accustomed to working in the nitty-gritty of my localized experience to find my answers, that I stopped considering the possibility that they could also be found in the great beyond — as long as we looked in its direction from within the uniquely embodied self.

I stepped into the store and went straight to the section that sells the meditation cushions. It felt familiar, like an old friend. I picked up the various cushions, finally landing on the perfect one. Not too rigid, and not too soft — the just-right balance. I bought one for me, and one for Susan. It was time to explore meditation again. Not as a way out, but as a way to more fully embody all that I am. Not as a bypass of my story, but to utilize every tool at my disposal to ensure that I continue to grow, and to reach toward a wider spectrum of ever-encompassing wholeness.

I don't feel as though I was a teacher to Michael, but I may well have helped to re-open the door to something he had long forgotten. And perhaps, he had done the same for me. Although the ultimate romance is with our own soul, it is our experiences together that give birth to the essential lessons. We join together in a dance of sacred imagination, stepping on each other's toes and turning each other toward wholeness, one clumsy step after another. If one of us steps off the dance floor, we postpone others' lessons too. Because we need each other. We are never alone on the dance floor of time. Our sacred purpose is always reciprocal in nature. We grow in unison, or not at all.

CALL TO ACTION!

Dear Friend,

I am pleased to meet you at this juncture of my path. If you've made it this far into the book—you know it's been quite a ride. As I move on from the laborious process of completing this book, into the next phase of my own sacred purpose journey—I would like to offer you some words of encouragement to carry with you, on your own journey. At our heart, we are all *souldiers* of sacred purpose.

As you may have gathered, through the years, I have gone through intense challenges on my personal journey, of actualizing my callings. It has never been an easy street—it has been more like a perpetual obstacle course. And as par for the course, I suffered extensively in the writing of this book. In order to write about both the raptures and difficulties of coming back into the body, I had to re-live my own embodiment journey. I had to go even deeper into my body, to find my voice, my creative rhythm, my fires of conviction. And if there was any part of me that imagined I could write from the memory of past victories, I was wrong. I had to wage the same internal battle for inclusivity that I advocated for. I had to step back on the battlefield of truth, and wrestle it out with my self-crafted limitations, along with the external forces that are invested in holding us back.

The journey of writing this book damn near killed me. This is the truth. It took all I had—physically, energetically, financially, emotionally—to stay inside of this creative process. It was gnarly, laborious, prolonged, and conflictual. I fought with my wife, I fought with my friends, I fought with my editor, and I fought—day after day, night after night—with my own personal demons. All manner of internal and external resistance reared up fiercely. Fear of speaking my voice, fear of standing my ground, fear of challenging man-made systems. There was a very real part of me that wanted nothing to do with this message, with sacred activism, with my need to ruthlessly examine established spiritualities and structures. I am 56 years old. I have fought a long hard battle for decades to overcome, to find my voice, to walk my path. I am tired, and at times secretly long for quiet respite and an uneventful road to retirement. And there are parts of me—and this is not easy to admit—that have gone to sleep, preferring complacency to confrontation, silence to activism, simplicity to the complexities of burning truth-speak.

And yet, there was this ever-persistent voice—the voice of sacred purpose—that again insisted on showing its full face to the world. It was merciless, it would not relent, no matter how determinedly I resisted. To humanifest it, I had to wage a battle with every remaining part of myself that was comfortably numb and disembodied, every avoidant part that preferred the comforts of falsity to the searing discomforts of truth, every piece of me that preferred the seeming safety of a fragmented consciousness to the rigors of true embodiment. By the end, I felt punch-drunk and battle-weary, like I had come back from a long and arduous war. I couldn't think straight. I could barely stand. My personal affairs were in a state of disarray. It was that gritty. And I don't regret it for a second. Because the path of sacred purpose is all of that—challenging, wild, ragged, and rugged. And it's worth every bead of sweat, every battle scar, to step back onto the path that is truly your own.

I did not endure this for personal gain. I did not do this for egoic or financial benefit. I did this because I am—at heart—a sacred activist with a sacred purpose, that demands I love humanity forward. I did this because sacred purpose is a fire that is inviolable and ravenous. The more you feed it—the more it rages, and consumes, and demands more from you. I did this because this is what it takes to fully express your voice in this quick-to-distract world. I made this offering because re-embodiment is the essential work that all of us must undertake to become strong, empowered, grounded, energetic, passionate and compassionate enough to evolve our world. And because I inherently know that we will never get there unless we are willing to fight for our right to the light. The energetic, ancestral, and cultural dark forces abound, feeding off our dissociation to secure their agendas. We must stand them down with fierce, pointed, and purposeful action.

The path of re-embodiment is a champion's path. It is rugged and rigorous, and riddled with resistance. You need to know this, so that you don't turn back when the growing gets tough. You need to know this—so you preserve it, and protect it, at all costs. You are the guardian of your sacred purpose. You must defend it with your life.

Because the journey is going to bring up everything. It is going to bring you face-to-face with every tangled trauma knot, with every self-imposed limitation, with every adaptation and disguise that has covered over your deepest truths. And yet there is no choice but to walk it. You will not be able to act in the challenging times that are upon us unless you are acting from the heart of the unified field. Before we can co-create a world of sacred possibility, we must become that, too. We must get *here*. If we aren't here, we won't see the ways we are being cradled into a half-hearted slumber. We won't see the paths that beckon us toward fulfilling our own uniquely encoded soul-scriptures. We won't see the map to collective transformation, and connective healing. We won't see what's happening in the world and feel inspired to do something about it. We won't see our species through to its heartfelt actualization.

We need you. Yes, YOU—the one who is reading these words. We need your unique blueprint, your one-of-a-kind gifts. Don't for one moment imagine yourself insignificant or not essential. We need your spirit, your authenticity, your intuition, your capacity for connection, your personally nuanced expression. We need your re-embodiment, your devotion, your reverence for sacred purpose. We need your passion, your bravery, your determination. We need your tender, quiet, subtle listening. We need your ferociousness—because it is only the fires of our conviction that can save our species from its own trappings.

The form your offering will take depends on the nature of your unique purpose. It is a personal road to discovery. Your sacred purpose may be subtle and calm, gently recalibrating your steps. Showing its face in your day-to-day micro-choices. Or it may be the fiery path of the activist—a visible force in this world. It may be the path of the vanguard on the front lines, or the humble servant in the background. It is for you to find that point of sacred balance, whether your purpose is subtly winding in the quieted recesses of your heart, or fiercely roaring like a lion. Or a combination of many faces, through the shifting and changing stages of your journey. Whatever expression your sacred purpose takes, it is essential in co-creating the magnificent world that we all long for.

There is much work to be done in this world on many different fronts. As this book highlights, we need your voice to call out any fragmented and dissociative spiritual teachings. If you feel that a consciousness model is doing damage to humanity, get angry about it. If you feel that a guru is abusing his authority, get angry about it. If you feel that spiritual materialism is out of control, get angry about it. Spirituality without conflict isn't spiritual at all. It's a flight from reality. The spiritual activist understands what has to be done. And (s)he does it.

And don't stop there. Make a determined effort to craft more humane and embodied models that encompass the broadest range of possibility. Not 'step one' models masquerading as 'step-everything,' but models that actually take us further into an inclusive consciousness—that embrace every aspect of our humanness in our awakening. I also invite you to co-create inter-relational models of consciousness that will serve us going forward. Models that speak to the stages of awakening that happen not merely within and among our individual aspects, but that also focus on what happens between us—in the connective field. We have far too many individually-centered models and far too few relational ones. We need maps, frameworks, and holarchies that speak to the stages of consciousness that arise at different stages of heart connection, and that elucidate the ways in which certain inter-personal relationships fuel our growth and deepen our individual and collective becoming. I may not have a chance to engage in that work this time around, but perhaps you can. Bring it, dear friends. Bring it fierce.

We also need you to develop somatic psychotherapies that move beyond band-aid approaches to healing, and plumb the roots of the traumas that plague and obstruct us. We need you to humanize and enhearten our political systems, supporting only those who are in genuine service to society as a whole. We need you to fight to make our legal system more inclusive and attuned to the very specific circumstances that befall a broad range of people from all walks of life. We need you to endeavor to make our medical system more heartfelt and wholistic. We need you to tear down the walls of artifice that frame our marketing structures, and create new paradigms for economic exchange. We need your efforts on an essential needs level: improving economic conditions, protecting basic rights, increasing dietary awareness, shielding others from aggressors in all their forms. We need you to encourage a reverential regard for this magnificent planet and eco-system, that is in our care. We need awakening men to rise up defiantly and stand down those men still locked inside patriarchal and sexist ways of being. It should not be women's work, alone, to shift patriarchal paradigms—men must boldly rally for their female counterparts. We need you to develop conscious media that uses its power to elevate rather than to alarm humanity. We need you to open centers and studios not just with traditional yoga classes, but also with radically expressive yoga classes, body-centered therapies, Holotropic Breathworks, Excavation Meditations, Sacred Purpose Inquiries, and as yet uninvented and unprecedented tools for healing, integration, and connection. We need you to take us from a culture rooted in dissociative survivalism to one rooted in wholesome integration and authenticity. We need you to make achievement a relational construct, where we lift one another in unison; where we work and rally for the whole of Us. We need you to normalize vulnerable self-revealing and compassionate interface. We need you to see beyond the veils to map out and humanifest as yet unseen visions of human possibility. This is the work of all spiritual warriors—to clear the path of debris, to infuse the path with so much lucid truth that others can find their way home. There is a mountain of good work to be done. And that's why we need each and every one of you.

As Andrew Harvey wrote in this book's Foreword, "What one does for diplomacy is not what one does for truth." The path of the spiritual warrior is not soft and sweet. It is not artificially blissful and feigned forgiving. It is not fearful of divisiveness. It is not afraid of its own shadow. It is not afraid of losing popularity when it speaks its truth. It will not beat around the bush where directness is required. It has no regard for vested interests that cause suffering. It is benevolent and it is fiery and it is cuttingly honest in its efforts to liberate itself and humanity from the egoic ties that bind. Shunning strong opinions in the name of spirituality is actually anti-spiritual. Spirituality that is only floaty soft is a recipe for disaster, allowing all manner of manipulation to run amok. Real spirituality is a quest for truth, in all its forms.

And don't imagine it less of a hero's or heroine's journey because you happen to be doing this work in Western society. The battleground for an authentic and embodied consciousness is everywhere. Don't be fooled by the shopping mall, the suburban malaise, or the numbing addiction to our phones, screens, and virtual realities. If anything, it's more evidence of our desperate need to humanize, re-purpose, and create new systems of communal and societal relations. It's a holy and wholly war between a survivalistic and a more inclusive consciousness. Everywhere.

So give it, all of it, wherever you can. Gift others with the sacred purpose that is encoded within you, coursing through your veins. Gift them with the gift that you are. But don't imagine that you are doing it for them alone. When we serve others, we are also serving ourselves. It's not an unselfish act of giving. It's reciprocal. By receiving our gift, they are also gifting us back. They are giving us an opportunity to embody and actualize all that we are. They are loving us forward, too.

Some spiritual paths emphasize: "don't just do something, sit there." I say the opposite: Don't just sit there, DO something. It's one thing to pray, meditate, dream, and visualize the sacred possibilities for our planet—it's quite another to ground our expansive intentions in lived action. It's quite another to get our hands in the dirt and actually make it happen. If you don't have a clear vision of your activism, don't hold back. Follow the tiniest thread, inkling, or intimation. Start with the little things. Advocate for something or someone. Be a lighthouse for those who have lost their way. A compassionate presence for those who have been treated unjustly. A voice for those who cannot speak for themselves. Look closely at what is still unfair in this world and speak it. Stand up for what you know to be right, and true. Stand up for each other, and not just those who share your lineage, or race, or religion. And identify your soulpod. You are going to need them along the way. And they will need you. Hold the light for them during their dark times. Carry their lantern. Hand them yours, when their own light flickers out. Or at times, give them a good kick in the ass. That's what our soulpod does. We are sacred advocates for each other. Revolutionaries for a common cause: our shared humanity.

This is a call to action. A call to authenticity. A call to dig yourself out from beneath the bushels of shame and self-doubt that have plagued humanity. A call to get off the dime and do the real work to confront your distraction patterns and excavate your own purpose in this lifetime. What are you here to learn? What are you here to overcome? What are you here to offer? What does your authentic face look like? Who are you beyond the inner static of inauthentic voices. This is about the real thing, the real deal, the vulnerable and courageous truth about who you are and why you are here. I ENCOURAGE you to take the question of sacred purpose seriously… to not postpone it for another hour, or week, or until you retire, until the next lifetime, until you finish school, or end your relationship… but to take it seriously now. To work like a dog to find out what lives inside of you, what you are here to express, what you are here to manifest, what you are here to give, to share, to learn, to create, to dance, to art, to walk… You don't know how long you have, it may be 80 years, it may be 80 seconds, you may not make it to retirement, you may not make it to tomorrow morning… But if you are questing for your purpose, living your truth, you will not suffer when it's time to leave your body in this lifetime. You will have made precious use of each moment through living in your authenticity. That is a life well-lived.

Whatever you do: Don't brand yourself—enreal yourself. Become so deeply and fully authentic that you can see into the next-step world that we cannot yet see—and then shout it from the trenches and the rooftops until others see it, too. Activate and energize every sinew of sacred possibility that courses through your soul-veins, in service of our evolving species. Emblazon our humanity with your own brilliant fire. And allow yourself to fail. The next evolutionary leap will not be made by those who think they know the way already. It will be made by those flawed and humble pioneers who are willing to fail and go on. It's going to be made by those who are deeply realistic about the difficulties and the joys, the setbacks and the unexpected surprises. Those with the passionate and fierce humanness required to re-shape this humanity in its most authentic, genuine, and wholesome image.

And recognize that it won't be easy. It requires the releasing of the emotional debris that encases our heart. The shedding of the false-identifications that obstruct our path. The bidding farewell to that which doesn't serve. The shifting from survivalism to authenticity as a way of being. It is hard, these steps. We may be the first authenticity-questing collective. We may be the first soulpod to consider the possibility that there is a sacred purpose at the heart of every birth. Our load, heavy. Our courage, essential. Our significance, profound. Our need for one another, irrefutable.

As difficult as it may be, the path of sacred purpose is remarkably glorious. Nothing can compare. There is no counterfeit accomplishment that can ever match the soul's truest expression in this human life, in this world. Nothing compares to the vigor, the vitality, the heart-thumping aliveness. Once you feed it some of your life, it becomes a raging fire that spreads and consumes more. The fire burning ardently within, that nourishes and keeps you warm. It's the light of truly living. And the gifts are immense. Sacred purpose pours and pours, until our cup runneth over. Once we start walking, our true-path becomes contagious. Witnessing the faces of the downtrodden become alight, by the nimble touch of kindness. Seeing those who live an elevated life come down to ground-level, to finally learn and grow. Sprinkling the seeds of awakening, and watching them sprout. Lighting each other's flames, along the way. Passing the torch of possibility to those who will follow. Lighting the world.

My greatest wish for you is that you arrive at the end of your journey feeling deeply aligned with your own true-path. With the knowledge that you did your best to honor all that you are, over the course of your lifetime. Few stones unturned, few gifts unopened, few offerings unextended. And with the knowledge that you have contributed to a profound conscious-ness shift on this planet. We are pioneers, we are. Pioneers of truth. We are laying down new tracks without a single footprint to follow. The next generations will be ever grateful for these giant steps. Let's give ourselves a bow. And then, get back to work...

— In Soulidarity,

Jeff Brown

Gratitudes

To the finest editor on Mother Earth, Amy Gallagher, who walked beside me with this book from the beginning. I am seldom at a loss for words, but your efforts were that remarkable. Such clarity, such creativity, such heartfelt dedication. I have little doubt—the Divine brought us together to love humanity forward.

To the ever-brilliant Andrew Harvey. Your faith in my voice enlivened me and illuminated my path. Just when I felt most worn down by this book process, there you were to pick me back up again. Thank you, Big Lion, for your deep love. Thank you for all the efforts that you made to become the brilliant being that you are. Your faith in humanity calls out to my own.

To the deeply courageous path traveler, Tarini Bresgi. You have been there, for years, enhancing my offerings with your tremendous talents and steady presence. Your contribution has had a genuine and profound impact on so many—including me. Deep bows to one of the bravest souls I have ever known.

To my wise and beautiful step-daughter, Lindsay Knapp. Your dedication to your studies, and to your own personal process, had a significant impact on this writing journey. Your focus called out to my own—particularly when I felt most depleted and discouraged. Thank you.

To my dear friend, Jody Bresgi. Thank you for your positivity, your wisdom, your reverence for my message. Your light is a rare and precious offering in this world. And to your sons—Friends Ryan and Lowen—for their energy, their intelligence, and their love of mischief.

To renaissance woman, Allyson Woodrooffe. Thank you for the many brilliant contributions you have made to my work over the years. You have been an instrumental part of this journey. And your set-up of this book was magnificent. Yet again, you saw something I didn't, and it made all the difference.

To Sophie Grégoire Trudeau. Thank you for your trust and friendship, and for blessing our world with your deep love and compassion. I am grateful for your presence on the planet at this significant moment in time. You are an essential messenger, inviting us toward the heartfelt world that awaits us. May your mission continue to heal and inspire humanity. May your hearticulations echo for all eternity.

To perhaps the most gifted Thai Massage therapist anywhere: Leslie

Macmillan. You have no idea how essential your brilliant work was to this book process. And to other wonderful healers who supported this journey: Dr. Tammy Grime (Wonder Woman), Juliana Salerno, Debbie Ingham, Tokyo Shiatsu Clinic, Diane Gordon, Russ Mater, Marika Pollak, Jennifer Song, Pak Man, Trinity Dempster, Sandra Finkelman, Omega Institute, Awareness Yoga, Yoga Space. Thank you, all.

To Jessie and Robert Frybort, Robert Frybort Jr., Susan's brothers and sisters (Barbara, John, Kathy, James, Peggy, Anita), Jill Angelo Birnbaum, Shayne Traviss, Ondrea Levine, David Sniderman, Seane Corn, Kathryn Beet, Jessie May Wolfe, Juliana Burbano, Linda Thornton, Shani Feldman, Elizabeth Lesser, Azure Gallagher Michalak, Debbie Jo, Sheena Grobb, Adiatmika and family, Bauble, Freeman Michaels, Tamar Geller, Tony Melaragni, Cory, Susan and Daniel Gallagher, Dawn Grimmer, Michael Gelbart, Kathryn Graham Wilson, Acacia Land, Adrian Sohn. You each contributed to this journey in your own unique way.

To my agent Johanna Maaghul (Waterside), Blackstone Audio, the whole crew at New Leaf Distribution. Thank you for your support and your efforts.

To Gloria Nye and the Eramosa Eden Center, Nirmala Nataraj, the librarians in Fergus, Rockwood, Acton, and Guelph Ontario. Thank you for your contribution.

Thank you to my beloved wife Susan, for being a dedicated reader, for the beautiful poetry she contributed, and for patiently enduring my grueling writing process the past two years.

To my chapter one readers: David Jurasek, Brad Rose, Carrie Richardson, Jessica Ann, Gabriel Keczan. Thank you for your generous feedback. It truly helped me to take the book dialogues down the right path.

To my social media supporters. You have rooted me, rooted for me, and kept me afloat through many creative phases. It has been a delight to share my words with you, and to learn from you. You have lifted me on your shoulders time and again, blessing me with your love and support. Thank you for all that you have brought.

To my brave and beautiful writing students. Your courage in-courage-d me to write to my growing edge while crafting this book. You wrote your way home—and inspired me to do the same. I am grateful for all of you.

To my dear friend Jackie Feldman. Thank you, I love you.

To Bubbi, Beela, Mom, Dad, Ova, Auntie Tilly, Gloria Robbins. Your love lives on. ☺

Selected Bibliography

Brown, Jeff. *Soulshaping: A Journey of Self-Creation*. Berkeley: North Atlantic Books, 2009.

Brown, Jeff. *An Uncommon Bond*. Toronto: Enrealment Press, 2015.

Dickens, Charles. *Great Expectations*. https://www.gutenberg.org/ebooks/1400.

Dyer, Wayne. *The Shift: Taking your Life from Ambition to Meaning*. Carlsbad, California: Hay House Inc., 2010.

Frybort, Susan. *Hope is a Traveler*. Toronto: Enrealment Press, 2015.

Frybort, Susan. *Open Passages*. Toronto: Enrealment Press, 2017.

Grof, Stanislav, and Grof, Christina. *Holotropic Breathwork: A New Approach to Self-Exploration and Therapy*. Albany: SUNY series in Transpersonal and Humanistic Psychology (Excelsior Editions), 2010.

Lowen, Alexander, and Lowen, Leslie. *The Way to Vibrant Health*. Vermont: The Alexander Lowen Foundation, 2012.

Maslow, Abraham. *Motivation and Personality* (2nd ed.). New York: Harper & Row, 1970.

Maslow, Abraham. *The Farther Reaches of Human Nature*. New York: Viking Press, 1971.

Maslow, Abraham. *Toward a Psychology of Being* (2nd ed.). Toronto: D. Van Nostrand Co., 1968.

Ram Dass. *Be Here Now*. New Mexico: Lama Foundation, 1978.

Saade, Chris. *At the Edge of Authenticity and Solidarity*. As yet unpublished.

Shepherd, Philip. *Radical Wholeness*. Berkeley: North Atlantic Books, 2017.

Tolle, Eckhart. *The Power of Now: A Guide to Spiritual Enlightenment*. Vancouver: Namaste Publishing Inc., 2002.

Welwood, John (1984). *"Principles of Inner Work: Psychological and Spiritual."* The Journal of Transpersonal Psychology, 1984, Vol. 16, 63-73.

Wilber, Ken. *Eye to Eye: The Quest for the New Paradigm* (Third edition, revised.) Boston: Shambhala, 2001.